Respiratory Disorders
SOURCEBOOK

Fourth Edition

Health Reference Series

Fourth Edition

Respiratory Disorders

SOURCEBOOK

Basic Consumer Health Information about the Risk Factors, Symptoms, Diagnosis, and Treatment of Lung and Respiratory Disorders, Including Asthma, Bronchitis, Chronic Obstructive Pulmonary Disease (COPD), Influenza, Lung Cancer, Pneumonia, and Other Infectious and Inflammatory Pulmonary Diseases

Along with Information about Pediatric Respiratory Disorders, Tips on Preventing Respiratory Problems and Living with Chronic Lung Disease, a Glossary of Related Terms, and a Directory of Resources for Additional Help and Information

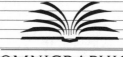

OMNIGRAPHICS

615 Griswold, Ste. 901, Detroit, MI 48226

Bibliographic Note
Because this page cannot legibly accommodate all the copyright notices, the Bibliographic
Note portion of the Preface constitutes an extension of the copyright notice.

* * *

Health Reference Series
Keith Jones, *Managing Editor*
***

OMNIGRAPHICS
A PART OF RELEVANT INFORMATION
***

Copyright © 2017 Omnigraphics
ISBN 978-0-7808-1536-0
E-ISBN 978-0-7808-1537-7

Library of Congress Cataloging-in-Publication Data

Title: Respiratory disorders sourcebook: basic consumer health information about
the risk factors, symptoms, diagnosis, and treatment of lung and respiratory
disorders, including asthma, bronchitis, chronic obstructive pulmonary
disease (COPD), influenza, lung cancer, pneumonia, and other infectious and
inflammatory pulmonary diseases: along with information about pediatric
respiratory disorders, tips on preventing respiratory problems and living with
chronic lung disease, a glossary of related terms, and a directory of resources for
additional help and information.

Description: Fourth edition. | Detroit, MI: Omnigraphics, [2017] | Series: Health
reference series | Includes bibliographical references and index. | Description
based on print version record and CIP data provided by publisher; resource not
viewed.

Identifiers: LCCN 2016041167 (print) | LCCN 2016039905 (ebook) | ISBN
9780780815377 (eBook) | ISBN 9780780815360 (hardcover: alk. paper) | ISBN
9780780815377 (ebook)

Subjects: LCSH: Respiratory organs--Diseases.

Classification: LCC RC731 (print) | LCC RC731. R468 2017 (ebook) | DDC 616.2--
dc23

LC record available at https://lccn.loc.gov/2016041167

This book is printed on acid-free paper meeting the ANSI Z39.48 Standard. The infinity
symbol that appears above indicates that the paper in this book meets that standard.

Printed in the United States

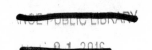

Table of Contents

Part II: Infectious Respiratory Disorders

Part V: Pediatric Respiratory Disorders

Part VI: Diagnosing and Treating Respiratory Disorders

Part VII: Living with Chronic Respiratory Problems

Part VIII: Additional Help and Information

Preface

About This Book

The average person can take in on average 12 to 16 breaths a minute, or approximately 17,000 to 23,000 breaths a day. When the respiratory system is working properly, most of this work is done automatically; however, for millions of people with respiratory disorders, meeting the body's vital need to take in life-sustaining oxygen and remove carbon dioxide becomes a challenge. Infections can cause mucus that narrows the airways and asthma triggers can cause muscles around the airways to tighten, restricting airflow. In addition, long-term exposure to toxins, such as cigarette smoke, air pollution, and chemical fumes, can lead to a condition called chronic obstructive pulmonary disease (COPD), a progressive disease that affects millions of Americans and is the third leading cause of death in the United States.

Respiratory Disorders Sourcebook, Fourth Edition, provides updated information about the causes, triggers, and treatments of infectious and inflammatory diseases of the respiratory system, including asthma, COPD, influenza, pneumonia, sinusitis, and tuberculosis. It also discusses other conditions that impair a person's ability to breathe, such as cystic fibrosis, lung cancer, and traumatic lung disorders. Lab and imaging tests used to diagnose respiratory disorders are explained, and a special section about pediatric concerns looks at the issues that arise when children experience breathing problems. The book also offers tips for living with chronic lung conditions, a glossary of related terms, and a directory of helpful organizations.

How to Use This Book

This book is divided into parts and chapters. Parts focus on broad areas of interest. Chapters are devoted to single topics within a part.

Part I: Understanding and Preventing Respiratory Problems describes the components of the respiratory system and how they work together to facilitate healthy breathing. It discusses factors that can impact respiratory functioning, including genetics, allergies, hormonal changes, the aging process, and exposure to toxins and irritants. The part concludes with statistical information about common respiratory disorders in the United States.

Part II: Infectious Respiratory Disorders discusses bacterial, viral, and fungal agents that lead to such illnesses as the common cold, bronchitis, influenza, ear infections, pertussis (whooping cough), pneumonia, sinusitis, tonsillitis, strep throat, aspergillosis, histoplasmosis, and inhalation anthrax. The part also offers tips for preventing the transmission of communicable respiratory diseases.

Part III: Inflammatory Respiratory Disorders begins with information about the most common chronic respiratory disorder—asthma. The part also describes other respiratory disorders that are characterized by inflammation. These include chronic obstructive pulmonary disease (COPD) and occupational lung diseases, such as those related to exposures to asbestos, silica, and mold.

Part IV: Other Conditions That Affect Respiration offers information about disorders and diseases that impact lung function and the ability to breath normally, including cystic fibrosis, hypersensitivity pneumonitis, lung cancer, amyotrophic lateral sclerosis, and muscular dystrophy. This part also discusses lung trauma and lung-related emergencies that can be life threatening, such as pulmonary embolism, pulmonary hypertension, and pneumothorax. The part concludes with information on how travel conditions can impact respiratory function.

Part V: Pediatric Respiratory Disorders discusses the effect of specific respiratory disorders on children. These include asthma, croup, meconium aspiration, and respiratory syncytial virus (bronchiolitis).

Part VI: Diagnosing and Treating Respiratory Disorders explains how pulmonologists and respiratory therapists treat and work with patients, and it describes common diagnostic tests, including pulmonary function tests and spirometry, bronchoscopy, chest CT and MRI scans, chloride sweat test, and others. Information about commonly used medications, surgical procedures, and pulmonary rehabilitation therapies is also included.

Part VII: Living with Chronic Respiratory Problems offers tips about minimizing triggers that contribute to asthma and other respiratory disorders, and it explains emergency action plans. Strategies for using common medical devices associated with respiratory care—including inhalers, peak flow monitors, and nebulizers—are also included.

Part VIII: Additional Help and Information provides a glossary of important terms related to respiratory disorders and a directory of organizations that offer information to patients with respiratory disorders and their families and caregivers.

Bibliographic Note

This volume contains documents and excerpts from publications issued by the following U.S. government agencies: Agency for Toxic Substances and Disease Registry (ATSDR); Bureau of Labor Statistics (BLS); Centers for Disease Control and Prevention (CDC); Federal Bureau of Prisons (BOP); Genetics Home Reference (GHR); National Cancer Institute (NCI); National Center for Biotechnology Information (NCBI); National Center for Complementary and Integrative Health (NCCIH); National Heart, Lung, and Blood Institute (NHLBI); National Institute of Allergy and Infectious Diseases (NIAID); National Institute of Environmental Health Sciences (NIEHS); National Institute on Aging (NIA); National Organization for Rare Disorders (NORD); Occupational Safety and Health Administration (OSHA); U.S. Environmental Protection Agency (EPA); and U.S. Food and Drug Administration (FDA).

In addition, this volume contains copyrighted documents from the following organization: The Nemours Foundation

It may also contain original material produced by Omnigraphics and reviewed by medical consultants.

About the Health Reference Series

The *Health Reference Series* is designed to provide basic medical information for patients, families, caregivers, and the general public. Each volume takes a particular topic and provides comprehensive coverage. This is especially important for people who may be dealing with a newly diagnosed disease or a chronic disorder in themselves or in a family member. People looking for preventive guidance, information about disease warning signs, medical statistics, and risk factors for health problems will also find answers to their questions in the *Health Reference Series*. The *Series*, however, is not intended to serve as a tool for diagnosing illness, in prescribing treatments, or as a substitute for the physician/patient relationship. All people concerned about medical symptoms or the possibility of disease are encouraged to seek professional care from an appropriate health care provider.

A Note about Spelling and Style

Health Reference Series editors use *Stedman's Medical Dictionary* as an authority for questions related to the spelling of medical terms and the *Chicago Manual of Style* for questions related to grammatical structures, punctuation, and other editorial concerns. Consistent adherence is not always possible, however, because the individual volumes within the *Series* include many documents from a wide variety of different producers, and the editor's primary goal is to present material from each source as accurately as is possible. This sometimes means that information in different chapters or sections may follow other guidelines and alternate spelling authorities.

Medical Review

Omnigraphics contracts with a team of qualified, senior medical professionals who serve as medical consultants for the *Health Reference Series*. As necessary, medical consultants review reprinted and originally written material for currency and accuracy. Citations including the phrase, "Reviewed (month, year)" indicate material reviewed by this team. Medical consultation services are provided to the *Health Reference Series* editors by:

Dr. Senthil Selvan, MBBS, DCH, MD
Dr. K. Sivanandham, MBBS, DCH, MS (Research), PhD

Our Advisory Board

We would like to thank the following board members for providing initial guidance on the development of this series:

- Dr. Lynda Baker, Associate Professor of Library and Information Science, Wayne State University, Detroit, MI

- Nancy Bulgarelli, William Beaumont Hospital Library, Royal Oak, MI

- Karen Imarisio, Bloomfield Township Public Library, Bloomfield Township, MI

- Karen Morgan, Mardigian Library, University of Michigan-Dearborn, Dearborn, MI

- Rosemary Orlando, St. Clair Shores Public Library, St. Clair Shores, MI

Health Reference Series *Update Policy*

The inaugural book in the *Health Reference Series* was the first edition of *Cancer Sourcebook* published in 1989. Since then, the *Series* has been enthusiastically received by librarians and in the medical community. In order to maintain the standard of providing high-quality health information for the layperson the editorial staff at Omnigraphics felt it was necessary to implement a policy of updating volumes when warranted.

Medical researchers have been making tremendous strides, and it is the purpose of the *Health Reference Series* to stay current with the most recent advances. Each decision to update a volume is made on an individual basis. Some of the considerations include how much new information is available and the feedback we receive from people who use the books. If there is a topic you would like to see added to the update list, or an area of medical concern you feel has not been adequately addressed, please write to:

Managing Editor
Health Reference Series
Omnigraphics
615 Griswold, Ste. 901
Detroit, MI 48226

Part One

Understanding and Preventing Respiratory Problems

Chapter 1

How the Lungs and Respiratory System Work

Breathing is so vital to life that it happens automatically. Each day, you breathe about 20,000 times, and by the time you're 70 years old, you'll have taken at least 600 million breaths.

Respiratory System Basics

All of this breathing couldn't happen without the respiratory system, which includes the nose, throat, voice box, windpipe, and lungs.

At the top of the respiratory system, the nostrils (also called nares) act as the air intake, bringing air into the nose, where it's warmed and humidified. Tiny hairs called cilia protect the nasal passageways and other parts of the respiratory tract, filtering out dust and other particles that enter the nose through the breathed air.

Air can also be taken in through the mouth. These two openings of the airway (the nasal cavity and the mouth) meet at the pharynx, or throat, at the back of the nose and mouth. The pharynx is part of the digestive system as well as the respiratory system because it carries both food and air. At the bottom of the pharynx, this pathway divides in two, one for food (the esophagus, which leads to the stomach) and the other for air. The epiglottis, a small flap of tissue, covers the air-only passage when we swallow, keeping food and liquid from going into the lungs.

The larynx, or voice box, is the uppermost part of the air-only pipe. This short tube contains a pair of vocal cords, which vibrate to make sounds.

The trachea, or windpipe, extends downward from the base of the larynx. It lies partly in the neck and partly in the chest cavity. The walls of the trachea are strengthened by stiff rings of cartilage to keep it open. The trachea is also lined with cilia, which sweep fluids and foreign particles out of the airway so that they stay out of the lungs.

At its bottom end, the trachea divides into left and right air tubes called bronchi, which connect to the lungs. Within the lungs, the bronchi branch into smaller bronchi and even smaller tubes called bronchioles. Bronchioles end in tiny air sacs called alveoli, where the exchange of oxygen and carbon dioxide actually takes place. Each lung houses about 300–400 million alveoli.

The lungs also contain elastic tissues that allow them to inflate and deflate without losing shape and are encased by a thin lining called the pleura. This network of alveoli, bronchioles, and bronchi is known as the bronchial tree.

The chest cavity, or thorax, is the airtight box that houses the bronchial tree, lungs, heart, and other structures. The top and sides of the thorax are formed by the ribs and attached muscles, and the bottom is formed by a large muscle called the diaphragm. The chest walls form a protective cage around the lungs and other contents of the chest cavity.

Separating the chest from the abdomen, the diaphragm plays a lead role in breathing. It moves downward when we breathe in, enlarging the chest cavity and pulling air in through the nose or mouth. When we breathe out, the diaphragm moves upward, forcing the chest cavity to get smaller and pushing the gases in the lungs up and out of the nose and mouth.

Respiration

The air we breathe is made up of several gases. Oxygen is the most important for keeping us alive because body cells need it for energy and growth. Without oxygen, the body's cells would die.

Carbon dioxide is the waste gas produced when carbon is combined with oxygen as part of the energy-making processes of the body. The lungs and respiratory system allow oxygen in the air to be taken into the body, while also enabling the body to get rid of carbon dioxide in the air breathed out.

Respiration is the set of events that results in the exchange of oxygen from the environment and carbon dioxide from the body's cells. The process of taking air into the lungs is inspiration, or inhalation, and the process of breathing it out is expiration, or exhalation.

Air is inhaled through the mouth or through the nose. Cilia lining the nose and other parts of the upper respiratory tract move back and forth, pushing foreign matter that comes in with air (like dust) either toward the nostrils to be expelled or toward the pharynx. The pharynx passes the foreign matter along to the stomach to eventually be eliminated by the body. As air is inhaled, the mucous membranes of the nose and mouth warm and humidify the air before it enters the lungs.

When you breathe in, the diaphragm moves downward toward the abdomen, and the rib muscles pull the ribs upward and outward. In this way, the volume of the chest cavity is increased. Air pressure in the chest cavity and lungs is reduced, and because gas flows from high pressure to low, air from the environment flows through the nose or mouth into the lungs.

In exhalation, the diaphragm moves upward and the chest wall muscles relax, causing the chest cavity to contract. Air pressure in the lungs rises, so air flows from the lungs and up and out of respiratory system through the nose or mouth.

Every few seconds, with each inhalation, air fills a large portion of the millions of alveoli. In a process called diffusion, oxygen moves from the alveoli to the blood through the capillaries (tiny blood vessels) lining the alveolar walls. Once in the bloodstream, oxygen gets picked up by the hemoglobin in red blood cells. This oxygen-rich blood then flows back to the heart, which pumps it through the arteries to oxygen-hungry tissues throughout the body.

In the tiny capillaries of the body tissues, oxygen is freed from the hemoglobin and moves into the cells. Carbon dioxide, which is produced during the process of diffusion, moves out of these cells into the capillaries, where most of it is dissolved in the plasma of the blood. Blood rich in carbon dioxide then returns to the heart via the veins. From the heart, this blood is pumped to the lungs, where carbon dioxide passes into the alveoli to be exhaled.

Lungs and Respiratory System Problems

The respiratory system is susceptible to a number of diseases, and the lungs are prone to a wide range of disorders caused by pollutants in the air.

The most common problems of the respiratory system are:

Asthma. More than 20 million people in the United States have asthma, and it's the #1 reason that kids frequently miss school. Asthma is a chronic inflammatory lung disease that causes airways to tighten and narrow. Often triggered by irritants in the air such as cigarette smoke, asthma flares involve contraction of the muscles and swelling of the lining of the tiny airways. The resulting narrowing of the airways prevents air from flowing properly, causing wheezing and difficulty breathing, sometimes to the point of being life-threatening. Controlling asthma starts with an asthma management plan, which usually involves avoiding asthma triggers and, sometimes, taking medicines.

Bronchiolitis. Not to be confused with bronchitis, bronchiolitis is an inflammation of the bronchioles, the smallest branches of the bronchial tree. Bronchiolitis affects mostly infants and young children, and can cause wheezing and serious difficulty breathing. It's usually caused by specific viruses in the wintertime, including respiratory syncytial virus (RSV).

Chronic obstructive pulmonary disease (COPD). COPD is a term that describes two lung diseases—emphysema and chronic bronchitis:

- Long-term smoking often causes **emphysema**, and although it seldom affects kids and teens, it can have its roots in the teen and childhood years. Talking to your kids about smoking is a key part of preventing smoking-related diseases. In emphysema, the lungs produce an excessive amount of mucus and the alveoli become damaged. It becomes difficult to breathe and get enough oxygen into the blood.

- In **bronchitis**, a common disease of adults and teens, the membranes lining the larger bronchial tubes become inflamed and an excessive amount of mucus is produced. The person develops a bad cough to get rid of the mucus. Cigarette smoking is a major cause of chronic bronchitis in teens.

Other Conditions

Common cold. Caused by more than 200 different viruses that cause inflammation in the upper respiratory tract, the common cold is the most common respiratory infection. Symptoms may include a mild fever, cough, headache, runny nose, sneezing, and sore throat.

Cough. A cough is a symptom of an illness, not an illness itself. There are many different types of cough and many different causes, ranging from not-so-serious to life-threatening. Some of the more common causes affecting kids are the common cold, asthma, sinusitis, seasonal allergies, croup, and pneumonia. Among the most serious causes of cough are tuberculosis (TB) and whooping cough (pertussis).

Cystic fibrosis (CF). Affecting more than 30,000 kids and young adults in the United States, cystic fibrosis is the most common inherited disease affecting the lungs. Affecting primarily the respiratory and digestive systems, CF causes mucus in the body to be abnormally thick and sticky. The mucus can clog the airways in the lungs and make a person more vulnerable to bacterial infections.

Lung cancer. Caused by an abnormal growth of cells in the lungs, lung cancer is a leading cause of death in the United States and is usually caused by smoking cigarettes. It starts in the lining of the bronchi and takes a long time to develop, so it's usually a disease in adults. Symptoms include a lasting cough that may bring up blood, chest pain, hoarseness, and shortness of breath. Radon gas (a gas that occurs in soil and rocks) exposure also might cause lung cancer. Radon is more likely to happen in certain parts of the United States. You can check your home's radon level with a radon kit available at your local home supply or hardware store.

Pneumonia. This inflammation of the lungs usually happens because of bacterial or viral infection. Pneumonia causes fever and inflammation of lung tissue, and makes breathing difficult because the lungs have to work harder to transfer oxygen into the bloodstream and remove carbon dioxide from the blood. Common causes of pneumonia are influenza (the flu) and infection with the bacterium *Streptococcus pneumoniae*.

Pulmonary hypertension. This is when the blood pressure in the arteries of the lungs is abnormally high, which means the heart has to work harder to pump blood against that high pressure. Pulmonary hypertension may happen in children because of a congenital (present at birth) heart defect or because of a health condition such as HIV infection.

Respiratory Diseases of Newborns

Several respiratory conditions can affect a newborn baby just starting to breathe for the first time. Premature babies are at increased risk for conditions such as:

- **Respiratory distress syndrome of the newborn.** Babies born prematurely may not have enough surfactant in the lungs. Surfactant helps to keep the baby's alveoli open; without surfactant, the lungs collapse and the baby is unable to breathe.

- **Apnea of prematurity (AOP).** Apnea is a medical term that means someone has stopped breathing. Apnea of prematurity (AOP) is a condition in which premature infants stop breathing for 15 to 20 seconds during sleep. AOP usually happens 2 days to 1 week after a baby is born. The lower the infant's weight and level of prematurity at birth, the more likely the baby is to have AOP spells.

- **Bronchopulmonary dysplasia (BPD).** BPD involves abnormal development of lung tissue. Sometimes called chronic lung disease, or CLD, it's a disease in infants characterized by inflammation and scarring in the lungs. It develops most often in premature babies who are born with underdeveloped lungs.

- **Meconium aspiration.** Meconium aspiration is when a newborn inhales (aspirates) a mixture of meconium (baby's first feces, ordinarily passed after birth) and amniotic fluid during labor and delivery. The inhaled meconium can cause a partial or complete blockage of the baby's airways.

- **Persistent pulmonary hypertension of the newborn (PPHN).** In the uterus, a baby's circulation bypasses the lungs. Normally, when a baby is born and begins to breathe air, his or her body quickly adapts and begins the process of respiration. PPHN is when a baby's body doesn't make that transition from fetal circulation to newborn circulation. This condition can cause symptoms such as rapid breathing, rapid heart rate, respiratory distress, and cyanosis (blue-tinged skin).

- **Transient tachypnea of the newborn (TTN).** Rapid breathing in a full-term newborn (more than 60 breaths a minute) is called transient tachypnea.

Although some respiratory diseases can't be prevented, many chronic lung and respiratory illnesses can be prevented by avoiding smoking, staying away from pollutants and irritants, washing hands often to avoid infection, and getting regular medical checkups.

Chapter 2

Improving Physical Activity and Lung Function

What Is Physical Activity?

Physical activity is any body movement that works your muscles and requires more energy than resting. Walking, running, dancing, swimming, yoga, and gardening are a few examples of physical activity.

According to the Department of Health and Human Services' (HHS) 2008 *Physical Activity Guidelines for Americans* physical activity generally refers to movement that enhances health.

Exercise is a type of physical activity that's planned and structured. Lifting weights, taking an aerobics class, and playing on a sports team are examples of exercise.

Physical activity is good for many parts of your body. This chapter focuses on the benefits of physical activity for your heart and lungs. The chapter also provides tips for getting started and staying active. Physical activity is one part of a heart-healthy lifestyle. A heart-healthy lifestyle also involves following a heart-healthy eating, aiming for a healthy weight, managing stress, and quitting smoking.

Benefits of Physical Activity

Physical activity has many health benefits. These benefits apply to people of all ages and races and both sexes.

This chapter includes text excerpted from "Physical Activity and Your Heart," National Heart, Lung, and Blood Institute (NHLBI), June 22, 2016.

For example, physical activity helps you maintain a healthy weight and makes it easier to do daily tasks, such as climbing stairs and shopping.

Physically active adults are at lower risk for depression and declines in cognitive function as they get older. (Cognitive function includes thinking, learning, and judgment skills.) Physically active children and teens may have fewer symptoms of depression than their peers.

Physical activity also lowers your risk for many diseases, such as coronary heart disease (CHD), diabetes, and cancer.

Many studies have shown the clear benefits of physical activity for your heart and lungs.

Physical Activity Strengthens Your Heart and Improves Lung Function

When done regularly, moderate- and vigorous-intensity physical activity strengthens your heart muscle. This improves your heart's ability to pump blood to your lungs and throughout your body. As a result, more blood flows to your muscles, and oxygen levels in your blood rise.

Capillaries, your body's tiny blood vessels, also widen. This allows them to deliver more oxygen to your body and carry away waste products.

Physical Activity Reduces Coronary Heart Disease (CHD) Risk Factors

When done regularly, moderate- and vigorous-intensity aerobic activity can lower your risk for CHD. CHD is a condition in which a waxy substance called plaque builds up inside your coronary arteries. These arteries supply your heart muscle with oxygen-rich blood.

Plaque narrows the arteries and reduces blood flow to your heart muscle. Eventually, an area of plaque can rupture (break open). This causes a blood clot to form on the surface of the plaque.

If the clot becomes large enough, it can mostly or completely block blood flow through a coronary artery. Blocked blood flow to the heart muscle causes a heart attack.

Certain traits, conditions, or habits may raise your risk for CHD. Physical activity can help control some of these risk factors because it:

- Can lower blood pressure and triglyceride. Triglycerides are a type of fat in the blood.

- Can raise HDL cholesterol levels. HDL sometimes is called "good" cholesterol.

- Helps your body manage blood sugar and insulin levels, which lowers your risk for type 2 diabetes.

- Reduces levels of C-reactive protein (CRP) in your body. This protein is a sign of inflammation. High levels of CRP may suggest an increased risk for CHD.

- Helps reduce overweight and obesity when combined with a reduced-calorie diet. Physical activity also helps you maintain a healthy weight over time once you have lost weight.

- May help you quit smoking. Smoking is a major risk factor for CHD.

Inactive people are more likely to develop CHD than people who are physically active. Studies suggest that inactivity is a major risk factor for CHD, just like high blood pressure, high blood cholesterol, and smoking.

For people who have CHD, aerobic activity done regularly helps the heart work better. It also may reduce the risk of a second heart attack in people who already have had heart attacks.

Vigorous aerobic activity may not be safe for people who have CHD. Ask your doctor what types of activity are safe for you.

Chapter 3

Factors That Affect Respiratory System Function

Chapter Contents

Section 3.1

Genetics and Lung Cancer

This section includes text excerpted from "Lung Cancer,"
Genetic Home Reference (GHR), October 2015.

Cancers occur when genetic mutations build up in critical genes, specifically those that control cell growth and division or the repair of damaged DNA. These changes allow cells to grow and divide uncontrollably to form a tumor. In nearly all cases of lung cancer, these genetic changes are acquired during a person's lifetime and are present only in certain cells in the lung. These changes, which are called somatic mutations, are not inherited. Somatic mutations in many different genes have been found in lung cancer cells.

Mutations in the *EGFR* and *KRAS* genes are estimated to be present in up to half of all lung cancer cases. These genes each provide instructions for making a protein that is embedded within the cell membrane. When these proteins are turned on (activated) by binding to other molecules, signaling pathways are triggered within cells that promote cell growth and division (proliferation).

Mutations in either the *EGFR* or *KRAS* gene lead to the production of a protein that is constantly turned on (constitutively activated). As a result, cells are signaled to constantly proliferate, leading to tumor formation. When these gene changes occur in cells in the lungs, lung cancer develops.

Mutations in many other genes have each been found in a small proportion of cases.

In addition to genetic changes, researchers have identified many personal and environmental factors that expose individuals to cancer-causing compounds (carcinogens) and increase the rate at which somatic mutations occur, contributing to a person's risk of developing lung cancer. The greatest risk factor is long-term tobacco smoking, which increases a person's risk of developing lung cancer 20-fold. Other risk factors include exposure to air pollution, radon, asbestos, or secondhand smoke; long-term use of hormone replacement therapy for menopause; and a history of lung disease such as tuberculosis, emphysema, or chronic bronchitis. A history of lung cancer in closely related family members is also an important risk factor; however, because relatives with lung cancer were likely smokers, it is unclear whether the increased risk of lung cancer is the result of genetic factors or exposure to secondhand smoke.

Inheritance Pattern

Most cases of lung cancer are not related to inherited gene changes. These cancers are associated with somatic mutations that occur only in certain cells in the lung.

When lung cancer is related to inherited gene changes, the cancer risk is inherited in an autosomal dominant pattern, which means one copy of the altered gene in each cell is sufficient to increase a person's chance of developing cancer. It is important to note that people inherit an increased risk of cancer, not the disease itself. Not all people who inherit mutations in these genes will develop lung cancer.

Section 3.2

Common Asthma Triggers

This section includes text excerpted from
"Asthma Triggers: Gain Control," U.S. Environmental
Protection Agency (EPA), April 27, 2016.

Americans spend up to 90 percent of their time indoors. Indoor allergens and irritants play a significant role in triggering asthma attacks. Triggers are things that can cause asthma symptoms, an episode or attack or make asthma worse. If you have asthma, you may react to just one trigger or you may find that several things act as triggers. Be sure to work with a doctor to identify triggers and develop a treatment plan that includes ways to reduce exposures to your asthma triggers.

Secondhand Smoke

Secondhand smoke is the smoke from a cigarette, cigar or pipe, and the smoke exhaled by a smoker. Secondhand smoke contains more than 4,000 substances, including several compounds that cause cancer.

Secondhand smoke can trigger asthma episodes and increase the severity of attacks. Secondhand smoke is also a risk factor for new cases of asthma in preschool-aged children. Children's developing bodies make them more susceptible to the effects of secondhand smoke and, due to their small size, they breathe more rapidly than adults, thereby taking in more secondhand smoke. Children receiving high doses of secondhand smoke, such as those with smoking parents, run the greatest relative risk of experiencing damaging health effects.

Actions You Can Take

- Don't let anyone smoke near your child.

- If you smoke—until you can quit, don't smoke in your home or car.

Dust Mites

Dust mites are tiny bugs that are too small to see. Every home has dust mites. They feed on human skin flakes and are found in mattresses, pillows, carpets, upholstered furniture, bedcovers, clothes, stuffed toys and fabric and fabric-covered items.

Body parts and droppings from dust mites can trigger asthma in individuals with allergies to dust mites. Exposure to dust mites can cause asthma in children who have not previously exhibited asthma symptoms.

Actions You Can Take

- Common house dust may also contain asthma triggers. These simple steps can help:
  - Wash bedding in hot water once a week. Dry completely.
  - Use dust proof covers on pillows and mattresses.
  - Vacuum carpets and furniture every week.
  - Choose stuffed toys that you can wash. Wash stuffed toys in hot water. Dry completely before your child plays with the toy.
  - Dust often with a damp cloth.

- Use a vacuum with a high efficiency particulate air (HEPA) filter on carpet and fabric-covered furniture to reduce dust build-up. People with asthma or allergies should leave the area being vacuumed.

Molds

Molds create tiny spores to reproduce, just as plants produce seeds. Mold spores float through the indoor and outdoor air continually. When mold spores land on damp places indoors, they may begin growing. Molds are microscopic fungi that live on plant and animal matter. Molds can be found almost anywhere when moisture is present. For people sensitive to molds, inhaling mold spores can trigger an asthma attack.

Actions You Can Take

- If mold is a problem in your home, you need to clean up the mold and eliminate sources of moisture.

- If you see mold on hard surfaces, clean it up with soap and water. Let the area dry completely.

- Use exhaust fans or open a window in the bathroom and kitchen when showering, cooking or washing dishes.

- Fix water leaks as soon as possible to keep mold from growing.

- Dry damp or wet things completely within one to two days to keep mold from growing.

- Maintain low indoor humidity, ideally between 30–50 percent relative humidity. Humidity levels can be measured by hygrometers, which are available at local hardware stores.

Cockroaches and Pests

Droppings or body parts of cockroaches and other pests can trigger asthma. Certain proteins are found in cockroach feces and saliva and can cause allergic reactions or trigger asthma symptoms in some individuals.

Cockroaches are commonly found in crowded cities and the southern regions of the United States. Cockroach allergens likely play a significant role in asthma in many urban areas.

Actions You Can Take

- Insecticides and pesticides are not only toxic to pests—they can harm people too. Try to use pest management methods that pose less of a risk. Keep counters, sinks, tables, and floors clean and free of clutter.

- Clean dishes, crumbs and spills right away.

- Store food in airtight containers.

- Seal cracks or openings around or inside cabinets.

Pets

Proteins in your pet's skin flakes, urine, feces, saliva, and hair can trigger asthma. Dogs, cats, rodents (including hamsters and guinea pigs), and other warm-blooded mammals can trigger asthma in individuals with an allergy to animal dander.

The most effective method to control animal allergens in the home is to not allow animals in the home. If you remove an animal from the home, it is important to thoroughly clean the floors, walls, carpets and upholstered furniture.

Some individuals may find isolation measures to be sufficiently effective. Isolation measures that have been suggested include keeping pets out of the sleeping areas, keeping pets away from upholstered furniture, carpets and stuffed toys, keeping the pet outdoors as much as possible and isolating sensitive individuals from the pet as much as possible.

Actions You Can Take

- Find another home for your cat or dog.

- Keep pets outside if possible.

- If you have to have a pet inside, keep it out of the bedroom of the person with asthma.

- Keep pets off of your furniture.

- Vacuum carpets and furniture when the person with asthma is not around.

Nitrogen Dioxide (NO$_2$)

Nitrogen dioxide (NO$_2$) is an odorless gas that can irritate your eyes, nose and throat and cause shortness of breath. NO$_2$ can come from appliances inside your home that burn fuels such as gas, kerosene and wood. NO_2 forms quickly from emissions from cars, trucks and buses, power plants and off-road equipment. Smoke from your stove or fireplace can trigger asthma.

In people with asthma, exposure to low levels of NO_2 may cause increased bronchial reactivity and make young children more susceptible to respiratory infections. Long-term exposure to high levels of NO_2 can lead to chronic bronchitis. Studies show a connection between breathing elevated short-term NO_2 concentrations, and increased visits to emergency departments and hospital admissions for respiratory issues, especially asthma.

Actions You Can Take

- If possible, use fuel-burning appliances that are vented to the outside. Always follow the manufacturer's instructions on how to use these appliances.

- Gas cooking stoves: If you have an exhaust fan in the kitchen, use it when you cook. Never use the stove to keep you warm or heat your house.

- Unvented kerosene or gas space heaters: Use the proper fuel and keep the heater adjusted the right way. Open a window slightly or use an exhaust fan when you are using the heater.

Outdoor Air Pollution

Outdoor air pollution is caused by small particles and ground level ozone that comes from car exhaust, smoke, road dust, and factory emissions. Outdoor air quality is also affected by pollen from plants, crops and weeds. Particle pollution can be high any time of year and are higher near busy roads and where people burn wood.

When inhaled, outdoor pollutants and pollen can aggravate the lungs, and can lead to:

- Chest pain
- Coughing
- Digestive problems
- Dizziness
- Fever
- Lethargy

- Shortness of breath
- Sneezing
- Throat irritation
- Watery eyes

Outdoor air pollution and pollen may also worsen chronic respiratory diseases, such as asthma.

Actions You Can Take

- Monitor the Air Quality Index (AQI) on your local weather report.
- Know when and where air pollution may be bad.
- Regular exercise is healthy. Check your local air quality to know when to play and when to take it a little easier.
- Schedule outdoor activities at times when the air quality is better. In the summer, this may be in the morning.
- Stay inside with the windows closed on high pollen days and when pollutants are high.
- Use your air conditioner to help filter the air coming into the home. Central air systems are the best.
- Remove indoor plants if they irritate or produce symptoms for you or your family.
- Pay attention to asthma warning signs. If you start to see signs, limit outdoor activity. Be sure to talk about this with your child's doctor.

Chemical Irritants

Chemical irritants are found in some products in your house and may trigger asthma. Your asthma or your child's asthma may be worse around products such as cleaners, paints, adhesives, pesticides, cosmetics or air fresheners. Chemical irritants are also present in schools and can be found in commonly used cleaning supplies and educational kits. Chemical irritants may exacerbate asthma. At sufficient concentrations in the air, many products can trigger a reaction.

Actions You Can Take

If you find that your asthma or your child's asthma gets worse when you use a certain product, consider trying different products. If you must use a product, then you should:

- Make sure your child is not around.

- Open windows or doors, or use an exhaust fan.

- Always follow the instructions on the product label.

Wood Smoke

Smoke from wood-burning stoves and fireplaces contain a mixture of harmful gases and small particles. Breathing these small particles can cause asthma attacks and severe bronchitis, aggravate heart and lung disease and may increase the likelihood of respiratory illnesses.

If you're using a wood stove or fireplace and smell smoke in your home, it probably isn't working as it should.

Actions You Can Take

- To help reduce smoke, make sure to burn dry wood that has been split, stacked, covered, and stored for at least 6 months.

- Have your stove and chimney inspected every year by a certified professional to make sure there are no gaps, cracks, unwanted drafts or to remove dangerous creosote build-up.

- If possible, replace your old wood stove with a new, cleaner heating appliance. Newer wood stoves are at least 50 percent more efficient and pollute 70 percent less than older models.

This can help make your home healthier and safer and help cut fuel costs.

Section 3.3

Asthma during Pregnancy

This section contains text excerpted from the following sources:
Text beginning with the heading "Discussing Current Medications"
is excerpted from "Medications and Pregnancy," Centers for
Disease Control and Prevention (CDC), August 18, 2016; Text
under the heading "Maternal Asthma Medication Use and the
Risk of Selected Birth Defects" is excerpted from "Key Findings:
Maternal Asthma Medication Use and the Risk of Selected Birth
Defects," Centers for Disease Control and Prevention (CDC),
October 22, 2014; Text under the heading "Treatment in Pregnancy"
is excerpted from "Management of Asthma," Federal Bureau of
Prisons (BOP), May 2013.

Discussing Current Medications

Some pregnant women must take medications to treat health conditions. For example, if a woman has asthma, epilepsy (seizures), high blood pressure, or depression, she might need to continue to take medication to stay healthy during pregnancy. If these conditions are not treated, a pregnant woman or her unborn baby could be harmed. It is important for a woman to discuss with her doctor which medications are needed during pregnancy. She also should talk to her doctor about which medications are likely to be the safest to take during pregnancy. It is important to balance the possible risks and benefits of any medication being considered. Suddenly stopping the use of a medication may be riskier than continuing to use the medication while under a doctor's care.

It also is important to know that dietary and herbal products, such as vitamins or herbs added to foods and drink, could be harmful to an unborn baby. These products can have other side effects when used during pregnancy. It's best for a woman to talk with her healthcare provider about everything she's taking or thinking about taking.

Accidental Exposure

Sometimes women take medication before they realize that they are pregnant. When this happens, they may worry about the effects of the medication on their unborn baby. The first thing a woman who is pregnant or who is planning on becoming pregnant should do is talk with her healthcare provider. Some medications are harmful when taken during pregnancy, but others are unlikely to cause harm.

Maternal Asthma Medication Use and the Risk of Selected Birth Defects

Recently, researchers used data from the National Birth Defects Prevention Study (NBDPS) to examine maternal asthma medication use during pregnancy and the risk of certain birth defects.

Asthma is a common disease during pregnancy, affecting about 4–12 percent of pregnant women. About 3 percent of pregnant women use asthma medications, including bronchodilators or anti-inflammatory drugs. Currently, guidelines recommend that women with asthma continue to use medication to control their condition during pregnancy. However, the safety data on using asthma medications during pregnancy are limited.

Main Findings from This Study

- Data from the study showed that using asthma medication during pregnancy

    - did not increase the risk for most of the birth defects studied

    - might increase the risk for some birth defects, such as esophageal atresia (birth defect of the esophagus or food tube), anorectal atresia (birth defect of the anus), and omphalocele (birth defect of the abdominal wall)

- The most commonly reported asthma medications used during pregnancy were

    - Albuterol (2–3 percent of women)

    - Fluticasone (about 1 percent of women)

- It was difficult to determine if asthma or other health problems related to having asthma increased the risk for these birth defects, or if the increased risk was from the medication use during pregnancy.

Treatment in Pregnancy

- Providers should monitor pregnant patients' asthma status during prenatal visits.

- Albuterol is the preferred short-acting beta$_2$-agonist (SABA) because it has an excellent safety profile; furthermore, the most data related to safety during human pregnancy are available for this medication.

- Inhaled corticosteroids (ICSs) are the preferred treatment for long-term control medication in pregnant patients. Budesonide is the preferred ICS, as it has been studied more in pregnant patients than other ICSs.

- For the treatment of comorbid conditions, intranasal corticosteroids are recommended for treating allergic rhinitis because they have a low risk of systemic effect.

Section 3.4

Effects of Aging on the Respiratory System

"Effects of Aging on the Respiratory System,"
© 2017 Omnigraphics. Reviewed September 2016.

Respiration, better known as breathing, is the process of inhaling oxygen from the air and exhaling carbon dioxide from the body. Inhaled air flows through the airways into the lungs, where it fills tiny sacs called alveoli. Blood vessels surrounding the alveoli carry oxygen into the bloodstream to be circulated among the organs and tissues. At the same time, the blood vessels empty carbon dioxide from the bloodstream into the alveoli to be removed from the body through exhalation.

The natural aging process affects respiration in a number of ways. Since the lungs stop producing new alveoli once people reach the age of about 20, their ability to exchange carbon dioxide and oxygen declines slowly from that point onward. Losses in muscle tone and changes in the nervous system also contribute to a gradual reduction in respiratory function as people age. Older people also face a higher risk of diminished lung capacity due to infections, diseases, and the destructive long-term effects of smoking and air pollution.

Changes in the Respiratory System

The aging process causes a gradual decline in the overall function of the lungs and respiratory tract. Some of the changes that occur during this process include the following:

- The diaphragm, a large muscle in the abdomen that pushes air in and out of the lungs, becomes weaker over time. As a result, the maximum force of inhalation and exhalation decreases with age.

- The intercostal muscles between the ribs grow weaker, decreasing the chest's ability to stretch during breathing.

- Bone mass decreases in the ribcage and spine, further reducing the capacity of the chest to expand and contract while breathing.

- Muscles and tissues in the airways lose elasticity over time, causing the airways to close more easily.

- The lungs' ability to expand and contract declines due to reduced levels of the protein elastin.

- Signals between the brain and the lungs lose strength and clarity, reducing the body's ability to respond to low oxygen levels or high carbon dioxide levels in the blood.

- Nerves in the airways that trigger the coughing reflex become less sensitive, allowing smoke, germs, or other foreign particles to build up and damage the lungs.

- Other bodily defenses designed to protect the lungs grow weaker, leaving the respiratory system more vulnerable to infections and diseases. For instance, the nose secretes fewer IgA antibodies to fight viruses, and the hair-like cilia lining the airways lose their ability to move mucus out of the body.

Effects of Age-Related Respiratory Changes

All of these age-related changes to the lungs cause a gradual decrease in maximum lung function. The rate of air flow declines, and the amount of oxygen in the bloodstream decreases. For some elderly people, low oxygen levels become chronic, causing persistent breathing difficulty, shortness of breath, and tiredness. But most generally healthy people maintain enough lung function to perform daily activities. They are most likely to notice symptoms of the gradual decrease in lung capacity during vigorous aerobic exercise, such as running, biking, or swimming. Other factors may contribute to a reduced ability to exercise as well, however, such as age-related changes in the heart, blood vessels, bones, and muscles.

The age-related changes to the respiratory system also make older people more susceptible to abnormal breathing patterns, such as sleep apnea. People with this condition stop breathing numerous times while they are asleep. Lung changes related to age also make elderly people more susceptible to infections, such as pneumonia and bronchitis, as well as diseases such as emphysema and lung cancer.

Preventing Age-Related Respiratory Problems

There are a number of measures people can take to minimize the impact of aging on the respiratory system. Some tips for maintaining good lung function include the following:

- Avoid smoking, which causes lung damage and speeds up the aging process.

- Exercise regularly to maintain peak lung capacity and function as long as possible.

- Avoid spending prolonged periods in bed during illness or recovery from surgery, which allows mucus to collect in the lungs and increases the risk of lung infections. Instead, get up and move around as much as possible and perform deep-breathing exercises to maintain lung function.

- Get annual vaccines to reduce the risk of respiratory infections such as influenza and pneumococcal pneumonia.

References

1. "Aging Changes in the Lungs," HealthCentral, 2015.

2. Lechtzin, Noah. "Effects of Aging on the Respiratory System," Merck Manuals, 2016.

3. Martin, Laura J. "Aging Changes in the Lungs," MedLine Plus, October 27, 2014.

Chapter 4

Toxins, Pollutants, and Respiratory Diseases

Chapter Contents

Section 4.1

Smoking and Respiratory Diseases

This section includes text excerpted from "Smoking and
Respiratory Diseases," Centers for Disease Control and
Prevention (CDC), October 15, 2014.

What You Should Know about Smoking and Lung Health

Toxins in tobacco smoke harm the body from the moment they
enter through the mouth and nose. They damage tissue and cells all
the way to the lungs. When cigarette smoke is inhaled, chemicals from
the smoke are absorbed in the lungs. As a result, smoking:

- causes lung diseases, including the majority of cases of chronic
  obstructive pulmonary disease (COPD)

- makes chronic lung diseases more severe; and

- increases the risk for respiratory infections

Genetic factors make some people more susceptible to lung disease
from smoking.

Although the lung has ways to protect itself from injury by inhaled
agents, these defenses are overwhelmed when cigarette smoke is
inhaled repeatedly over time. After years of exposure to cigarette
smoke, lung tissue becomes scarred, loses its elasticity, and can no
longer exchange air efficiently.

Smoking and Lung Growth

Adults who smoked as teenagers can have lungs that never grow to
their potential size and never perform at full capacity. This happens
because the lungs of young people are still growing, but the chemicals
in cigarette smoke slow down lung growth. Such damage is permanent,
and increases the risk of COPD later in life.

Tuberculosis

Tuberculosis (TB) is a common bacterial infection that usually
attacks the lungs and is spread through the air when people with the

disease cough or sneeze. Although TB in the United States has been dramatically reduced over the past decades, TB remains a serious health problem elsewhere in the world. There is now sufficient evidence to conclude that smoking increases a person's risk of getting TB. Smokers who have had TB are more likely than nonsmokers to have a recurrence of their TB and smokers with active TB are more likely to die from it than are nonsmokers who have the disease.

Chronic Obstructive Pulmonary Disease (COPD)

Lung injury from tobacco smoke leads to the development of chronic obstructive pulmonary disease (COPD), the nation's third largest killer. People with COPD have damaged airways and slowly die from lack of oxygen. Eight out of 10 cases of COPD are caused by smoking. The number of Americans suffering from COPD is increasing and there is no cure for this disease.

Recent studies show that risks for COPD are increasing, especially in women. Their risk for COPD is now similar to the risk among men. Women smokers in certain age groups are more than 38 times as likely to develop COPD, compared with women who have never smoked. Also, more women are dying from COPD than men, and women appear more likely to develop severe COPD at younger ages.

Asthma

Asthma is the most common chronic disease of childhood and is also very common among adults. The disease usually begins during childhood, but can start at any age. Asthma restricts airways and obstructs air flow, which results in wheezing and coughing.

More than 1 in 10 high school students in the United States have asthma, and studies suggest that youth who smoke may be more likely to develop asthma. Exposure to secondhand smoke can trigger an asthma attack in both children and adults. A severe asthma attack can put a child's life in danger.

Lung Cancer

Lung cancer is the number one cancer killer of both men and women in the United States. The first Surgeon General's Report on smoking and health in 1964 found that smoking was a cause of lung cancer in men. Since that time, risks for developing lung cancer have risen steadily among smokers, and have risen dramatically among women smokers. Changes in the design and contents of cigarettes over the last 50 years have contributed to higher lung cancer risks among smokers.

Quit Smoking—for Healthy Lungs!

Although we don't know exactly which smokers may develop lung disease from smoking, smoking is very dangerous to lung health, and many serious chronic diseases of the lung are caused by smoking. Children and teens who smoke can damage their lungs for life. Quitting smoking improves lung function and reduces the risk of lung infections.

Section 4.2

Secondhand Smoke and Respiratory Health

This section contains text excerpted from the following sources: Text in this section begins with excerpts from "Smoking and Tobacco Use," Centers for Disease Control and Prevention (CDC), February 17, 2016; Text under the heading "How Can I Protect my Loved Ones from Secondhand Smoke?" is excerpted from "Tips from Former Smokers: Quit Guide," Centers for Disease Control and Prevention (CDC), March 15, 2015.

Secondhand smoke is the combination of smoke from the burning end of a cigarette and the smoke breathed out by smokers. Secondhand smoke contains more than 7,000 chemicals. Hundreds are toxic and about 70 can cause cancer.

Since the 1964 Surgeon General's Report, 2.5 million adults who were nonsmokers died because they breathed secondhand smoke.

There is no risk-free level of exposure to secondhand smoke.

- Secondhand smoke causes numerous health problems in infants and children, including more frequent and severe asthma attacks, respiratory infections, ear infections, and sudden infant death syndrome (SIDS).

- Smoking during pregnancy results in more than 1,000 infant deaths annually.

- Some of the health conditions caused by secondhand smoke in adults include coronary heart disease, stroke, and lung cancer.

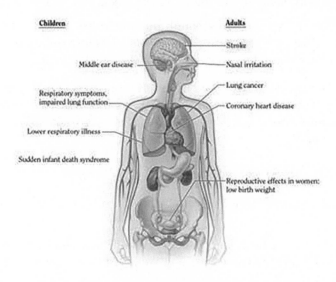

Figure 4.1. *Health Consequences Causally Linked to Exposure to Second-hand Smoke*

Secondhand Smoke Causes Cardiovascular Disease

Exposure to secondhand smoke has immediate adverse effects on the cardiovascular system and can cause coronary heart disease and stroke.

- Secondhand smoke causes nearly 34,000 premature deaths from heart disease each year in the United States among nonsmokers.

- Nonsmokers who are exposed to secondhand smoke at home or at work increase their risk of developing heart disease by 25–30 percent.

- Secondhand smoke increases the risk for stroke by 20–30 percent.

- Secondhand smoke exposure causes more than 8,000 deaths from stroke annually.

Breathing secondhand smoke can have immediate adverse effects on your blood and blood vessels, increasing the risk of having a heart attack.

- Breathing secondhand smoke interferes with the normal functioning of the heart, blood, and vascular systems in ways that increase the risk of having a heart attack.

- Even brief exposure to secondhand smoke can damage the lining of blood vessels and cause your blood platelets to become stickier. These changes can cause a deadly heart attack.

People who already have heart disease are at especially high risk of suffering adverse effects from breathing secondhand smoke and should take special precautions to avoid even brief exposures.

Secondhand Smoke Causes Lung Cancer

Secondhand smoke causes lung cancer in adults who have never smoked.

- Nonsmokers who are exposed to secondhand smoke at home or at work increase their risk of developing lung cancer by 20–30%.

- Secondhand smoke causes more than 7,300 lung cancer deaths among U.S. nonsmokers each year.

- Nonsmokers who are exposed to secondhand smoke are inhaling many of the same cancer-causing substances and poisons as smokers.

- Even brief secondhand smoke exposure can damage cells in ways that set the cancer process in motion.

- As with active smoking, the longer the duration and the higher the level of exposure to secondhand smoke, the greater the risk of developing lung cancer.

Secondhand Smoke Causes SIDS

Sudden infant death syndrome (SIDS) is the sudden, unexplained, unexpected death of an infant in the first year of life. SIDS is the leading cause of death in otherwise healthy infants. Secondhand smoke increases the risk for SIDS.

- Smoking by women during pregnancy increases the risk for SIDS.

- Infants who are exposed to secondhand smoke after birth are also at greater risk for SIDS.

- Chemicals in secondhand smoke appear to affect the brain in ways that interfere with its regulation of infants' breathing.

- Infants who die from SIDS have higher concentrations of nicotine in their lungs and higher levels of cotinine (a biological marker for secondhand smoke exposure) than infants who die from other causes.

Parents can help protect their babies from SIDS by taking the following three actions:

1. Do not smoke when pregnant.

2. Do not smoke in the home or around the baby.

3. Put the baby down to sleep on its back.

Secondhand Smoke Harms Children

Secondhand smoke can cause serious health problems in children.

- Studies show that older children whose parents smoke get sick more often. Their lungs grow less than children who do not breathe secondhand smoke, and they get more bronchitis and pneumonia.

- Wheezing and coughing are more common in children who breathe secondhand smoke.

- Secondhand smoke can trigger an asthma attack in a child. Children with asthma who are around secondhand smoke have more severe and frequent asthma attacks. A severe asthma attack can put a child's life in danger.

- Children whose parents smoke around them get more ear infections. They also have fluid in their ears more often and have more operations to put in ear tubes for drainage.

Parents can help protect their children from secondhand smoke by taking the following actions:

- Do not allow anyone to smoke anywhere in or near your home.

- Do not allow anyone to smoke in your car, even with the window down.

- Make sure your children's day care centers and schools are tobacco-free.

- If your state still allows smoking in public areas, look for restaurants and other places that do not allow smoking. "No-smoking sections" do not protect you and your family from secondhand smoke.

How Can I Protect my Loved Ones from Secondhand Smoke?

The best thing you can do to protect your family from secondhand smoke is to quit smoking. Right away, you get rid of their exposure to secondhand smoke in your home and car, and reduce it anywhere else you go together.

Another important step is to make sure your house and car remain smokefree. Kids breathe in secondhand smoke at home more than any other place. The same goes for many adults. Set "smokefree rules" for anyone in your home or car. Setting these rules can:

- reduce the amount of secondhand smoke your family breathes in

- help you quit smoking and stay smokefree

- lower the chance of your child becoming a smoker

Whether at home or on the go, there are steps you can take to protect your family from secondhand smoke. These include:

- asking people not to smoke in your home or car

- making sure people looking after your children (e.g., nannies, babysitters, day care) do not smoke

- choosing smokefree restaurants

- avoiding indoor public places that allow smoking

- teaching your children to stay away from secondhand smoke

Section 4.3

Indoor Air Pollution and Respiratory Health

> This section contains text excerpted from the following sources: Text beginning with the heading "Indoor Air Pollution and Health" is excerpted from "Indoor Air Quality (IAQ)—An Introduction to Indoor Air Quality," U.S. Environmental Protection Agency (EPA), July 21, 2016; Text beginning with the heading "Diagnostic Quick Reference" is excerpted from "Indoor Air Quality (IAQ)—Indoor Air Pollution: An Introduction for Health Professionals," U.S. Environmental Protection Agency (EPA), September 6, 2016.

Indoor Air Pollution and Health

Indoor Air Quality (IAQ) refers to the air quality within and around buildings and structures, especially as it relates to the health and comfort of building occupants. Understanding and controlling common pollutants indoors can help reduce your risk of indoor health concerns.

Health effects from indoor air pollutants may be experienced soon after exposure or, possibly, years later.

Immediate Effects

Some health effects may show up shortly after a single exposure or repeated exposures to a pollutant. These include irritation of the eyes, nose, and throat, headaches, dizziness, and fatigue. Such immediate effects are usually short-term and treatable. Sometimes the treatment is simply eliminating the person's exposure to the source of the pollution, if it can be identified. Soon after exposure to some indoor air pollutants, symptoms of some diseases such as asthma may show up, be aggrevated or worsened.

The likelihood of immediate reactions to indoor air pollutants depends on several factors including age and preexisting medical conditions. In some cases, whether a person reacts to a pollutant depends on individual sensitivity, which varies tremendously from person to person. Some people can become sensitized to biological or chemical pollutants after repeated or high level exposures.

35

Certain immediate effects are similar to those from colds or other viral diseases, so it is often difficult to determine if the symptoms are a result of exposure to indoor air pollution. For this reason, it is important to pay attention to the time and place symptoms occur. If the symptoms fade or go away when a person is away from the area, for example, an effort should be made to identify indoor air sources that may be possible causes. Some effects may be made worse by an inadequate supply of outdoor air coming indoors or from the heating, cooling or humidity conditions prevalent indoors.

Long-Term Effects

Other health effects may show up either years after exposure has occurred or only after long or repeated periods of exposure. These effects, which include some respiratory diseases, heart disease and cancer, can be severely debilitating or fatal. It is prudent to try to improve the indoor air quality in your home even if symptoms are not noticeable.

While pollutants commonly found in indoor air can cause many harmful effects, there is considerable uncertainty about what concentrations or periods of exposure are necessary to produce specific health problems. People also react very differently to exposure to indoor air pollutants. Further research is needed to better understand which health effects occur after exposure to the average pollutant concentrations found in homes and which occurs from the higher concentrations that occur for short periods of time.

Diagnostic Quick Reference

Table 4.1. Signs and Symptoms of Exposure to Indoor Air Pollution

Signs and Symptoms	Environmental Tobacco Smoke	Other Combustion Products	Biological Pollutants	Volatile Organics	Heavy Metals	Sick Building Syndrome
Respiratory						
Rhinitis, nasal congestion	Yes	Yes	Yes	Yes	No	Yes
Epistaxis	No	No	No	Yes[1]	No	No
Pharyngitis, cough	Yes	Yes	Yes	Yes	No	Yes

Table 4.1. Continued

Signs and Symptoms	Environmental Tobacco Smoke	Other Combustion Products	Biological Pollutants	Volatile Organics	Heavy Metals	Sick Building Syndrome
Wheezing, worsening asthma	Yes	Yes	No	Yes	No	Yes
Dyspnea	Yes[2]	No	Yes	No	No	Yes
Severe lung disease	No	No	No	No	No	Yes[3]

1. Associated especially with formaldehyde.
2. In asthma.
3. Hypersensitivity pneumonitis, Legionnaires Disease.

Section 4.4

Outdoor Air Quality and Health

This section includes text excerpted from "Air," Agency for Toxic Substances and Disease Registry (ATSDR), January 1, 2009. Reviewed September 2016.

All around the earth there is a thick blanket of air called the atmosphere. Air, like other gases, does not have a fixed shape. It spreads out to fill any available space so nothing is really empty. But air cannot escape from the atmosphere as the force of gravity keeps it from floating away from the earth.

Air Pollution

Ever since people first gathered in settlements there has been pollution. Pollution usually refers to the presence of substances that are either present in the environment where it doesn't belong or at levels greater than it should be.

Air pollution is caused by any undesirable substance, which enters the atmosphere. Air pollution is a major problem in modern society. Even though air pollution is usually a greater problem in cities, pollutants contaminate air everywhere. These substances include various gases and tiny particles, or particulates that can harm human health and damage the environment. They may be gases, liquids, or solids. Many pollutants are given off into the air as a result of human behavior. Pollution occurs on different levels: personal, national, and global. Some pollutants come from natural sources.

- Forest fires emit particulates, gases, and VOCs (volatile organic compounds).

- Ultra-fine dust particles created by soil erosion when water and weather loosen layers of soil, increase airborne particulate levels.

- Volcanoes spew out sulfur dioxide and large amounts of pulverized lava rock known as volcanic ash.

The major types of air pollution are:

Gaseous pollutants: A different mix of vapors and gaseous air pollutants is found in outdoor and indoor environments. The most common gaseous pollutants are carbon dioxide, carbon monoxide, hydrocarbons, nitrogen oxides, sulfur oxides and ozone. A number of sources produce these chemical compounds but the major man-made source is the burning of fossil fuel. Indoor air pollution is caused by cigarette smoking, the use of certain construction materials, cleaning products, and home furnishings. Outdoor gaseous pollutants come from volcanoes, fires, and industry, and in some areas may be substantial. The most commonly recognized type of air pollution is smog. Smog generally refers to a condition caused by the action of sunlight on exhaust gases from motor vehicles and factories.

The **Greenhouse effect** prevents the sun's heat from rising out of the atmosphere and flowing back into space. This warms the earth's surface causing the green house effect. While a certain amount of green house gases in the atmosphere are necessary to make the earth warm, activities such as the burning of fossil fuels are creating a gaseous layer that is too dense to allow the heat to escape. Many scientists believe this is causing global warming. Other gases contributing to the problem include chlorofluorocarbons (CFC), methane, nitrous oxides, and ozone.

Acid rain forms when moisture in the air interacts with nitrogen oxide and sulfur dioxide released by factories, power plants, and motor vehicles that burn coal or oil. This interaction of gases with water vapor forms sulfuric acid and nitric acids. Eventually these chemicals fall to earth as precipitation, or acid rain. Acid rain pollutants may travel long distances, with winds carrying them thousands of miles before they fall as dew, drizzle, fog, snow or rain.

Damage to the ozone layer is primarily caused by the use of chloroflurocarbons (CFCs). Ozone is a form of oxygen found in the earth's upper atmosphere. The thin layer of ozone molecules in the atmosphere absorb some of the sun's ultraviolet (UV) rays before it reaches the earth's surface, making life on earth possible. The depletion of ozone is causing higher levels of UV radiation on earth, endangering both plants and animals.

Particulate matter is the general term used for a mixture of solid particles and liquid droplets found in the air. Some particles are large or dark enough to be seen as soot or smoke. Others are so small they can be detected only with an electron microscope. When particulate matter is breathed in, it can irritate and damage the lungs causing breathing problems. Fine particles are easily inhaled deeply into the lungs where they can be absorbed into the blood stream or remain embedded for long periods of time.

Climatic effects: Normally pollutants rise or flow away from their sources without building up to unsafe levels. Wind patterns, clouds, rain, and temperature can affect how quickly pollutants move away from an area. Weather patterns that can trap air pollution in valleys or move it across the globe may be able to damage pristine environments far from the original sources.

Air Quality Index (AQI)

The air quality index (AQI) is a tool used by U.S. Environmental Protection Agency (EPA) and other agencies to provide the public with timely and easy-to-understand information on local air quality and whether air pollution levels pose a health concern. The AQI tells the public how clean the air is and whether or not they should be concerned for their health. The AQI is focused on health effects that can happen within a few hours or days after breathing polluted air.

Table 4.2. Air Quality Index

Air Quality Index (AQI) Values	Levels of Health Concerns	Colors
When the AQI is in this range	air quality conditions are	as symbolized by this color
0 to 50:	Good	Green
51 to 100:	Moderate	Yellow
101 to 150:	Unhealthy for Sensetive Groups	Orange
151 to 200:	Unhealthy	Red
201 to 300:	Very unhealthy	Purple
301 to 500:	Hazardous	Maroon

How Does Air Pollution Affect Me?

Many studies have shown links between pollution and health effects. Increases in air pollution have been linked to decreases in lung function and increases in heart attacks. High levels of air pollution according to the EPA Air Quality Index directly affect people with asthma and other types of lung or heart disease. Overall air quality has improved in the last 20 years but urban areas are still a concern. The elderly and children are especially vulnerable to the effects of air pollution.

The level of risk depends on several factors:

• the amount of pollution in the air

• the amount of air we breathe in a given time

• our overall health

Other, less direct ways people are exposed to air pollutants are:

• eating food products contaminated by air toxins that have been deposited where they grow

• drinking water contaminated by air pollutants

• ingesting contaminated soil, and

• touching contaminated soil, dust or water

Section 4.5

Climate Change and Airway Diseases

This section includes text excerpted from "Health Impacts of Climate Change," National Institute of Environmental Health Sciences (NIEHS), September 9, 2015.

Changes in the greenhouse gas concentrations and other drivers alter the global climate and bring about myriad human health consequences. Environmental consequences of climate change, such as extreme heat waves, rising sea-levels, changes in precipitation resulting in flooding and droughts, intense hurricanes, and degraded air quality, affect directly and indirectly the physical, social, and psychological health of humans. For instance, changes in precipitation are creating changes in the availability and quantity of water, as well as resulting in extreme weather events such as intense hurricanes and flooding. Climate change can be a driver of disease migration, as well as exacerbate health effects resulting from the release of toxic air pollutants in vulnerable populations such as children, the elderly, and those with asthma or cardiovascular disease.

Asthma, Respiratory Allergies, and Airway Diseases

Health Impacts

Climate change is expected to affect air quality through several pathways, including production and allergenicity of allergens and increase regional concentrations of ozone, fine particles, and dust. Some of these pollutants can directly cause respiratory disease or exacerbate existing conditions in susceptible populations, such as children or the elderly. Some of the impacts that climate change can have on air quality include:

- Increase ground level ozone and fine particle concentrations, which can trigger a variety of reactions including chest pains, coughing, throat irritation, and congestion, as well as reduce lung function and cause inflammation of the lungs.

41

- Increase carbon dioxide concentrations and temperatures, thereby affecting the timing of aeroallergen distribution and amplifying the allergenicity of pollen and mold spores.

- Increase precipitation in some areas leading to an increase in mold spores.

- Increase in rate of ozone formation due to higher temperatures and increased sunlight.

- Increase the frequency of droughts, leading to increased dust and particulate matter.

Adaptation and Mitigation

- Mitigating short-lived contamination species that both air pollutants and green house gases, such as ozone or black carbon. Examples include urban tree covers or rooftop gardens in urban settings.

- Decreasing the use of vehicle miles traveled to reduce ozone precursors.

- Utilizing alternative transportation options, such as walking or biking, which have the co-benefit of reducing emissions while increasing cardiovascular fitness and contributing to weight loss. However, these activities also have the potential to increase exposure to harmful outdoor air pollutants, particularly in urban areas.

- Increasing the use of air conditioning can alleviate the health effects of exposure to chronic or acute heat. However, this can potentially result in higher greenhouse gas emissions depending on the method of power generation.

Research Needs

- Developing and validating real-time remote sensing and other in *situ* monitoring techniques to evaluate air quality, aeroallergens, aerosolized pathogens, dust burdens, and other climate-sensitive exposures directly linked to asthma and airway diseases.

- Understanding and modeling the impact of climate change on air quality, aeroallergens, and aerosolized marine toxins, and the resulting effects on asthma and airway diseases including in vulnerable populations.

- Identifying and mapping populations and communities at increased risk of climate-related respiratory disease, which will also help to identify populations at risk for other climate-related health impacts as many environmentally mediated diseases share common risk factors.

- Studying the health effects of airborne and indoor dust on asthma exacerbation, including changes in dust composition resulting from climate change.

- Understanding the acute and long-term impacts of wild fires on asthma and other respiratory diseases.

- Examining chemicals used in energy efficient technologies to ensure that they do not contribute to lung sensitization, asthma, or other respiratory diseases.

- Examining the relative risks for respiratory disease based on chemicals with lower global warming potential than existing greenhouse gases.

Chapter 5

Avoiding Smoke Exposure

Chapter Contents

Section 5.1

Smoking Cessation Tips

This section contains text excerpted from the following sources:
Text beginning with the heading "Steps to Prepare" is excerpted
from "Tips from Former Smokers," Centers for Disease Control and
Prevention (CDC), March 15, 2015; Text under the heading "Nicotine
Replacement Products" is excerpted from "FDA 101: Smoking
Cessation Products," U.S. Food and Drug Administration (FDA),
February 19, 2016.

Steps to Prepare

Prepare to Quit

Quitting is hard. But quitting can be a bit easier if you have a plan.
When you think you're ready to quit, here are a few simple steps you
can take to put your plan into action.

Know Why You're Quitting

Before you actually quit, it's important to know why you're doing
it. Do you want to be healthier? Save money? Keep your family safe?
If you're not sure, ask yourself these questions:

- What do I dislike about smoking?
- What do I miss out on when I smoke?
- How is smoking affecting my health?
- What will happen to me and my family if I keep smoking?
- How will my life get better when I quit?

Learn How to Handle Your Triggers and Cravings

Triggers are specific persons, places, or activities that make you
feel like smoking. Knowing your smoking triggers can help you learn
to deal with them.

Cravings are short but intense urges to smoke. They usually only
last a few minutes. Plan ahead and come up with a list of short activities you can do when you get a craving.

Find Ways to Handle Nicotine Withdrawal

During the first few weeks after you quit, you may feel uncomfortable and crave a cigarette. This is because of nicotine withdrawal. During withdrawal, your body is getting used to not having nicotine from cigarettes. For most people, the worst symptoms of withdrawal last a few days to a few weeks. During this time, you may:

• feel a little depressed

• be unable to sleep

• become cranky, frustrated, or mad

• feel anxious, nervous, or restless

• have trouble thinking clearly

You may be tempted to smoke to relieve these feelings. Just remember that they are temporary, no matter how powerful they feel at the time.

One of the best ways to deal with nicotine withdrawal is to try nicotine replacement therapy (NRT). NRT can reduce withdrawal symptoms. And NRT can double your chances of quitting smoking for good. NRT comes in several different forms, including gum, patch, nasal spray, inhaler, and lozenge. Many are available without a prescription.

A lot of research has been done on NRT. It has been shown to be safe and effective for almost all smokers who want to quit, including teens. But if you have a severe medical condition or are pregnant, talk to your doctor about using NRT.

If you plan to use NRT, remember to have it available on your quit day. Read the instructions on the NRT package and follow them carefully. NRT will give you the most benefit if you use it as recommended.

Explore Your Quit Smoking Options

It is difficult to quit smoking on your own, but quitting "cold turkey" is not your only choice. In fact, choosing another option may improve your chances of success. Check out:

• SmokefreeTXT text message program

• QuitGuide app

• Quitlines like 1-800-QUIT-NOW (1-800-784-8669) and 1-877-44U-QUIT (1-877-448-7848)

Find a quit method that might be right for you.

Tell Your Family and Friends You Plan to Quit

Quitting smoking is easier when the people in your life support you. Let them know you are planning to quit and explain how they can help. Here are a few tips:

- Tell your family and friends your reasons for quitting.

- Ask them to check in with you to see how things are going.

- Ask them to help you think of smokefree activities you can do together (like going to the movies or a nice restaurant).

- Ask a friend or family member who smokes to quit with you, or at least not smoke around you.

- Ask your friends and family not to give you a cigarette—no matter what you say or do.

- Alert your friends and family that you may be in a bad mood while quitting. Ask them to be patient and help you through it.

Support is one of the keys to successfully quitting. Find more ways to get support to help you quit.

Make a Quit Plan

Having a plan can make quitting easier. Create your personalized plan to help you stay focused, confident, and motivated to quit.

Nicotine Replacement Products

Nicotine replacement is one category of smoking cessation product. Designed to wean your body off cigarettes, they supply you with nicotine in controlled amounts while sparing you from other chemicals found in tobacco products.

As you go about quitting smoking, you may experience symptoms of nicotine withdrawal. These symptoms—which include a craving, or urge, to smoke, depression, trouble sleeping, irritability, anxiety, and increased appetite—may occur no matter which method of stopping you choose.

Available over the counter and by prescription, nicotine replacement products should usually be used for a short time to help you manage nicotine cravings and withdrawal. However, the U.S. Food and Drug Administration (FDA) recognizes that some people may find that they need to use these products longer to stay smoke-free.

FDA has determined that there do not appear to be significant safety concerns if smokers use nicotine replacement products in combination with another product, for example, a long-acting skin patch with a short-acting gum or if they do not stop smoking completely before beginning to use such products. You may want to talk with your health-care professional to find your best strategy to quit.

If you are under 18 years of age and want to quit smoking, you should talk to a healthcare professional about potential use of nicotine replacement therapies.

OTC nicotine replacement products are approved for sale to persons 18 years of age and older. These products are available under brand names and sometimes as generic products. They include:

- **skin patches** known as transdermal nicotine patches. These patches are affixed to the skin, similar to how you would apply an adhesive bandage

- **chewing gum** also known as nicotine gum

- **lozenges** also known as nicotine lozenges. Lozenges are taken by dissolving in the mouth

Prescription-only nicotine replacement products are available only under the brand name Nicotrol and are available both as a nasal spray and an oral inhaler.

There is important advice to consider before beginning a nicotine replacement therapy.

Women who are pregnant or breast-feeding should use these products only with approval from their healthcare professional.

Talk to your healthcare professional before using these products if you have

- diabetes, heart disease, asthma, or stomach ulcers

- had a recent heart attack

- high blood pressure that is not controlled with medicine

- a history of irregular heartbeat

- been prescribed medication to help you quit smoking

If you take prescription medication for depression or asthma, let your healthcare professional know if you are quitting smoking; your prescription dose may need to be adjusted.

Stop using a nicotine replacement product and call your healthcare professional if you experience any of the following symptoms: nausea, dizziness, weakness, vomiting, fast or irregular heartbeat, mouth problems with the lozenge or gum, or redness or swelling of the skin around the patch that does not go away.

Section 5.2

Where to Get Help to Quit Smoking

This section contains text excerpted from the following sources:
Text beginning with the heading "What Resources Are Available to
Help Someone Quit Smoking?" is excerpted from "FAQs for Helping
Someone Quit," Smokefree.gov, National Cancer Institute (NCI),
June 29, 2016; Text beginning with the heading "12 Tips to Get
Support as You Quit" is excerpted from "Tips from Former Smokers,"
Centers for Disease Control and Prevention (CDC), March 15, 2015.

What Resources Are Available to Help Someone Quit Smoking?

Suggest to someone who is trying to quit that they use the online tips, tools, and support on Smokefree (smokefree.gov). Encourage them to talk to their doctor or check out other ways to talk to experts about quitting smoking.

How Long Does Nicotine Withdrawal Usually Last?

For most people, the worst symptoms of withdrawal last a few days to a few weeks. Be extra mindful of the things that could trigger their urge to smoke during this time. Have a distraction or backup plan ready in case a craving hits.

What If My Friend or Family Member Is Pregnant?

Many smokers get strong pressure to quit smoking when they become pregnant. Many of them also want to quit smoking. But being

50

pregnant doesn't magically make it easier. While many women do succeed in quitting smoking before their baby is born, many others have a hard time staying quit after their baby is born.

Pregnant women who quit smoking can have withdrawal and cravings just like women who aren't pregnant. Having a baby can be very stressful. Many women use smoking as a way to deal with it. Your support is important to helping someone quit and stay quit.

What If the Person Doesn't Want to Quit Smoking Right Now?

Quitting smoking is the best thing a person can do for their health. But the decision to quit is one they have to make for themselves. You can't force them if they're not ready. However, you should continue to come back to the topic, and let them know that you'll be there to support them when they are ready.

What If I Smoke?

If your friend or family member is quitting and you've also been thinking about it, now could be a good time to quit. But if you aren't ready to quit smoking, decide how you will handle your own smoking around them. You don't want to trigger their urge to reach for a cigarette. Be sure to ask yourself whether you can be supportive while continuing to smoke.

- Don't smoke around them or buy cigarettes when you're together.
- Use mouthwash, wash your hands, and change your clothes to avoid smelling like cigarettes when you're together.
- Create a "no smoking" rule for your home and car if you live together.
- Keep your ashtrays, lighters, and cigarettes out of sight.
- Be supportive of spending time in smokefree places like at the movies.

12 Tips to Get Support as You Quit

Getting support from the important people in your life can make a big difference as your quit. In fact, two out of five former smokers felt that support from others mattered a lot in their success. Remember

51

that you are not in this alone. Your friends and family are there for you, in both good times and bad.

Follow These 12 Tips to Get the Support You Need

1. Surround Yourself with People You Trust

Think of the people you trust the most—people you can talk to about anything and who have been there for you when you needed them. They could be friends, significant others, parents, co-workers, or other family members. Whoever they are, spend more time with them.

Tip: Bring friends along for your daily activities. Grab lunch with a friend, get a group together to go shopping, or meet up at a sporting event.

2. Focus on People Who Can Help

If a friendship doesn't feel right anymore, it might be time to let it go. Don't be afraid to try a little distance with people who aren't giving you the support you need. Letting go can be hard, but it is sometimes for the best.

Tip: Focus your energy on spending time with people who make you feel good about yourself and want you to succeed.

3. Invest in Your Relationships

Make a point to invest time and effort in important relationships. People are more willing to provide support when they know you are there for them. You will also feel more comfortable calling on them for support if the relationship is strong.

Tip: Go to that movie your friend really wants to see, even if it's not your top choice. Or go out of your way to call a friend just to chat and see how things are going.

4. Ask for Help

You might like to solve problems on your own, but the truth is we all need a little help from time to time. Go ahead and ask the people you trust. It doesn't mean you're weak. Your true friends will be there, ready and willing to help.

Tip: Not sure how to ask? Send a text or email to get the conversation started (e.g., I want to quit smoking. Can you help me?). Know an ex-smoker? Ask them why and how they quit.

5. **Be Specific About Your Wants**

    Your friends and family won't always be able to predict what you need during your quit. Be specific about what support you want (and don't want). Try to be nice about it. They are just trying to do what is best for you.

    Tip: Feeling stressed after a long day at work and craving a cigarette? Tell a friend and ask them to help plan a smokefree night out to distract you.

6. **Say Thank You**

    Don't let acts of kindness go unnoticed. Tell your friends you appreciate them, whether you speak it, text it, or show it with your actions. Saying thanks doesn't take a lot of time, so do it in the moment before you forget.

    Tip: Have a friend who gave up their last piece of gum to help you beat a cigarette craving? Buy some gum and give it to them with a note that says, "Thanks for helping me stay quit!"

7. **Avoid Stressful Situations**

    Steer clear of the things that add unneeded stress to your day and look for more positive things to do.

    Tip: Identify what stresses you out and come up with ways to deal with that stress. Stress can make you feel like you want to smoke. Ask friends and family to be aware of your stressors. They can help make your life easier during your quit.

8. **Grow Your Social Circle**

    Give your social circle a boost by connecting with other people who share your interests. Start by thinking about the things you like to do. Then look for ways to get more involved in them. Get talking with the people around you, and chances are, you'll find you have stuff in common.

    Tip: Strike up a conversation with someone new at work, join an intramural sport league, or volunteer. You never know who you will meet!

9. **Be Approachable**

    How you present yourself to others is a big part of branching out and strengthening friendships. Make yourself approachable by making eye contact when talking with others. Smile.

Sit and stand straight. Give compliments. People will be drawn to your confidence and positive attitude.

Tip: Say hi and smile to co-workers as you pass them at work, compliment a family member on how great their shirt looks, or tell your friend you like their new haircut.

10. Be Hands-on

Don't wait around for others to come to you. Create opportunities to spend time with friends by suggesting things to do. Join in conversations and give your opinion.

Tip: Reach out to the people you care about. Have lunch with a co-worker or friend. Invite friends over to your place for a game night.

11. Listen

Listening is a great way to strengthen and build friendships. Get people to open up by asking questions that can't be answered in just one word, like yes or no. Let them talk. Resist the urge to interrupt with your own comments and stories.

Tip: Are your friend's eyes glazing over when you talk? Take a breath and give them a chance to say something. Ask what they think of a new song you heard or if they have any plans for the weekend.

12. Support Others

Support is a two-way street. If you want others to be there for you, you have to be there for them, too. Check in with your friends and help them out when you can. Sometimes small favors mean the most.

Tip: Do something small to brighten someone's day. Make a friend smile by emailing or texting them a joke, get someone a small treat for their birthday, or call a family member to see how they are doing.

Chapter 6

Preventing Indoor Air Pollution

Chapter Contents

Section 6.1

Improving Air Quality at Home

This section includes text excerpted from "Improving Indoor Air Quality," U.S. Environmental Protection Agency (EPA), November 19, 2015.

There are three basic strategies to improve indoor air quality:

1. Source control

2. Improved ventilation

3. Air cleaners

Source Control

Usually the most effective way to improve indoor air quality is to eliminate individual sources of pollution or to reduce their emissions.

Some sources, like those that contain asbestos, can be sealed or enclosed; others, like gas stoves, can be adjusted to decrease the amount of emissions. In many cases, source control is also a more cost-efficient approach to protecting indoor air quality than increasing ventilation because increasing ventilation can increase energy costs.

Ventilation Improvements

Another approach to lowering the concentrations of indoor air pollutants in your home is to increase the amount of outdoor air coming indoors.

For most indoor air quality problems in the home, source control is the most effective solution.

Most home heating and cooling systems, including forced air heating systems, do not mechanically bring fresh air into the house. Opening windows and doors, operating window or attic fans, when the weather permits, or running a window air conditioner with the vent control open increases the outdoor ventilation rate. Local bathroom or kitchen fans that exhaust outdoors remove contaminants directly from the room where the fan is located and also increase the outdoor air ventilation rate.

It is particularly important to take as many of these steps as possible while you are involved in short-term activities that can generate high levels of pollutants—for example, painting, paint stripping, heating with kerosene heaters, cooking, or engaging in maintenance and hobby activities such as welding, soldering, or sanding. You might also choose to do some of these activities outdoors, if you can and if weather permits.

Advanced designs of new homes are starting to feature mechanical systems that bring outdoor air into the home. Some of these designs include energy-efficient heat recovery ventilators (also known as air-to-air heat exchangers).

Ventilation and shading can help control indoor temperatures. Ventilation also helps remove or dilute indoor airborne pollutants coming from indoor sources. This reduces the level of contaminants and improves indoor air quality (IAQ). Carefully evaluate using ventilation to reduce indoor air pollutants where there may be outdoor sources of pollutants, such as smoke or refuse, nearby.

The introduction of outdoor air is one important factor in promoting good air quality. Air may enter a home in several different ways, including:

- through natural ventilation, such as through windows and doors

- through mechanical means, such as through outdoor air intakes associated with the heating, ventilation and air conditioning (HVAC) system

- through infiltration, a process by which outdoor air flows into the house through openings, joints and cracks in walls, floors and ceilings, and around windows and doors.

Infiltration occurs in all homes to some extent.

Natural ventilation describes air movement through open windows and doors. If used properly natural ventilation can at times help moderate the indoor air temperature, which may become too hot in homes without air-conditioning systems or when power outages or brownouts limit or make the use of air conditioning impossible.

Natural ventilation can also improve indoor air quality by reducing pollutants that are indoors. Examples of natural ventilation are:

- opening windows and doors

- window shading such as closing the blinds

Most residential forced air-heating systems and air-conditioning systems do not bring outdoor air into the house mechanically, and infiltration and natural ventilation are relied upon to bring outdoor air into the home. Advanced designs for new homes are starting to add a mechanical feature that brings outdoor air into the home through the HVAC system. Some of these designs include energy efficient heat recovery ventilators to mitigate the cost of cooling and heating this air during the summer and winter.

Air Cleaners

There are many types and sizes of air cleaners on the market, ranging from relatively inexpensive table-top models to sophisticated and expensive whole-house systems. Some air cleaners are highly effective at particle removal, while others, including most table-top models, are much less so. Air cleaners are generally not designed to remove gaseous pollutants.

The effectiveness of an air cleaner depends on how well it collects pollutants from indoor air (expressed as a percentage efficiency rate) and how much air it draws through the cleaning or filtering element (expressed in cubic feet per minute).

A very efficient collector with a low air-circulation rate will not be effective, nor will a cleaner with a high air-circulation rate but a less efficient collector. The long-term performance of any air cleaner depends on maintaining it according to the manufacturer's directions.

Another important factor in determining the effectiveness of an air cleaner is the strength of the pollutant source. Table-top air cleaners, in particular, may not remove satisfactory amounts of pollutants from strong nearby sources. People with a sensitivity to particular sources may find that air cleaners are helpful only in conjunction with concerted efforts to remove the source.

Over the past few years, there has been some publicity suggesting that houseplants have been shown to reduce levels of some chemicals in laboratory experiments. There is currently no evidence, however, that a reasonable number of houseplants remove significant quantities of pollutants in homes and offices. Indoor houseplants should not be over-watered because overly damp soil may promote the growth of microorganisms which can affect allergic individuals.

At present, U.S. Environmental Protection Agency (EPA) does not recommend using air cleaners to reduce levels of radon and its decay products. The effectiveness of these devices is uncertain because they only partially remove the radon decay products and do not diminish the amount of radon entering the home. EPA plans to do additional research on whether air cleaners are, or could become, a reliable means of reducing the health risk from radon.

Section 6.2

Indoor Air Quality in Schools

This section includes text excerpted from "Managing Asthma in the School Environment," U.S. Environmental Protection Agency (EPA), September 8, 2016.

Asthma Management: A Priority for Schools

- An average of one out of every 10 school-age children has asthma.

- Asthma is a leading cause of school absenteeism.

- Each year, 10.5 million school days are missed due to asthma.

- Asthma can be controlled through medical treatment and management of environmental triggers.

- Asthma is a serious, sometimes life-threatening respiratory disease that affects 24.6 million Americans, including 7.1 million children. Although there is no cure for asthma, it can be controlled through medical treatment and management of environmental triggers.

Asthma and Absenteeism

Asthma has reached epidemic proportions in the United States, affecting millions of people of all ages and races. An average of one out of every 10 school-age children now has asthma, and the percentage of children with asthma is rising more rapidly in preschool-age children than in any other age group.

Asthma is a leading cause of school absenteeism due to a chronic condition, accounting for nearly **13 million** missed school days per year. Asthma also accounts for many nights of interrupted sleep, limits activity and disrupts family and caregiver routines.

Asthma symptoms that are not severe enough to require a visit to an emergency room or to a physician can still be serious enough to prevent a child with asthma from living a fully active life.

Asthma is a long-term, inflammatory disease that causes the airways of the lungs to tighten and constrict, leading to wheezing, breathlessness, chest tightness and coughing. The inflammation also causes the airways of the lungs to become especially sensitive to a variety of asthma triggers. The particular trigger or triggers and the severity of symptoms can differ for each person with asthma.

Because Americans spend up to 90 percent of their time indoors, exposure to indoor allergens and irritants may play a significant role in triggering asthma episodes. Some of the most common asthma triggers found in schools, as well as techniques to mitigate them, are addressed in this section.

Each day, one in five Americans occupies a school building. The majority of these occupants are children. Environmental asthma triggers commonly found in school buildings include:

- respiratory viruses
- cockroaches and other pests
- mold resulting from excess moisture in the building
- dander from animals in the classroom
- dander brought in on clothing from animals at home

Secondhand smoke and dust mites are other known environmental asthma triggers found in schools. Children with asthma may be affected by other pollutants from sources found inside schools, such as:

- unvented stoves or heaters
- common products including:
  - chemicals
  - cleaning agents
  - perfumes
  - pesticides
  - sprays

In addition, outdoor environmental asthma triggers, like ozone and particle pollution, or bus exhaust, can affect children with asthma while at school.

Students with uncontrolled asthma often miss more school and have poorer academic performance than healthy students. With the help of strong school asthma management programs, students with asthma can have equally good school attendance. When asthma is well controlled, students are ready to learn.

Effectively managing a child's asthma is best accomplished through a comprehensive plan that addresses both the medical management of the disease and the avoidance of environmental triggers. Because children spend most of their time in schools, day care facilities or at home, it is important to reduce their exposure to environmental asthma triggers as much as possible in each of these environments.

Develop an Asthma Management Plan in Your School or District

As you develop your district's or school's Asthma Management Plan, consider incorporating the following activities for quality asthma management:

- Use the *IAQ Tools for Schools* action kit.
- Identify all students with asthma.
- Provide school-based asthma education programs.
- Communicate with parents.

An indoor air quality (IAQ) management program that does not address asthma will not be able to address environmental health risks comprehensively, because IAQ and asthma are inextricably linked. By managing IAQ, you are already taking an important first step to managing asthma in your school or district. However, IAQ is only one component of effective asthma management.

To address asthma on all fronts, it is important to have an asthma management plan. If you are using the *IAQ Tools for Schools* Program and "Framework for Effective School IAQ Management," you most likely have the sustainable programmatic infrastructure in place to address this critical need in a more measurable, targeted and intentional way.

The components of Centers for Disease Control and Prevention's (CDC) "Strategies for Addressing Asthma within a Coordinated School Health Program," described below, form the foundation for an effective asthma management plan.

1. Establish management and support systems for asthma-friendly schools.

2. Provide appropriate school health and mental health services for students with asthma.

3. Provide asthma education and awareness programs for students and school staff.

4. Provide a safe and healthy school environment to reduce asthma triggers.

5. Provide safe, enjoyable physical education and activity opportunities for students with asthma.

6. Coordinate school, family and community efforts to better manage asthma symptoms and reduce school absences among students with asthma.

It is important to identify all students with asthma through monitoring morbidity associated with asthma, for example, frequent episodes at school, health room visits, limited physical activity, needing to leave school early or absenteeism. This can help to assess which programs or monitoring activities your school or district should implement. Focus resources on students whose asthma is not well controlled in order to promote improved school attendance and performance.

In order to identify what works and how you can improve the design and delivery of your school asthma management plan, it is essential to monitor program effectiveness. CDC and U.S. Environmental Protection Agency (EPA) offer resources on evaluation guidance specifically for asthma programs.

Controlling Common Asthma Triggers Found in Schools

Many factors found in the indoor and outdoor environment can cause, trigger, or exacerbate asthma symptoms. Some common environmental asthma triggers found in schools are listed below, along with suggestions for managing each common trigger:

Table 6.1. Environmental Asthma Triggers

Asthma Triggers Found in Schools	Asthma Management Tips for Schools
Environmental Tobacco Smoke— Environmental tobacco smoke is a mixture of smoke from the burning end of a cigarette, pipe, or cigar and the smoke exhaled by the smoker.	**Eliminate Exposure to Environmental Tobacco Smoke** Enforce no-smoking policies in schools.

Table 6.1. Continued

Asthma Triggers Found in Schools	Asthma Management Tips for Schools
Pests—Cockroach body parts, secretions, and droppings, as well as the urine, droppings, and saliva of other pests (such as rodents) are often found in areas where food and water are present.	**Control Pest Problems** Use Integrated Pest Management (IPM) to prevent cockroach and other pest problems (e.g., store food in tightly sealed containers and place dumpsters away from the building).
Mold—Mold can grow indoors when mold spores land on wet or damp surfaces. In schools, mold is most commonly found in bathrooms, kitchens, basements, around roof seams and plumbing, and in portable classrooms and trailers. Mold can grow anywhere that moisture is present.	**Clean Up Mold and Moisture** Fix leaks and moisture problems and thoroughly dry wet areas within 24–48 hours to prevent mold growth. Clean hard, moldy surfaces with water and detergent, then dry thoroughly.
Dust mites—Dust mites are too small to be seen but can be found in almost every home, school, and building. Dust mites can be found in school carpeting, upholstered furniture, stuffed animals or toys, and pillows.	**Reduce Dust Mite Exposure** Make sure schools are dusted and vacuumed thoroughly and regularly, and keep classrooms free of clutter. If stuffed toys are present, ensure they are washable and wash them regularly in hot water.
Animal dander—Pets' skin flakes, urine, and saliva are often found in classrooms and science labs. Any warm-blooded animal, including cats and dogs, may trigger asthma.	**Control Animal Allergens** Remove classroom animals from the school, if possible. If not, locate animals away from sensitive students and ventilation systems.

Other Sources of Indoor Air Pollutants

Usually the most effective way to improve IAQ is to eliminate individual sources of pollution or to reduce their emissions. Common sources of indoor pollution include secondhand smoke, school bus diesel exhaust coming into the school building, the off-gassing of furnishings and flooring, and chemicals from cleaning products. The following pollutant sources are especially important to control:

- **School Bus Exhaust.** Passing no-idling policies near the school building can reduce the indoor air pollution from school bus exhaust.

- **Cleaning Products.** Choosing the least-toxic cleaning methods and selecting appropriate products are important components of pollutant control. Fumes from cleaning products can linger long after they have been applied, which can exacerbate asthma symptoms and expose students and staff to potentially harmful substances.

- **Chemical Management.** The School Chemical Cleanout Campaign gives K-12 schools information and tools to responsibly manage chemicals. A successful chemical management program meets the unique needs of each school and ensures that all schools are free from hazards associated with mismanaged chemicals.

Section 6.3

Using a Respirator at Work

This section includes text excerpted from "Respiratory Protection in General Industry: An Overview of Hazards and OSHA's Program Requirements," Occupational Safety and Health Administration (OSHA), January 27, 2012. Reviewed September 2016.

Respiratory hazards can exist in various forms at general industry worksites. They may be gases, vapors, dusts, mists, fumes, smoke, sprays, and fog. Some of these substances can make you sick or kill you if you breathe them in. Certain respiratory hazards act quickly, like carbon monoxide—an invisible, odorless gas—which can make you unconscious or kill you in minutes. Other respiratory hazards can take years to make you sick, like asbestos which can cause lung cancer years or even decades after you breathe it in. More examples of respiratory hazards in general industry include, but are not limited to:

- dusts, such as those found when adding dry ingredients to a mixture;

- metal fumes from welding, cutting, and smelting of metals;

- solvent vapors from spray coatings, adhesives, paints, strippers, and cleaning solvents;

- infectious agents, such as tuberculosis bacteria in healthcare settings;

- chemical hazards, such as chlorine gas and anhydrous ammonia in chemical processing and use operations;

- sensitizing vapors or dusts, such as isocyanates, certain epoxies, and beryllium;

- oxygen deficiency, which might be found in confined spaces; and

- pharmaceuticals during the production of prescription drugs.

When there are respiratory hazards in your workplace, your employer must use several methods to reduce your exposure to them, including:

- engineering controls (such as local exhaust ventilation);

- work practice controls (such as applying coatings using a brush rather than a spray); and

- administrative controls (such as minimizing the exposure time or the number of workers exposed to the hazard).

When you and your co-workers cannot be adequately protected from respiratory hazards through use of these methods, then your employer must provide you with an appropriate respirator to protect your health.

Respiratory protection must be selected based on the hazard you will be exposed to on the job. Not every respirator will protect you against every hazard, so it's important for your employer to select the right one.

For example, filtering facepiece respirators may protect you against particulate hazards, such as dusts. However, a filtering facepiece respirator will not protect you against gas and vapor hazards, such as solvent vapors. If you are exposed to airborne hazards that are not particulates, you will need a different type of respirator. For example, you could use an air-purifying respirator with chemical cartridges or an atmosphere-supplying respirator, such as an airline respirator or a self-contained breathing apparatus—also known as an SCBA.

In addition, atmosphere-supplying respirators are the only respirators that will protect you against hazardous atmospheres, like carbon monoxide and lack of oxygen.

Remember, selecting an appropriate respirator is your employer's responsibility.

When respirators must be used in your workplace, your employer must have a respiratory protection program. This program must meet the requirements of either the Federal Occupational Safety and Health Administration (OSHA) or your State OSHA respiratory protection standard.

The standard requires your employer to do the following:

- develop and implement a written respiratory protection program;
- evaluate the respiratory hazards in the workplace;
- select and provide appropriate respirators;
- provide worker medical evaluations and respirator fit testing;
- provide for the maintenance, storage, and cleaning of respirators;
- provide worker training about respiratory hazards and proper respirator use;
- evaluate workers' use of respirators and correct any problems;
- provide you with access to specific records and documents, such as a written copy of your employer's respiratory protection program; and
- conduct a periodic program review.

Because each workplace is different, it is very important that your employer's respiratory protection program address your specific workplace. For example, workplaces may differ in the following ways:

- the types and amount of respiratory hazards present;
- the people who manage the program;
- the policies and procedures for tasks, such as respirator selection, maintenance, and use; and
- other exposure control methods, such as using local exhaust ventilation.

Workplace conditions that affect respiratory hazards and respirator use may change over time. Therefore, the written program must be updated as necessary to account for those changes in workplace conditions that affect respiratory hazards and respirator use. For example, changes in workplace conditions related to respiratory hazards could include:

- new work processes or techniques, such as installing a new electroplating line;
- the use of new or different materials or chemicals;
  - changes in the amount of a respiratory hazard in the workplace; or
  - changes in the types of respirators being used.

Notify your supervisor if something changes in your workplace that conflicts with, or may not be covered by, your respirator training or established workplace policies or procedures.

Your employer's respiratory protection program must be managed by a qualified, trained program administrator. This person must monitor the program and make sure that you and your co-workers are adequately protected. The program administrator will know a lot about your workplace respiratory protection program and should be able to answer any questions you may have about respirator use. The program administrator must know about the requirements of the OSHA or State OSHA Respiratory Protection Standard and evaluate the program periodically and make any necessary changes.

Section 6.4

Improving Indoor Air Quality at Work

This section includes text excerpted from "An Office Building Occupants Guide to Indoor Air Quality," U.S. Environmental Protection Agency (EPA), September 6, 2016.

Why Is Indoor Air Quality Important?

Indoor air quality is a major concern to businesses, building managers, tenants and employees because it can impact the health, comfort, well being and productivity of building occupants.

Most Americans spend up to 90 percent of their time indoors and many spend most of their working hours in an office environment. Studies conducted by the U.S. Environmental Protection Agency (EPA) and others show that indoor environments sometimes can have levels of pollutants that are actually higher than levels found outside.

Pollutants in our indoor environment can increase the risk of illness. Several studies by EPA, states, and independent scientific panels have consistently ranked indoor air pollution as an important environmental health problem. While most buildings do not have severe indoor air quality problems, even well-run buildings can sometimes experience episodes of poor indoor air quality.

A 1989 EPA Report to Congress concluded that improved indoor air quality can result in higher productivity and fewer lost work days. EPA estimates that poor indoor air may cost the nation tens of billions of dollars each year in lost productivity and medical care.

Factors That Contribute to Indoor Air Quality

Indoor air quality is not a simple, easily defined concept like a desk or a leaky faucet. It is a constantly changing interaction of complex factors that affect the types, levels and importance of pollutants in indoor environments. These factors include: sources of pollutants or odors; design, maintenance and operation of building ventilation systems; moisture and humidity; and occupant perceptions and susceptibilities. In addition, there are many other factors that affect comfort or perception of indoor air quality.

Controlling indoor air quality involves integrating three main strategies. First, manage the sources of pollutants either by removing them from the building or isolating them from people through physical barriers, air pressure relationships, or by controlling the timing of their use. Second, dilute pollutants and remove them from the building through ventilation. Third, use filtration to clean the air of pollutants.

Management of Pollutant Sources, Both inside and outside the Building

Pollutants can be generated by outdoor or indoor sources, including building maintenance activities, pest control, housekeeping, renovation or remodeling, new furnishings or finishes, and building occupant activities.

One important goal of an indoor air quality program is to minimize people's exposure to pollutants from these sources. Some of the key pollutant categories include:

- **Biological contaminants.** Excessive concentrations of bacteria, viruses, fungi (including molds), dust mite allergen, animal dander and pollen may result from inadequate maintenance and housekeeping, water spills, inadequate humidity control, condensation, or may be brought into the building by occupants, infiltration, or ventilation air. Allergic responses to indoor biological pollutant exposures cause symptoms in allergic individuals and also play a key role in triggering asthma episodes for an estimated 15 million Americans.

- **Chemical pollutants.** Sources of chemical pollutants include tobacco smoke, emissions from products used in the building (e.g., office equipment; furniture, wall and floor coverings; and cleaning and consumer products) accidental spill of chemicals, and gases such as carbon monoxide and nitrogen dioxide, which are products of combustion.

- **Particles.** Particles are solid or liquid substances which are light enough to be suspended in the air, the largest of which may be visible in sunbeams streaming into a room. However, smaller particles that you cannot see are likely to be more harmful to health. Particles of dust, dirt, or other substances may be drawn into the building from outside and can also be produced by activities that occur in buildings, like sanding wood or drywall, printing, copying, operating equipment and smoking.

Type of Pollutant

Many different factors influence how indoor air pollutants impact occupants. Some pollutants, like radon, are of concern because exposure to high levels of the pollutant over long periods of time increases risk of serious, life threatening illnesses, such as lung cancer. Other contaminants, such as carbon monoxide at very high levels, can cause death within minutes. Some pollutants can cause both short and long term health problems. Prolonged exposure to environmental tobacco smoke can cause lung cancer, and short term exposures can result in irritation and significant respiratory problems for some people, particularly young children.

People can react very differently when exposed to the same contaminants at similar concentrations. For example, some people can develop severe allergic reactions to biological contaminants to which other people will not react. Similarly, exposure to very low levels of chemicals may be irritating to some people but not others. For people with asthma and other pre-existing conditions, exposure to irritants like environmental tobacco smoke or gases or particles from various indoor sources may cause more severe reactions than the same exposure would in others.

Moisture and Humidity

It is important to control moisture and relative humidity in occupied spaces. The presence of moisture and dirt can cause molds and other biological contaminants to thrive. Relative humidity levels that are too high can contribute to the growth and spread of unhealthy biological pollutants, as can failure to dry water-damaged materials promptly (usually within 24 hours) or to properly maintain equipment with water reservoirs or drain pans (e.g., humidifiers, refrigerators and ventilation equipment). Humidity levels that are too low, however, may contribute to irritated mucous membranes, dry eyes and sinus discomfort.

Design, Maintenance, and Operation of Building Ventilation Systems

Maintaining good indoor air quality requires attention to the building's heating, ventilation and air conditioning (HVAC) system; the design and layout of the space; and pollutant source management. HVAC systems include all of the equipment used to ventilate, heat and cool the building; to move the air around the building (ductwork); and to filter and clean the air. These systems can have a significant impact on how pollutants are distributed and removed. HVAC systems can even act as sources of pollutants in some cases, such as when ventilation air filters become contaminated with dirt and/or moisture and when microbial growth results from stagnant water in drip pans or from uncontrolled moisture inside of air ducts. Because of the HVAC system's importance, good indoor air quality management includes attention to:

- **Ventilation system design**. The air delivery capacity of an HVAC system is based in part on the projected number of people and amount of equipment in a building. When areas in a building are used differently than their original purpose, the HVAC system may require modification to accommodate these changes. For example, if a storage area is converted into space occupied by people, the HVAC system may require alteration to deliver enough conditioned air to the space.

- **Outside air supply**. Adequate supply of outside air, typically delivered through the HVAC system, is necessary in any office environment to dilute pollutants that are released by equipment, building materials, furnishings, products and people. Distribution of ventilation air to occupied spaces is essential for comfort.

- **Outdoor air quality.** When present, outdoor air pollutants such as carbon monoxide, pollen and dust may affect indoor conditions when outside air is taken into the building's ventilation system. Properly installed and maintained filters can trap many of the particles in this outdoor supply air. Controlling gaseous or chemical pollutants may require more specialized filtration equipment.

- **Space planning**. The use and placement of furniture and equipment may affect the delivery of air to an occupied space. For instance, the placement of heat generating equipment, like a computer, directly under an HVAC control device such as a thermostat may cause the HVAC system to deliver too much cool air, because the thermostat senses that the area is too warm. Furniture or partitions that block supply or return air registers can affect IAQ as well, and need to be positioned with attention to air flow.

- **Equipment maintenance.** Diligent maintenance of HVAC equipment is essential for the adequate delivery and quality of building air. All well-run buildings have preventive maintenance programs that help ensure the proper functioning of HVAC systems.

- **Controlling other pollutant pathways.** Pollutants can spread throughout a building by moving through stairwells, elevator shafts, wall spaces and utility chases. Special ventilation or other control measures may be needed for some sources.

Factors That Affect Occupant Comfort and Productivity

Besides the factors that *directly impact the levels of pollutants* to which people are exposed, a number of environmental and personal factors can affect how people *perceive* air quality. Some of these factors affect both the levels of pollutants *and* perceptions of air quality:

- odors

- temperature—too hot or cold

- air velocity and movement—too drafty or stuffy

- heat or glare from sunlight

- glare from ceiling lights, especially on monitor screens

- furniture crowding

- stress in the workplace or home

- feelings about physical aspects of the workplace: location, work environment, availability of natural light and the aesthetics of office design, such as color and style

- work space ergonomics, including height and location of computer, and adjustability of keyboards and desk chairs

- noise and vibration levels

- selection, location and use of office equipment

Ask your supervisor or office manager who to talk with if you have a concern about any of these factors.

Indoor Air Quality Is a Shared Responsibility

Some of the factors that contribute to poor indoor air quality may originate from inadequate HVAC design. Some may be solely in the control of the building management, such as maintenance of the HVAC system and the amount of outside air being mechanically brought into the building. Others are largely in the control of building tenants and occupants, such as materials used in renovations and products and furnishings brought into or used in the building by occupants. Some, like cleanliness and general housekeeping of the building, require the cooperation of both the building management as well as all of the individuals who work in the building. For these reasons, indoor air quality is a shared responsibility.

Good indoor air quality management practices can make a big difference. However, some factors, like reactions to indoor air contaminants among highly susceptible individuals, or the quality of the outside air, may not be within anyone's immediate control. It is also important to remember that any building, no matter how well operated, may experience periods of unacceptable indoor air quality due to equipment breakdown, inadequate maintenance, or in some cases, the actions of building occupants.

It is also important to keep in mind that many perceived indoor air quality problems are often comfort problems, such as temperature, humidity, or air movement in the space being too low or too high. In addition, many symptoms, such as headaches, can have causes that are not related to factors in the building.

The Good News...

Even though the factors that affect the quality of the indoor environment are numerous, the good news is that most indoor environmental problems can be prevented or corrected easily and inexpensively through the application of common sense and vigilance on the part of everyone in the building. Success depends on cooperative actions taken by building management and occupants to improve and maintain indoor air quality. By becoming knowledgeable about indoor air quality, tenants and occupants are in a good position to help building managers maintain a comfortable and healthy building environment. Work with management any time you:

- identify or suspect an indoor air problem

- need cleaning and maintenance service

- plan to install new office equipment

- plan for renovations and/or remodeling with a professional interior designer and/or an architect

- experience leaks, spills, or accidents

Things Everyone in the Building Can Do

All of the occupants of a building can have a great influence on indoor air quality. Everyday activities like heating food in a microwave and using the photocopier can generate odors and pollutants. By being aware of indoor air issues, occupants can help prevent problems. Here are some things you can do:

- **Do not block air vents or grilles.** Keep supply vents or return air grilles unblocked, so you won't unbalance the HVAC system or affect the ventilation of a neighboring office. Furniture, boxes or other materials near supply vents or return air grilles may also affect air flow. Follow your office's procedures to notify building management if your space is too hot, too cold, stuffy or drafty.

- **Comply with the office and building smoking policy.** Smoke in designated areas only.

- **Clean up all water spills promptly, water and maintain office plants properly and report water leaks right away.** Water creates a hospitable environment for the growth of micro-organisms such as molds or fungi. Some of these microbes, if they become airborne, can cause health problems.

- **Dispose of garbage promptly and properly.** Dispose of garbage in appropriate containers that are emptied daily to prevent odors and biological contamination.

- **Store food properly.** Food attracts pests. Some foods, if left unrefrigerated, can spoil and generate unpleasant odors. Never store perishable food products in your desk or on shelves. Refrigerators should be cleaned on a regular basis to prevent odors. Keep kitchens and dining areas clean and sanitize as necessary to prevent pests and maintain hygiene.

- **Notify your building or facility manager immediately if you suspect an IAQ problem.** This helps management determine the cause of the problem quickly so that a timely solution can be reached.

Chapter 7

Outdoor Air Pollution: Minimizing the Effects

Why Is Air Quality Important?

Local air quality affects how you live and breathe. Like the weather, it can change from day to day or even hour to hour. The U.S. Environmental Protection Agency (EPA) and your local air quality agency have been working to make information about outdoor air quality as easy to find and understand as weather forecasts. A key tool in this effort is the air quality index, or AQI. EPA and local officials use the AQI to provide simple information about your local air quality, how unhealthy air may affect you, and how you can protect your health.

How Can I Avoid Being Exposed to Unhealthy Air?

You can take simple steps to reduce your exposure to unhealthy air. First, you need to find out whether AQI levels are a concern in your area. You can do this, as described previously, by visiting the AIRNow website (www.airnow.gov), signing up for EnviroFlash, or checking your local media. If the AQI for ozone, particle pollution, carbon monoxide, or sulfur dioxide is a concern in your area, you can learn what

---

This chapter includes text excerpted from "Air Quality Index—A Guide to Air Quality and Your Health," U.S. Environmental Protection Agency (EPA), January 26, 2016.

steps to take to protect your health by checking the charts on the following pages. Two important terms you will need to understand are:

- **Prolonged exertion.** This means any outdoor activity that you'll be doing intermittently for several hours and that makes you breathe slightly harder than normal. A good example of this is working in the yard for part of a day. When air quality is unhealthy, you can protect your health by reducing how much time you spend on this type of activity.

- **Heavy exertion.** This means intense outdoor activities that cause you to breathe hard. When air quality is unhealthy, you can protect your health by reducing how much time you spend on this type of activity, or by substituting a less intense activity—for example, go for a walk instead of a jog. Be sure to reduce your activity level if you experience any unusual coughing, chest discomfort, wheezing, breathing difficulty, or unusual fatigue.

Ozone

What Is Ozone?

Ozone is a gas found in the air we breathe. Ozone can be good or bad, depending where it occurs:

Good ozone is present naturally in the earth's upper atmosphere—approximately 6 to 30 miles above the earth's surface. This natural ozone shields us from the sun's harmful ultraviolet rays.

Bad ozone forms near the ground when pollutants (emitted by sources such as cars, power plants, industrial boilers, refineries, and chemical plants) react chemically in sunlight. Ozone pollution is more likely to form during warmer months. This is when the weather conditions normally needed to form ground-level ozone—lots of sun—occur.

Who Is Most at Risk?

Several groups of people are particularly sensitive to ozone, especially when they are active outdoors. This is because ozone levels are higher outdoors, and physical activity causes faster and deeper breathing, drawing more ozone into the body.

- **People with lung diseases, such as asthma, chronic bronchitis, and emphysema,** can be particularly sensitive to ozone. They will generally experience more serious health effects at lower levels. Ozone can aggravate their diseases, leading to increased medication use, doctor and emergency room visits, and hospital admissions.

- **Children,** including teenagers, are at higher risk from ozone exposure because they often play outdoors in warmer weather when ozone levels are higher, they are more likely to have asthma (which may be aggravated by ozone exposure), and their lungs are still developing.

- **Older adults** may be more affected by ozone exposure, possibly because they are more likely to have pre-existing lung disease.

- **Active people** of all ages who exercise or work vigorously outdoors are at increased risk.

- **Some healthy people** are more sensitive to ozone. They may experience health effects at lower ozone levels than the average person even though they have none of the risk factors listed above. There may be a genetic basis for this increased sensitivity.

In general, as concentrations of ground-level ozone increase, more people begin to experience more serious health effects. When levels are very high, everyone should be concerned about ozone exposure.

What Are the Health Effects?

Ozone affects the lungs and respiratory system in many ways. It can:

- **Irritate the respiratory system,** causing coughing, throat soreness, airway irritation, chest tightness, or chest pain when taking a deep breath.

- **Reduce lung function,** making it more difficult to breathe as deeply and vigorously as you normally would, especially when exercising. Breathing may start to feel uncomfortable, and you may notice that you are taking more rapid and shallow breaths than normal.

- **Inflame and damage the cells that line the lungs.** Within a few days, the damaged cells are replaced and the old cells are shed—much like the way your skin peels after sunburn. Studies suggest that if this type of inflammation happens repeatedly, lung tissue may become permanently scarred and lung function may be permanently reduced.

- **Make the lungs more susceptible to infection.** Ozone reduces the lung's defenses by damaging the cells that move particles and bacteria out of the airways and by reducing the number and effectiveness of white blood cells in the lungs.

- **Aggravate asthma.** When ozone levels are unhealthy, more people with asthma have symptoms that require a doctor's attention or the use of medication. Ozone makes people more sensitive to allergens—the most common triggers for asthma attacks. Also, asthmatics may be more severely affected by reduced lung function and airway inflammation. People with asthma should ask their doctor for an asthma action plan and follow it carefully when ozone levels are unhealthy.

- **Aggravate other chronic lung diseases** such as emphysema and bronchitis. As concentrations of ground-level ozone increase, more people with lung disease visit doctors or emergency rooms and are admitted to the hospital.

- **Cause permanent lung damage.** Repeated short-term ozone damage to children's developing lungs may lead to reduced lung function in adulthood. In adults, ozone exposure may accelerate the natural decline in lung function that occurs with age.

How Can I Protect My Health at Different AQI Values?

Table 7.1. Actions to Protect Your Health from Ozone

AQI Values	Actions to Protect Your Health From Ozone
Good (0–50)	None
Moderate (51–100*)	Unusually sensitive people should consider reducing prolonged or heavy outdoor exertion.
Unhealthy for Sensitive Groups (101–150)	The following groups should reduce prolonged or heavy outdoor exertion: • people with lung disease, such as asthma • children and older adults • people who are active outdoors
Unhealthy (151–200)	The following groups should avoid prolonged or heavy outdoor exertion: • people with lung disease, such as asthma • children and older adults • people who are active outdoors Everyone else should limit prolonged outdoor exertion.

Table 7.1. Continued

AQI Values	Actions to Protect Your Health From Ozone
Very Unhealthy (201–300)	The following groups should avoid all outdoor exertion: • people with lung disease, such as asthma • children and older adults • people who are active outdoors Everyone else should limit outdoor exertion.

* An AQI of 100 for ozone corresponds to an ozone level of 0.075 parts per million (averaged over 8 hours).

Particle Pollution

What Is Particle Pollution?

Particle pollution (also known as "particulate matter") consists of a mixture of solids and liquid droplets. Some particles are emitted directly; others form when pollutants emitted by various sources react in the atmosphere. Particle pollution levels can be very unhealthy and even hazardous during events such as forest fires. Particle levels can be elevated indoors, especially when outdoor particle levels are high.

Particles come in a wide range of sizes. Those less than 10 micrometers in diameter (smaller than the width of a single human hair) are so small that they can get into the lungs, where they can cause serious health problems.

- **Fine particles.** The smallest particles (those 2.5 micrometers or less in diameter) are called "fine" particles. These particles are so small they can be detected only with an electron microscope. Major sources of fine particles include motor vehicles, power plants, residential wood burning, forest fires, agricultural burning, some industrial processes, and other combustion processes.

- **Coarse particles.** Particles between 2.5 and 10 micrometers in diameter are referred to as "coarse." Sources of coarse particles include crushing or grinding operations, and dust stirred up by vehicles traveling on roads.

What Are the Health Effects and Who Is Most at Risk?

Particles smaller than 10 micrometers in diameter can cause or aggravate a number of health problems and have been linked with illnesses and deaths from heart or lung disease. These effects have been associated with both short-term exposures (usually over 24 hours, but possibly as short as one hour) and long-term exposures (years).

Sensitive groups for particle pollution include people with heart or lung disease (including heart failure and coronary artery disease, or asthma and chronic obstructive pulmonary disease), older adults (who may have undiagnosed heart or lung disease), and children. The risk of heart attacks, and thus the risk from particle pollution, may begin as early as the mid-40s for men and mid-50s for women.

• When exposed to particle pollution, people with heart or lung diseases and older adults are more likely to visit emergency rooms, be admitted to hospitals, or in some cases, even die.

• Exposure to particle pollution may cause people with heart disease to experience chest pain, palpitations, shortness of breath, and fatigue. Particle pollution has also been associated with cardiac arrhythmia and heart attacks.

• When exposed to high levels of particle pollution, people with existing lung disease may not be able to breathe as deeply or vigorously as they normally would. They may experience symptoms such as coughing and shortness of breath. Healthy people also may experience these effects, although they are unlikely to experience more serious effects.

• Particle pollution also can increase susceptibility to respiratory infections and can aggravate existing respiratory diseases, such as asthma and chronic bronchitis, causing more use of medication and more doctor visits.

How Can I Protect My Health at Different AQI Values?

Table 7.2. Actions to Protect Your Health from Particle Pollution

AQI Value	Actions to Protect Your Health From Particle Pollution
Good (0–50)	None
Moderate (51–100*)	Unusually sensitive people should consider reducing prolonged or heavy exertion.
Unhealthy for Sensitive Groups (101–150)	The following groups should reduce prolonged or heavy outdoor exertion: • people with heart or lung disease • children and older adults

Table 7.2. Continued

AQI Value	Actions to Protect Your Health From Particle Pollution
Unhealthy (151–200)	The following groups should avoid prolonged or heavy exertion: • people with heart or lung disease • children and older adults Everyone else should reduce prolonged or heavy exertion.
Very Unhealthy (201–300)	The following groups should avoid all physical activity outdoors: • people with heart or lung disease • children and older adults Everyone else should avoid prolonged or heavy exertion.

For particles up to 2.5 micrometers in diameter: An AQI of 100 corresponds to 35 micrograms per cubic meter (averaged over 24 hours).
For particles up to 10 micrometers in diameter: An AQI of 100 corresponds to 150 micrograms per cubic meter (averaged over 24 hours).

Carbon Monoxide

What Is Carbon Monoxide?

Carbon monoxide is an odorless, colorless gas. It forms when the carbon in fuels does not completely burn. Vehicle exhaust contributes roughly 75 percent of all carbon monoxide emissions nationwide, and up to 95 percent in cities. Other sources include fuel combustion in industrial processes and natural sources such as wildfires. Carbon monoxide levels typically are highest during cold weather, because cold temperatures make combustion less complete and cause inversions that trap pollutants close to the ground.

What Are the Health Effects and Who Is Most at Risk?

Carbon monoxide enters the bloodstream through the lungs and binds to hemoglobin, the substance in blood that carries oxygen to cells. It reduces the amount of oxygen reaching the body's organs and tissues.

- People with cardiovascular disease, such as coronary artery disease, are most at risk. They may experience chest pain and other cardiovascular symptoms if they are exposed to carbon monoxide, particularly while exercising.

- People with marginal or compromised cardiovascular and respiratory systems (for example, individuals with congestive heart failure, cerebrovascular disease, anemia, or chronic obstructive lung disease), and possibly young infants and fetuses, also may be at greater risk from carbon monoxide pollution.

• In healthy individuals, exposure to higher levels of carbon monoxide can affect mental alertness and vision.

How Can I Protect My Health at Different AQI Values?

Table 7.3. Actions to Protect Your Health from Carbon Monoxide

AQI Value	Actions to Protect Your Health From Carbon Monoxide
Good (0–50)	None
Moderate (51–100*)	None
Unhealthy for Sensitive Groups (101–150)	People with heart disease, such as angina, should reduce heavy exertion and avoid sources of carbon monoxide, such as heavy traffic.
Unhealthy (151–200)	People with heart disease, such as angina, should reduce moderate exertion and avoid sources of carbon monoxide, such as heavy traffic.
Very Unhealthy (201–300)	People with heart disease, such as angina, should avoid exertion and sources of carbon monoxide, such as heavy traffic.

* An AQI of 100 for carbon monoxide corresponds to a level of 9 parts per million (averaged over 8 hours).

Sulfur Dioxide

What Is Sulfur Dioxide?

Sulfur dioxide, a colorless, reactive gas, is produced when sulfur-containing fuels such as coal and oil are burned. Generally, the highest levels of sulfur dioxide are found near large industrial complexes. Major sources include power plants, refineries, and industrial boilers.

What Are the Health Effects and Who Is Most at Risk?

Sulfur dioxide is an irritant gas that is removed by the nasal passages. Moderate activity levels that trigger mouth breathing, such as a brisk walk, are needed for sulfur dioxide to cause health effects in most people.

• People with asthma who are physically active outdoors are most likely to experience the health effects of sulfur dioxide. The main effect, even with very brief exposure (minutes), is a narrowing of the airways (called bronchoconstriction). This may be accompanied by wheezing, chest tightness, and shortness of breath, which may require use of medication that opens the airways. Symptoms increase as sulfur dioxide levels or breathing rate increases. When exposure to sulfur dioxide ceases, lung function typically returns to normal within an hour, even without medication.

- At very high levels, sulfur dioxide may cause wheezing, chest tightness, and shortness of breath even in healthy people who do not have asthma.

- Long-term exposure to sulfur dioxide may cause respiratory symptoms and illness, and aggravate asthma. People with asthma are the most susceptible to sulfur dioxide. However, people with other chronic lung diseases or cardiovascular disease, as well as children and older adults, may also be susceptible to these effects.

How Can I Protect My Health at Different AQI Values?

Table 7.4. Actions to Protect Your Health from Sulfur Dioxide

AQI Value	Actions to Protect Your Health From Sulfur Dioxide
Good (0–50)	None
Moderate (51–100*)	None
Unhealthy for Sensitive Groups (101–150)	People with asthma should consider reducing exertion outdoors.
Unhealthy (151–200)	Children, asthmatics, and people with heart or lung disease should reduce exertion outdoors.
Very Unhealthy (201–300)	Children, asthmatics, and people with heart or lung disease should avoid outdoor exertion. Everyone else should reduce exertion outdoors.

* An AQI of 100 for sulfur dioxide corresponds to a level of 75 parts per billion (averaged over one hour).

Chapter 8

Statistics on
Respiratory Disorders

Chapter Contents

Section 8.1

Lung Cancer

This section includes text excerpted from "Lung Cancer,"
Centers for Disease Control and Prevention (CDC),
August 20, 2015.

Lung Cancer Statistics

More people in the United States die from lung cancer than any other type of cancer. This is true for both men and women.

In 2013—

- 212,584 people in the United States were diagnosed with lung cancer, including 111,907 men and 100,677 women.[*†]

- 156,176 people in the United States died from lung cancer, including 85,658 men and 70,518 women.[*†]

[*]Incidence counts cover about 99 percent of the U.S. population; death counts cover about 100 percent of the U.S. population. Use caution when comparing incidence and death counts.

[†]Source: U.S. Cancer Statistics Working Group. U.S. Cancer Statistics: 1999–2013 Incidence and Mortality Web-based Report. Atlanta (GA): Department of Health and Human Services, Centers for Disease Control and Prevention, and National Cancer Institute; 2016.

Risk by Age

The risk of getting lung cancer increases with age and is greater in men than in women. The tables below shows the percentage of men or women (how many out of 100) who will get lung cancer over different time periods. The time periods are based on the person's current age.

For example, go to the men's current age 60. The table 8.1 shows 1.96 percent of men who are now 60 years old will get lung cancer sometime during the next 10 years. That is, 1 or 2 out of every 100 men who are 60 years old today will get lung cancer by the age of 70.

Table 8.1. Percent of U.S. Men Who Develop Lung Cancer

Current Age	10 Years	20 Years	30 Years
30	0.02	0.16	0.82
40	0.14	0.81	2.58
50	0.69	2.51	5.34
60	1.96	5.01	7.04
70	3.57	5.93	N/A

Source: Howlader N, Noone AM, Krapcho M, Garshell J, Miller D, Altekruse SF, Kosary CL, Yu M, Ruhl J, Tatalovich Z, Mariotto A, Lewis DR, Chen HS, Feuer EJ, Cronin KA (eds). SEER Cancer Statistics Review, 1975–2012. National Cancer Institute. Bethesda, MD, based on November 2014 SEER data submission, posted to the SEER website, April 2015.

Table 8.2. Percent of U.S. Women Who Develop Lung Cancer

Current Age	10 Years	20 Years	30 Years
30	0.02	0.17	0.72
40	0.15	0.71	2.11
50	0.57	2	4.28
60	1.5	3.89	5.49
70	2.64	4.42	N/A

Source: Howlader N, Noone AM, Krapcho M, Garshell J, Miller D, Altekruse SF, Kosary CL, Yu M, Ruhl J, Tatalovich Z, Mariotto A, Lewis DR, Chen HS, Feuer EJ, Cronin KA (eds). SEER Cancer Statistics Review, 1975–2012, National Cancer Institute. Bethesda, MD, based on November 2014 SEER data submission, posted to the SEER ewbsite, April 2015.

Trends

Note: The word "significantly" below refers to statistical significance. 2012 is the latest year for which data are available.

Incidence Trends

From 2003 to 2012 in the United States, the incidence rate of lung cancer—

Men

- Decreased significantly by 2.5 percent per year among men.

- Decreased significantly by 2.5 percent per year among white men.

- Decreased significantly by 2.8 percent per year among black men.

- Decreased significantly by 3.1 percent per year among Hispanic men.

- Decreased significantly by 2.6 percent per year among American Indian/Alaska Native men.

- Decreased significantly by 1.8 percent per year among Asian/Pacific Islander men.

Women

- Decreased significantly by 0.9 percent per year among women.

- Decreased significantly by 0.9 percent per year among white women.

- Decreased significantly by 1 percent per year among black women.

- Decreased significantly by 1.3 percent per year among Hispanic women.

- Remained level among American Indian/Alaska Native women.

- Remained level among Asian/Pacific Islander women.

Mortality Trends

From 2003 to 2012 in the United States, the death rate from lung cancer—

Men

- Decreased significantly by 2.7 percent per year among men.

- Decreased significantly by 2.6 percent per year among white men.

- Decreased significantly by 3.4 percent per year among black men.

- Decreased significantly by 3.1 percent per year among Hispanic men.

- Remained level among American Indian/Alaska Native men.

- Decreased significantly by 2 percent per year among Asian/ Pacific Islander men.

Women

- Decreased significantly by 1.4 percent per year among women.

- Decreased significantly by 1.3 percent per year among white women.

- Decreased significantly by 1.8 percent per year among black women.

- Decreased significantly by 1.4 percent per year among Hispanic women.

- Decreased significantly by 1.3 percent per year among American Indian/Alaska Native women.

- Decreased significantly by 0.5 percent per year among Asian/ Pacific Islander women.

Data source: *Ryerson AB, Eheman CR, Altekruse SF, Ward JW, Jemal A, Sherman RL, Henley SJ, Holtzman D, Lake A, Noone AM, Anderson RN, Ma J, Ly KN, Cronin KA, Penberthy L, Kohler BA. Annual Report to the Nation on the Status of Cancer, 1975–2012, featuring the increasing incidence of liver cancer.*

Note: *Hispanic origin is not mutually exclusive from race categories (white, black, Asian/Pacific Islander, American Indian/Alaska Native).*

Section 8.2

Asthma

This section contains text excerpted from the following sources:
Text under the heading "Asthma FastStats" is excerpted from
"FastStats—Statistics by Topic," Centers for Disease Control and
Prevention (CDC), October 5, 2015; Text beginning with the heading
"Asthma Prevalence" is excerpted from "Most Recent Asthma Data,"
Centers for Disease Control and Prevention (CDC), March 2016.

Asthma FastStats

- Number of adults who currently have asthma: 17.7 million

- Percent of adults who currently have asthma: 7.4%

- Number of children who currently have asthma: 6.3 million

- Percent of children who currently have asthma: 8.6%

- Number of visits to physician offices with asthma as primary diagnosis: 10.5 million

- Number of visits to emergency departments with asthma as primary diagnosis: 1.8 million

- Number of deaths: 3,630

- Deaths per 100,000 population: 1.1

Asthma Prevalence

Table 8.3. National Current Asthma Prevalence (2014)

Characteristic*	Number with Current Asthma (in thousands)	Percent with Current Asthma
Total	24,009	7.70%
Child (Age <18)	6,292	8.60%
Adult (Age 18+)	17,717	7.40%
All Age Groups		

Table 8.3. Continued

Characteristic*	Number with Current Asthma (in thousands)	Percent with Current Asthma
0–4 years	849	4.30%
5–14 years	4,244	10.30%
15–19 years	1,912	9.10%
20–24 years	1,890	8.90%
25–34 years	3,133	7.50%
35–64 years	8,897	7.30%
65+ years	3,084	6.90%
Child Age Group		
0–4 years	849	4.30%
5–11 years	3,021	10.60%
12–17 years	2,422	9.70%
Young Teens (12–14 years)	1,223	9.70%
Teenagers (15–17 years)	1,199	9.70%
Adolescents (11–21 years)	4,236	9.30%
Young Adults (22–39 years)	5,634	7.60%
Sex		
Males	9,659	6.30%
Boys (Age <18)	3,770	10.10%
Men (Age 18+)	5,889	5.10%
Females	14,350	9.00%
Girls (Age <18)	2,522	7.00%
Women (Age 18+)	11,828	9.60%
Race/Ethnicity		
White NH	14,852	7.60%
Child (Age <18)	2,910	7.60%
Adult (Age 18+)	11,942	7.60%
Black NH	3,760	9.90%
Child (Age <18)	1,332	13.40%
Adult (Age 18+)	2,428	8.70%
Other NH	1,746	7.00%
Child (Age <18)	533	7.60%
Adult (Age 18+)	1,213	6.80%
Hispanic	3,651	6.70%

Table 8.3. Continued

Characteristic*	Number with Current Asthma (in thousands)	Percent with Current Asthma
Child (Age <18)	1,516	8.50%
Adult (Age 18+)	2,135	5.80%
Puerto Rican†	817	16.50%
Child (Age <18)	365	23.50%
Adult (Age 18+)	452	13.30%
Mexican/Mexican American†	1,952	5.70%
Child (Age <18)	857	7.10%
Adult (Age 18+)	1,095	4.90%
Federal Poverty Threshold		
Below 100% of poverty level	5,180	10.40%
100% to less than 250% of poverty level	6,746	7.60%
250% to less than 450% of poverty level	6,237	7.60%
450% of poverty level or higher	5,846	6.30%

Note: NH = Non-Hispanic

*Numbers within selected characteristics may not sum to total due to rounding

†As a subset of Hispanic

Asthma Mortality

Table 8.4. National Asthma Mortality (2014)

Characteristic	Number of Deaths*	Death Rate*,** per million
Total	**3,651**	**10.6**
Child (Age <18)	187	2.5†
Adult (Age 18+)	3,464	14.1†

Note: NH = Non-Hispanic

*Underlying cause of death is asthma

**Population-based rates are age-adjusted to the 2000 standard population

†Rates not age-adjusted

Section 8.3

Chronic Obstructive Pulmonary Disease (COPD)

This section includes text excerpted from "FastStats: Chronic Obstructive Pulmonary Disease (COPD)," Centers for Disease Control and Prevention (CDC), October 7, 2015.

Morbidity

- Number of adults with diagnosed chronic bronchitis in the past year: 8.7 million
- Percent of adults with diagnosed chronic bronchitis in the past year: 3.6%
- Number of adults who have ever been diagnosed with emphysema: 3.4 million
- Percent of adults who have ever been diagnosed with emphysema: 1.4%

Emergency Department Visits

Number of visits to emergency departments with chronic and unspecified bronchitis as the primary hospital discharge diagnosis: 285,000

Assisted Living and Other Residential Care

Percent of residents with COPD: 10.8%

Mortality

- Number of deaths from chronic lower respiratory diseases (including asthma): 149,205
- Chronic lower respiratory diseases (including asthma) deaths per 100,000 population: 47.2

- Cause of death rank: 3

- Number of bronchitis (chronic and unspecified) deaths: 664

- Bronchitis (chronic and unspecified) deaths per 100,000 population: 0.2

- Number of emphysema deaths: 8,284

- Emphysema deaths per 100,000 population: 2.6

- Number of deaths from other chronic lower respiratory diseases (excluding asthma): 136,627

- Other chronic lower respiratory diseases (excluding asthma) deaths per 100,000 population: 43.2

Section 8.4

Tuberculosis (TB)

This section includes text excerpted from "Tuberculosis (TB)," Centers for Disease Control and Prevention (CDC), October 9, 2014.

Trends in Tuberculosis (TB), 2014

How Many Cases of Tuberculosis (TB) Were Reported in the United States in 2014?

A total of 9,421 TB cases (a rate of 2.96 cases per 100,000 persons) were reported in the United States in 2014. Both the number of TB cases reported and the case rate decreased; this represents a 1.5 percent and 2.2 percent decline, respectively, compared to 2013*. This is the smallest decline in more than a decade.

Ratio calculation is based on unrounded data values.

Is the Rate of TB Declining in the United States?

Yes. Since the 1992 peak of TB resurgence in the United States, the number of TB cases reported each year has decreased.

How Do the TB Rates Compare between U.S.-Born Persons and Foreign-Born Persons Living in the United States?

In 2014, a total of 66 percent of reported TB cases in the United States occurred among foreign-born persons. The case rate among foreign-born persons (15.4 cases per 100,000 persons) in 2014 was approximately 13 times higher than among U.S.-born persons (1.2 cases per 100,000 persons).

How Many People Died from TB in the United States?

There were 555 deaths from TB in 2013, the most recent year for which these data are available. This is an 8 percent increase from the 510 TB deaths in 2012. Overall, the number of TB deaths reported annually has decreased by 67 percent since 1992.

What Are the Rates of TB for Different Racial and Ethnic Populations?

- American Indians or Alaska Natives: 5 TB cases per 100,000 persons
- Asians: 17.8 TB cases per 100,000 persons
- Blacks or African Americans: 5.1 TB cases per 100,000 persons
- Native Hawaiians and other Pacific Islanders: 16.9 TB cases per 100,000 persons
- Hispanics or Latinos: 5 TB cases per 100,000 persons
- Whites: 0.6 TB cases per 100,000 persons

For this report, persons identified as white, black, Asian, American Indian/Alaska Native, native Hawaiian or other Pacific Islander, or of multiple races are all non-Hispanic. Persons identified as Hispanic may be of any race.

Is Multidrug-Resistant Tuberculosis (MDR TB) on the Rise?

Overall, the percentage of MDR TB cases decreased slightly from 1.4 percent (96 cases) in 2013 to 1.3 percent (91 cases) in 2014.**

Of the total number of reported MDR TB cases, the proportion occurring among foreign-born persons increased from 31 percent (149 of 484) in 1993 to 88 percent (80 of 91) in 2014.

* MDR TB is defined as TB disease that is resistant to at least isoniazid and rifampin.
** Among culture-positive TB cases in the United States with initial drug-susceptibility testing results.

Part Two

Infectious
Respiratory Disorders

Chapter 9

Preventing Infectious Diseases

Chapter Contents

Section 9.1

Tips to Prevent Seasonal Flu

This section contains text excerpted from the following sources:
Text beginning with heading "Actions to Fight the Flu" is excerpted
from "Seasonal Influenza (Flu): Preventive Steps," Centers for
Disease Control and Prevention (CDC), September 1, 2016; Text
under the heading "Preventing the Flu: Good Health Habits Can
Help Stop Germs" is excerpted from "Seasonal Influenza (Flu):
Good Health Habits," Centers for Disease Control and
Prevention (CDC), August 2, 2016.

Flu is a serious contagious disease that can lead to hospitalization
and even death.

Actions to Fight the Flu

Take Time to Get a Flu Vaccine

- Centers for Disease Control and Prevention (CDC) recommends
  a yearly flu vaccine as the first and most important step in protecting against flu viruses.

- While there are many different flu viruses, a flu vaccine protects against the viruses that research suggests will be most
  common.

- Flu vaccination can reduce flu illnesses, doctors' visits, and
  missed work and school due to flu, as well as prevent flu-related
  hospitalizations.

- Everyone 6 months of age and older should get a flu vaccine by
  the end of October, if possible.

- CDC recommends use of injectable influenza vaccines (including inactivated influenza vaccines and recombinant influenza
  vaccines). The nasal spray flu vaccine (live attenuated influenza
  vaccine or LAIV) should not be used.

- Vaccination of high risk persons is especially important to
  decrease their risk of severe flu illness.

- People at high risk of serious flu complications include young children, pregnant women, people with certain chronic health conditions like asthma, diabetes or heart and lung disease and people 65 years and older.

- Vaccination also is important for healthcare workers, and other people who live with or care for high risk people to keep from spreading flu to them.

- Children younger than 6 months are at high risk of serious flu illness, but are too young to be vaccinated. People who care for infants should be vaccinated instead.

Take Everyday Preventive Actions to Stop the Spread of Germs

- Try to avoid close contact with sick people.

- While sick, limit contact with others as much as possible to keep from infecting them.

- If you are sick with flu-like illness, CDC recommends that you stay home for at least 24 hours after your fever is gone except to get medical care or for other necessities. (Your fever should be gone for 24 hours without the use of a fever-reducing medicine.)

- Cover your nose and mouth with a tissue when you cough or sneeze. Throw the tissue in the trash after you use it.

- Wash your hands often with soap and water. If soap and water are not available, use an alcohol-based hand rub.

- Avoid touching your eyes, nose and mouth. Germs spread this way.

- Clean and disinfect surfaces and objects that may be contaminated with germs like the flu.

Take Flu Antiviral Drugs If Your Doctor Prescribes Them

- If you get the flu, antiviral drugs can be used to treat your illness.

- Antiviral drugs are different from antibiotics. They are prescription medicines (pills, liquid or an inhaled powder) and are not available over-the-counter.

- Antiviral drugs can make illness milder and shorten the time you are sick. They may also prevent serious flu complications. For people with high-risk factors, treatment with an antiviral drug can mean the difference between having a milder illness versus a very serious illness that could result in a hospital stay.

- Studies show that flu antiviral drugs work best for treatment when they are started within 2 days of getting sick, but starting them later can still be helpful, especially if the sick person has a high-risk health condition or is very sick from the flu. Follow your doctor's instructions for taking this drug.

- Flu-like symptoms include fever, cough, sore throat, runny or stuffy nose, body aches, headache, chills and fatigue. Some people also may have vomiting and diarrhea. People may be infected with the flu, and have respiratory symptoms without a fever.

Preventing the Flu: Good Health Habits Can Help Stop Germs

The **single best way to prevent seasonal flu is to get vaccinated** each year, but good health habits like covering your cough and washing your hands often can help stop the spread of germs and prevent respiratory illnesses like the flu. There also are flu antiviral drugs that can be used to treat and prevent flu.

1. **Avoid close contact**

   Avoid close contact with people who are sick. When you are sick, keep your distance from others to protect them from getting sick too.

2. **Stay home when you are sick**

   If possible, stay home from work, school, and errands when you are sick. This will help prevent spreading your illness to others.

3. **Cover your mouth and nose**

   Cover your mouth and nose with a tissue when coughing or sneezing. It may prevent those around you from getting sick.

4. **Clean your hands**

   Washing your hands often will help protect you from germs. If soap and water are not available, use an alcohol-based hand rub.

5. **Avoid touching your eyes, nose or mouth**

   Germs are often spread when a person touches something that is contaminated with germs and then touches his or her eyes, nose, or mouth.

6. **Practice other good health habits**

   Clean and disinfect frequently touched surfaces at home, work or school, especially when someone is ill. Get plenty of sleep, be physically active, manage your stress, drink plenty of fluids, and eat nutritious food.

Section 9.2

Handwashing Prevents Infectious Diseases

This section includes text excerpted from "CDC Features: Healthy Living," Centers for Disease Control and Prevention (CDC), April 11, 2016.

Wash Your Hands

Handwashing is one of the best ways to protect yourself and your family from getting sick.
Handwashing is easy to do and it's one of the most effective ways to prevent the spread of many types of infection and illness in all settings—from your home and workplace to child care facilities and hospitals. Clean hands can stop germs from spreading from one person to another and throughout an entire community.

When Should You Wash Your Hands?

Feces (poop) from people or animals is an important sources of germs. A single gram of human feces—which is about the weight of a paper clip—can contain one trillion germs. Help stop the spread of germs by washing your hands often, especially during key times listed below.

- **Before**, during, and after preparing food
- **Before** eating food
- **Before** and after caring for someone who is sick
- **Before** and after treating a cut or wound
- **After** using the toilet
- **After** changing diapers or cleaning up a child who has used the toilet
- **After** blowing your nose, coughing, or sneezing
- **After** touching an animal, animal feed, or animal waste
- **After** touching garbage

What Is the Right Way to Wash Your Hands?

Follow the five steps below to wash your hands the right way every time.

- **Wet** your hands with clean, running water (warm or cold), turn off the tap, and apply soap.
- **Lather** your hands by rubbing them together with the soap. Be sure to lather the backs of your hands, between your fingers, and under your nails.
- **Scrub** your hands for at least 20 seconds. Need a timer? Hum the "Happy Birthday" song from beginning to end twice.
- **Rinse** your hands well under clean, running water.
- **Dry** your hands using a clean towel or air dry them.

What Should You Do If You Don't Have Soap and Clean, Running Water?

Washing hands with soap and water is the best way to reduce the number of germs on them in most situations. If soap and water are not available, use an alcohol-based hand sanitizer that contains at least 60 percent alcohol. Alcohol-based hand sanitizers can quickly reduce the number of germs on hands in some situations, but sanitizers do NOT eliminate all types of germs.

Hand sanitizers may not be as effective when hands are visibly dirty or greasy. Furthermore, hand sanitizers might not remove harmful chemicals like pesticides and heavy metals from hands. Be cautious when using hand sanitizers around children; swallowing alcohol-based hand sanitizers can cause alcohol poisoning if a person swallows more than a couple mouthfuls. How do you use hand sanitizers?

- Apply the product to the palm of one hand (read the label to learn the correct amount).

- Rub your hands together.

- Rub the product over all surfaces of your hands and fingers until your hands are dry.

Section 9.3

Pneumococcal Vaccination

This section includes text excerpted from "Pneumococcal Vaccination: What Everyone Should Know," Centers for Disease Control and Prevention (CDC), June 19, 2015.

Vaccine Information

The pneumococcal conjugate vaccine, **PCV13** or Prevnar 13®, is currently recommended for all children younger than 5 years old, all adults 65 years or older, and people 6 through 64 years old with certain medical conditions.

Pneumovax® is a 23-valent pneumococcal polysaccharide vaccine (**PPSV23**) that is currently recommended for use in all adults 65 years or older and for people who are 2 years or older and at high risk for pneumococcal disease (e.g., those with sickle cell disease, HIV infection, or other immunocompromising conditions). PPSV23 is also recommended for use in adults 19 through 64 years old who smoke cigarettes or who have asthma.

Does My Child Need the PCV13 Vaccine?

- **Infants and Children younger than 2 Years Old**

  - PCV13 is routinely given to infants as a series of 4 doses, one dose at each of these ages: 2 months, 4 months, 6 months, and 12 through 15 months.

- Children who miss their shots or start the series later should still get the vaccine. The number of doses recommended and the intervals between doses will depend on the child's age when vaccination begins. Ask your healthcare provider for details.

- **Children 2 through 5 Years Old**

  - Healthy children 24 months through 4 years old who are unvaccinated or have not completed the PCV13 series should get 1 dose.

  - Children 24 months through 5 years old with medical conditions such as the following should get 1 or 2 doses of PCV13 if they have not already completed the 4-dose series. Ask your healthcare provider for details.

  - sickle cell disease

  - a damaged spleen or no spleen

  - cochlear implant(s)

  - cerebrospinal fluid (CSF) leaks

  - HIV/AIDS or other diseases that affect the immune system (such as diabetes, cancer, or liver disease)

  - chronic heart or lung disease

  - children who take medications that affect the immune system, such as chemotherapy or steroids

- **Children 6 through 18 Years Old**

  - A single dose of PCV13 should be given to children 6 through 18 years old with certain medical conditions (i.e., sickle cell disease, HIV-infection, or other immunocompromising condition, cochlear implant, or cerebrospinal fluid (CSF) leaks) who have not previously received PCV13, regardless of whether they have previously received the 7-valent pneumococcal conjugate vaccine (PCV7) or the 23-valent pneumococcal polysaccharide vaccine (PPSV23). Ask your healthcare provider for details.

PCV13 may be given at the same time as other vaccines. However, PCV13 should not be given with PPSV23 nor with meningococcal conjugate vaccine. For children who are recommended to receive PPSV23 in addition to PCV13, PPSV23 should be administered at least 8 weeks after the child has received the final dose of PCV13. Children with a damaged spleen or no spleen should complete the PCV13 recommended series before getting meningococcal conjugate vaccine.

Which Adults Need the PCV13 Vaccine?

- All adults 65 years or older who have not previously received PCV13.

- Adults 19 years or older with certain medical conditions, and who have not previously received PCV13. Medical conditions include:
  - cerebrospinal fluid (CSF) leaks
  - cochlear implant(s)
  - sickle cell disease and other hemaglobinopathies
  - functional or anatomic asplenia
  - congenital or acquired immunodeficiencies
  - HIV infection
  - chronic renal failure
  - nephrotic syndrome
  - leukemia
  - Hodgkin disease
  - generalized malignancy
  - long-term immunosuppressive therapy
  - solid organ transplant
  - multiple myeloma

When Should Adults Get the PCV13 Vaccine?

- Adults who are 65 years or older and who have not previously received PCV13, should receive a dose of PCV13 first, followed 6 to 12 months later by a dose of PPSV23. If you have already received one or more doses of PPSV23, the dose of PCV13 should be given at least 1 year after you got your most recent dose of PPSV23.

- Adults 19 years or older with one of the above listed conditions who have not received any pneumococcal vaccine, should get a dose of PCV13 first and should also continue to receive the recommended doses of PPSV23. Ask your healthcare provider for details.

- Adults 19 years or older who have previously received one or more doses of PPSV23, and have one of the above listed conditions should also receive a dose of PCV13 and should continue to receive the remaining recommended doses of PPSV23. Ask your healthcare provider for details.

Which Children and Adults Need the PPSV23 Vaccine?

- All adults 65 years or older.

- Anyone 2 through 64 years old who has a long-term health problem such as: heart disease, lung disease, sickle cell disease, diabetes, alcoholism, cirrhosis, leaks of cerebrospinal fluid or cochlear implant.

- Anyone 2 through 64 years old who has a disease or condition that lowers the body's resistance to infection, such as: Hodgkin disease; lymphoma or leukemia; kidney failure; multiple myeloma; nephrotic syndrome; HIV infection or AIDS; damaged spleen, or no spleen; organ transplant.

- Anyone 2 through 64 years old who is taking a drug or treatment that lowers the body's resistance to infection, such as: long-term steroids, certain cancer drugs, radiation therapy.

- Any adult 19 through 64 years old who is a smoker or has asthma.

Residents of long-term care facilities should be evaluated for indications to receive PCV13 and/or PPSV23.

PPSV23 may be less effective for some people, especially those with lower resistance to infection. But these people should still be vaccinated, because they are more likely to have serious complications if they get pneumococcal disease.

Children who often get ear infections, sinus infections, or other upper respiratory diseases, but who are otherwise healthy, do not need to get PPSV23 because it is not effective against those conditions.

Are Pneumococcal Vaccines Effective?

Yes. Studies done on 7-valent pneumococcal conjugate vaccine (PCV7), which was licensed by U.S. Food and Drug Administration (FDA) in late 2000, showed the vaccine to be highly effective in preventing invasive pneumococcal disease in young children. The 13-valent pneumococcal conjugate vaccine, also known as Prevnar 13® or PCV13, which was licensed by FDA in February 2010, provides protection against infections caused by a greater variety of pneumococcal serotypes ("strains"). PCV13 is similar to PCV7 but includes 6 additional serotypes. This means that it provides protection against infections caused by a greater variety of pneumococcal serotypes. Studies have shown that PCV13 causes the body's immune system to create protective antibodies, which help fight the pneumococcal bacteria, similar to PCV7.

Pneumovax®, the pneumococcal polysaccharide vaccine that includes 23 serotypes, has been shown to be 50–85 percent effective in preventing invasive disease caused by those 23 serotypes in adults with healthy immune systems.

Questions and Answers for Parents and People Considering Immunization

What Pneumococcal Conjugate Vaccines Are Available in the United States?

Prevnar 13®, or PCV13, is a vaccine that covers 13 pneumococcal serotypes, which cause the majority of pneumococcal infections. PCV13 replaced the previous version of Prevnar®, known as PCV7, which included 7 pneumococcal serotypes.

Why Was PCV13 Developed?

There are more than 90 strains (serotypes) of pneumococcal bacteria and the first pneumococcal conjugate vaccine (PCV7) protects against 7 of them. Before PCV7 was introduced, these 7 serotypes were responsible for over 80 percent of severe pneumococcal infections among children. Since PCV7 introduction in 2000, there is significantly less pneumococcal disease. Even though there is less disease, other strains of pneumococcal bacteria have become more common-particularly one serotype, 19A. PCV13 includes the original 7 serotypes in PCV7 **plus** the 6 additional serotypes, including 19A. This gives us a vaccine that protects against the most common strains of pneumococcal bacteria currently responsible for severe pneumococcal infections.

Will PCV13 Be given to Children and Adults Who Already Received PCV7 or PPSV23?

Yes, depending on your child's situation and age. Ask your healthcare provider for details.

Is PCV13 Safe?

The first pneumococcal conjugate vaccine (PCV7) was extensively tested in more than 18,000 children before being licensed by the U.S. Food and Drug Administration (FDA) as safe and effective. After the vaccine was licensed, PCV7 safety was evaluated in more than 65,900 children and no major safety problems were identified.

The safety of PCV13 was assessed in 13 studies in which over 4,700 healthy infants and toddlers were administered at least 1 dose of PCV13 and over 2,700 children received at least 1 dose of PCV7 with other routine pediatric vaccines. The most commonly reported (more than 20 percent of subjects) adverse reactions were injection-site reactions, fever, decreased appetite, irritability, and increased or decreased sleep. The frequency and severity of local reactions at the injection site (pain/tenderness, redness of the skin, and induration/swelling) and systemic reactions (irritability, drowsiness/increased sleep, decreased appetite, fever, and restless sleep/decreased sleep) were similar in the PCV13 and PCV7 groups. These data suggest that the safety profile of PCV13 is comparable to PCV7.

Safety of PCV13 was evaluated in approximately 6,000 PPSV23-naïve and PPSV23-experienced adults 50 years or older. Common adverse reactions reported with PCV13 were pain, redness, and swelling at the injection site; limitation of movement of the injected arm; fatigue; headache; chills; decreased appetite; generalized muscle pain; and joint pain. Similar reactions were observed in adults who received PPSV23.

Ongoing surveillance for PCV7-associated adverse events has been conducted since 2000 by Centers for Disease Control and Prevention (CDC) and FDA using the Vaccine Adverse Event Reporting System as well as by the vaccine manufacturer. This monitoring of PCV13 safety will continue. Any adverse events can be reported by healthcare providers or patients to VAERS at 1-800-822-7967.

Has PCV13 Been Linked to Any Serious Condition at All?

PCV13 continues to be monitored, like all vaccines, for any safety concerns. Monitoring that was done during the 2010–11 flu season suggested that when flu vaccine and PCV13 are given on the same day, there may be an association with febrile seizures in children 12–23 months old. CDC is committed to further analyses and assessments to monitor the safety of PCV13. For PCV7, a considerable body of scientific evidence found it to be safe and effective against a very serious pathogen. Unfounded claims can cause harm to children if they result in less protection for them against potentially serious diseases.

Can I (Safely) Wait to Give PCV13 until My Child Is a Year Old in Order to Reduce the Number of Shots?

Because the risk of invasive pneumococcal disease is greatest for children less than one year old, the greatest advantage in disease prevention can be obtained by vaccinating your child at 2, 4 and 6 months old.

Does PCV13 Contain Thimerosal, a Mercury-Containing Preservative?

No. PCV13 does not contain thimerosal.

Chapter 10

Colds

Chapter Contents

Section 10.1

Common Cold

This section includes text excerpted from "Common Colds:
Protect Yourself and Others," Centers for Disease Control and
Prevention (CDC), February 8, 2016.

Common colds are the main reason that children miss school and
adults miss work. Each year in the United States, there are millions
of cases of the common cold. Adults have an average of 2–3 colds per
year, and children have even more.

Most people get colds in the winter and spring, but it is possible to
get a cold any time of the year. Symptoms usually include sore throat,
runny nose, coughing, sneezing, watery eyes, headaches and body
aches. Most people recover within about 7–10 days. However, people
with weakened immune systems, asthma, or respiratory conditions
may develop serious illness, such as pneumonia.

How to Protect Yourself and Others

You can help reduce your risk of getting a cold:

- **Wash your hands often with soap and water**

  Wash them for 20 seconds, and help young children do the
  same. If soap and water are not available, use an alcohol-based
  hand sanitizer. Viruses that cause colds can live on your hands,
  and regular handwashing can help protect you from getting
  sick.

- **Avoid touching your eyes, nose, and mouth with
  unwashed hands**

  Viruses that cause colds can enter your body this way and make
  you sick.

- **Stay away from people who are sick**

  Sick people can spread viruses that cause the common cold
  through close contact with others.

If you have a cold, you should follow these tips to prevent spreading it to other people:

- Stay at home while you are sick
- Avoid close contact with others, such as hugging, kissing, or shaking hands
- Move away from people before coughing or sneezing
- Cough and sneeze into a tissue then throw it away, or cough and sneeze into your upper shirt sleeve, completely covering your mouth and nose
- Wash your hands after coughing, sneezing, or blowing your nose
- Disinfect frequently touched surfaces, and objects such as toys and doorknobs

There is no vaccine to protect you against the common cold.

How to Feel Better

There is no cure for a cold. To feel better, you should get lots of rest and drink plenty of fluids. Over-the-counter medicines may help ease symptoms but will not make your cold go away any faster. Always read the label and use medications as directed. Talk to your doctor before giving your child nonprescription cold medicines, since some medicines contain ingredients that are not recommended for children.

Antibiotics will not help you recover from a cold. They do not work against viruses, and they may make it harder for your body to fight future bacterial infections if you take them unnecessarily.

When to See a Doctor

You should call your doctor if you or your child has one or more of these conditions:

- a temperature higher than 100.4° F
- symptoms that last more than 10 days
- symptoms that are severe or unusual

If your child is younger than 3 months of age and has a fever, you should always call your doctor right away. Your doctor can determine if you or your child has a cold and can recommend therapy to help with symptoms.

Causes of the Common Cold

Many different viruses can cause the common cold, but rhinoviruses are the most common. Rhinoviruses can also trigger asthma attacks and have been linked to sinus and ear infections. Other viruses that can cause colds include respiratory syncytial virus, human parainfluenza viruses, and human metapneumovirus.

Viruses that cause colds can spread from infected people to others through the air and close personal contact. You can also get infected through contact with stool (poop) or respiratory secretions from an infected person. This can happen when you shake hands with someone who has a cold, or touch a doorknob that has viruses on it, then touch your eyes, mouth, or nose.

Section 10.2

Bronchitis (Chest Cold)

This section includes text excerpted from "Bronchitis (Chest Cold),"
Centers for Disease Control and Prevention (CDC), April 17, 2015.

Acute bronchitis, or chest cold, often occurs after an upper respiratory infection like a cold, and is usually caused by a viral infection. The most common viruses that cause acute bronchitis include:

- Respiratory syncytial virus (RSV)

- Adenovirus

- Influenza viruses

- Parainfluenza

Risk Factors

There are many things that can increase your risk for acute bronchitis, including:

- Contact with another person with bronchitis

- Exposure to secondhand smoke, chemicals, dust, or air pollution

- A weakened immune system or taking drugs that weaken the immune system

Signs and Symptoms

Signs and symptoms of acute bronchitis include:

- coughing that produces mucus (you may not see mucus during the first few days you are sick)
- soreness in the chest
- fatigue (being tired)
- mild headache
- mild body aches
- fever (usually less than 101 °F)
- watery eyes
- sore throat

Most symptoms of acute bronchitis last for up to 2 weeks, but the cough can last up to 8 weeks in some people.

When to Seek Medical Care

See a healthcare professional if you or your child has any of the following:

- temperature higher than 100.4 °F
- a fever and cough with thick or bloody mucus
- shortness of breath or trouble breathing
- symptoms that last more than 3 weeks
- repeated episodes of bronchitis

In addition, people with chronic heart or lung problems should see a healthcare professional if they experience any new symptoms of acute bronchitis.

If your child is younger than three months of age and has a fever, it's important to always call your healthcare professional right away.

Diagnosis and Treatment

Acute bronchitis is diagnosed based on the signs and symptoms a patient has when they visit their healthcare professional.

Acute bronchitis almost always gets better on its own and is almost never caused by bacteria, so antibiotics are not needed. Antibiotic treatment in these cases may even cause harm in both children and adults. Your healthcare professional may prescribe other medicine or give you tips to help with symptoms like sore throat and coughing.

If your healthcare professional diagnoses you or your child with another type of respiratory infection, such as pneumonia or whooping cough (pertussis), antibiotics will most likely be prescribed.

Symptom Relief

Rest, over-the-counter (OTC) medicines and other self-care methods may help you or your child feel better. For more information about symptomatic relief, talk to your healthcare professional, including your pharmacist. Remember, always use OTC products as directed. Many over-the-counter products are not recommended for children of certain ages.

Prevention

There are several steps you can take to help prevent bronchitis, including:

- Avoid smoking and avoid exposure to secondhand smoke

- Practice good hand hygiene

- Keep you and your child up to date with recommended immunizations

Chapter 11

Influenza

Chapter Contents

Section 11.1

Key Facts about Seasonal Influenza

This section includes text excerpted from "Key Facts about
Influenza (Flu)," Centers for Disease Control and
Prevention (CDC), August 25, 2016.

What Is Influenza (Also Called Flu)?

The flu is a contagious respiratory illness caused by influenza
viruses that infect the nose, throat, and lungs. It can cause mild to
severe illness, and at times can lead to death. The best way to prevent
the flu is by getting a flu vaccine each year.

Signs and Symptoms of Flu

People who have the flu often feel some or all of these signs and
symptoms:

- Fever* or feeling feverish/chills

- Cough

- Sore throat

- Runny or stuffy nose

- Muscle or body aches

- Headaches

- Fatigue (very tired)

- Some people may have vomiting and diarrhea, though this is
  more common in children than adults.

It's important to note that not everyone with flu will have a fever.

How Flu Spreads

Most experts believe that flu viruses spread mainly by droplets
made when people with flu cough, sneeze or talk. These droplets can

land in the mouths or noses of people who are nearby. Less often, a person might also get flu by touching a surface or object that has flu virus on it and then touching their own mouth, eyes or possibly their nose.

Period of Contagiousness

You may be able to pass on the flu to someone else before you know you are sick, as well as while you are sick. Most healthy adults may be able to infect others beginning 1 day **before** symptoms develop and up to 5 to 7 days **after** becoming sick. Some people, especially young children and people with weakened immune systems, might be able to infect others for an even longer time.

Onset of Symptoms

The time from when a person is exposed to flu virus to when symptoms begin is about 1 to 4 days, with an average of about 2 days.

Complications of Flu

Complications of flu can include bacterial pneumonia, ear infections, sinus infections, dehydration, and worsening of chronic medical conditions, such as congestive heart failure, asthma, or diabetes.

People at High Risk from Flu

Anyone can get the flu (even healthy people), and serious problems related to the flu can happen at any age, but some people are at high risk of developing serious flu-related complications if they get sick. This includes people 65 years and older, people of any age with certain chronic medical conditions (such as asthma, diabetes, or heart disease), pregnant women, and young children.

Preventing Flu

The first and most important step in preventing flu is to get a flu vaccination each year. Centers for Disease Control and Prevention (CDC) also recommends everyday preventive actions (like staying away from people who are sick, covering coughs and sneezes and frequent handwashing) to help slow the spread of germs that cause respiratory (nose, throat, and lungs) illnesses, like flu.

Diagnosing Flu

It is very difficult to distinguish the flu from other viral or bacterial causes of respiratory illnesses on the basis of symptoms alone. There are tests available to diagnose flu.

Treating

There are influenza antiviral drugs that can be used to treat flu illness.

Section 11.2

Types of Influenza Viruses

This section includes text excerpted from "Influenza Viruses," Centers for Disease Control and Prevention (CDC), August 19, 2014.

There are three types of influenza viruses: A, B and C. Human influenza A and B viruses cause seasonal epidemics of disease almost every winter in the United States. The emergence of a new and very different influenza virus to infect people can cause an influenza pandemic. Influenza type C infections cause a mild respiratory illness and are not thought to cause epidemics.

Influenza A viruses are divided into subtypes based on two proteins on the surface of the virus: the hemagglutinin (H) and the neuraminidase (N). There are 18 different hemagglutinin subtypes and 11 different neuraminidase subtypes. (H1 through H18 and N1 through N11 respectively.)

Influenza A viruses can be further broken down into different strains. Current subtypes of influenza A viruses found in people are influenza A (H1N1) and influenza A (H3N2) viruses. In the spring of 2009, a new influenza A (H1N1) virus emerged to cause illness in people. This virus was very different from the human influenza A (H1N1) viruses circulating at that time. The new virus caused the first influenza pandemic in more than 40 years. That virus (often called "2009 H1N1") has now replaced the H1N1 virus that was previously circulating in humans.

Influenza B viruses are not divided into subtypes, but can be further broken down into lineages and strains. Currently circulating influenza B viruses belong to one of two lineages: B/Yamagata and B/Victoria.

Centers for Disease Control and Prevention (CDC) follows an internationally accepted naming convention for influenza viruses. The approach uses the following components:

- The antigenic type (e.g., A, B, C)

- The host of origin (e.g., swine, equine, chicken, etc. For human-origin viruses, no host of origin designation is given.)

- Geographical origin (e.g., Denver, Taiwan, etc.)

- Strain number (e.g., 15, 7, etc.)

- Year of isolation (e.g., 57, 2009, etc.)

- For influenza A viruses, the hemagglutinin and neuraminidase antigen description in parentheses (e.g., (H1N1), (H5N1))

For example:

- A/duck/Alberta/35/76 (H1N1) for a virus from duck origin

- A/Perth/16/2009 (H3N2) for a virus from human origin

Influenza A (H1N1), A (H3N2), and one or two influenza B viruses (depending on the vaccine) are included in each year's influenza vaccine. Getting a flu vaccine can protect against flu viruses that are the same or related to the viruses in the vaccine. The seasonal flu vaccine does not protect against influenza C viruses. In addition, flu vaccines will NOT protect against infection and illness caused by other viruses that also can cause influenza-like symptoms. There are many other non-flu viruses that can result in influenza-like illness (ILI) that spread during flu season.

Section 11.3

Avian Influenza

This section includes text excerpted from "Avian Influenza A
Virus Infections in Humans," Centers for Disease Control and
Prevention (CDC), May 25, 2016.

Avian Influenza A Virus Infections in Humans

Although avian influenza A viruses usually do not infect humans,
rare cases of human infection with these viruses have been reported.
Infected birds shed avian influenza virus in their saliva, mucous and
feces. Human infections with bird flu viruses can happen when enough
virus gets into a person's eyes, nose or mouth, or is inhaled. This can
happen when virus is in the air (in droplets or possibly dust) and a person breathes it in, or when a person touches something that has virus
on it then touches their mouth, eyes or nose. Rare human infections
with some avian viruses have occurred most often after unprotected
contact with infected birds or surfaces contaminated with avian influenza viruses. However, some infections have been identified where
direct contact was not known to have occurred. Illness in humans has
ranged from mild to severe.

Signs and Symptoms of Avian Influenza A Virus Infections in Humans

The reported signs and symptoms of low pathogenic avian influenza* (LPAI) A virus infections in humans have ranged from conjunctivitis to influenza-like illness (e.g., fever, cough, sore throat, muscle
aches) to lower respiratory disease (pneumonia) requiring hospitalization. Highly pathogenic avian influenza (HPAI) A virus infections in
people have been associated with a wide range of illness from conjunctivitis only, to influenza-like illness, to severe respiratory illness (e.g.,
shortness of breath, difficulty breathing, pneumonia, acute respiratory
distress, viral pneumonia, respiratory failure) with multi-organ disease, sometimes accompanied by nausea, abdominal pain, diarrhea,
vomiting and sometimes neurologic changes (altered mental status,

seizures). LPAI H7N9 and HPAI Asian H5N1 have been responsible for most human illness worldwide to date, including the most serious illnesses and deaths.

Avian influenza A viruses are designated as highly pathogenic avian influenza (HPAI) or low pathogenicity avian influenza (LPAI) based on molecular characteristics of the virus and the ability of the virus to cause disease and mortality in chickens in a laboratory setting.

Detecting Avian Influenza A Virus Infection in Humans

Avian influenza A virus infection in humans cannot be diagnosed by clinical signs and symptoms alone; laboratory testing is required. Avian influenza A virus infection is usually diagnosed by collecting a swab from the nose or throat of the sick person during the first few days of illness. This specimen is sent to a lab; the laboratory looks for avian influenza A virus either by using a molecular test, by trying to grow the virus, or both. (Growing avian influenza A viruses should only be done in laboratories with high levels of protection).

For critically ill patients, collection and testing of lower respiratory tract specimens may lead to diagnosis of avian influenza virus infection. For some patients who are no longer very sick or who have fully recovered, it may be difficult to find the avian influenza A virus in the specimen, using these methods. Sometimes it may still be possible to diagnose avian influenza A virus infection by looking for evidence of the body's immune response to the virus infection by detecting specific antibodies the body has produced in response to the virus. This is not always an option because it requires two blood specimens (one taken during the first week of illness and another taken 34 weeks later). Also, it can take several weeks to verify the results, and testing must be performed in a special laboratory, such as at Centers for Disease Control and Prevention (CDC).

Treating Avian Influenza A Virus Infections in Humans

CDC currently recommends oseltamivir, peramivir, or zanamivir for treatment of human infection with avian influenza A viruses. Analyses of available avian influenza viruses circulating worldwide suggest that most viruses are susceptible to oseltamivir, peramivir, and zanamivir. However, some evidence of antiviral resistance has been reported in HPAI Asian H5N1 viruses and influenza A H7N9 viruses isolated from some human cases. Monitoring for antiviral resistance among avian influenza A viruses is crucial and ongoing. These data directly inform CDC and WHO antiviral treatment recommendations.

Preventing Human Infection with Avian Influenza A Viruses

The best way to prevent infection with avian influenza A viruses is to avoid sources of exposure. Most human infections with avian influenza A viruses have occurred following direct or close contact with infected poultry.

People who have had contact with infected birds may be given influenza antiviral drugs preventatively. While antiviral drugs are most often used to treat flu, they also can be used to prevent infection in someone who has been exposed to influenza viruses. When used to prevent seasonal influenza, antiviral drugs are 70 percent to 90 percent effective.

Seasonal influenza vaccination will not prevent infection with avian influenza A viruses, but can reduce the risk of co-infection with human and avian influenza A viruses. It's also possible to make a vaccine that can protect people against avian influenza viruses. For example, the U.S. government maintains a stockpile of vaccine to protect against avian influenza A H5N1 vaccine. The stockpiled vaccine could be used if a similar H5N1 virus were to begin transmitting easily from person to person. Creating a candidate vaccine virus is the first step in producing a vaccine.

Section 11.4

Influenza Vaccination

This section includes text excerpted from "Seasonal Influenza (Flu): Vaccination," Centers for Disease Control and Prevention (CDC), September 7, 2016.

Who Should Get Vaccinated?

All persons 6 months and older should be vaccinated annually.

Vaccination to prevent influenza is particularly important for persons who are at increased risk for severe complications from influenza as well as those people who live with or care for persons at higher risk for influenza-related complications, including healthcare personnel.

There are special considerations regarding vaccination of persons with history of egg allergy.

What Are the Influenza Vaccine Options This Season?

Centers for Disease Control and Prevention (CDC) recommends use of injectable influenza vaccines (including inactivated influenza vaccines and recombinant influenza vaccines). The nasal spray flu vaccine (live attenuated influenza vaccine or LAIV) should not be used.

Both trivalent (three-component) and quadrivalent (four-component) flu vaccines will be available.

Trivalent flu vaccines include:

- Standard-dose trivalent shots (IIV3) that are manufactured using virus grown in eggs. Different flu shots are approved for different age groups. Most flu shots are given in the arm (muscle) with a needle. One trivalent vaccine formulation can be given with a jet injector, for persons aged 18 through 64 years.

- A high-dose trivalent shot, approved for people 65 and older.

- A recombinant trivalent shot that is egg-free, approved for people 18 years and older.

- A trivalent flu shot made with adjuvant (an ingredient of a vaccine that helps create a stronger immune response in the patient's body), approved for people 65 years of age and older.

Quadrivalent flu vaccines include:

- Quadrivalent flu shots approved for use in different age groups.

- An intradermal quadrivalent flu shot, which is injected into the skin instead of the muscle and uses a much smaller needle than the regular flu shot. It is approved for people 18 through 64 years of age.

- A quadrivalent flu shot containing virus grown in cell culture, which is approved for people 4 years of age and older.

Package inserts should be consulted for recommended age groups and possible contraindications for each vaccine in addition to information regarding additional components of various vaccine formulations.

In addition, the *Advisory Committee on Immunization Practices (ACIP), Influenza Vaccine Recommendations, 2014–15* should be consulted.

Are Any of the Available Flu Vaccines Recommended over Others?

The Advisory Committee on Immunization Practices (ACIP) recommends annual influenza vaccination for everyone 6 months and older with either the inactivated influenza vaccine (IIV) or the recombinant influenza vaccine (RIV). The nasal spray flu vaccine (live attenuated influenza vaccine or LAIV) should not be used. There is no preference for one vaccine over another among the recommended, approved injectable influenza vaccines. There are many vaccine options to choose from, but the most important thing is for all people 6 months and older to get a flu vaccine every year. If you have questions about which vaccine is best for you, talk to your doctor or other healthcare professional.

When Should Vaccination Occur?

Optimally, vaccination should occur before onset of influenza activity in the community. Healthcare providers should offer vaccination by the end of October, if possible. Vaccination should continue to be offered as long as influenza viruses are circulating. While seasonal influenza outbreaks can happen as early as October, most of the time influenza activity peaks between December and March, although activity can last as late as May. Since it takes about two weeks after vaccination for antibodies to develop in the body that protect against influenza virus infection, it is best that people get vaccinated so they are protected before influenza begins spreading in their community.

Vaccination for Children

Children younger than 6 months old are the pediatric group at highest risk of serious influenza complications, but they are too young to get an influenza vaccine. The best way to protect young children is to make sure members of their household and their caregivers are vaccinated.

Influenza vaccination is recommended for all children 6 months of age and older.

Children 6 months through 8 years who have previously received 2 or more total doses of any influenza vaccine only need one dose. The two previous doses do not need to have been given during the same season or consecutive seasons.

Children 6 months through 8 years who have previously received only 1 dose of influenza vaccine, or who have never received influenza vaccine previously, need two doses of vaccine to be fully protected.

2 Dose Vaccination Instructions

The first dose should be given as soon as vaccine becomes available, and the second dose should be given at least 4 weeks after the first dose. The first dose "primes" the immune system; the second dose provides immune protection. Children who only get one dose but need two doses can have reduced or no protection from a single dose of flu vaccine. Two doses are necessary to protect these children. If a child needs the two doses, begin the process early, so that they are protected before influenza starts circulating in your community. Make sure to follow up to get the child a second dose if they need one. It usually takes about two weeks after the second dose for protection to begin.

Children who require two doses of flu vaccine do not need to receive the same flu vaccine both times; live or inactivated vaccine can be used for either dose. (Within approved indications and recommendations, no preferential recommendation is made for any type or brand of licensed influenza vaccine over another.)

Vaccination for Adults

Everyone 6 months of age and older are recommended to get the flu vaccine, including even the healthiest adults. Vaccination is especially important for people at high risk of serious influenza complications or people who live with or care for people at higher risk for serious complications.

Persons working in healthcare settings also should be vaccinated annually against influenza. Vaccination of healthcare professionals has been associated with reduced work absenteeism and with fewer deaths among nursing home patients.

People Who Should Not Be Vaccinated

People who have had a severe reaction to an influenza vaccination, and children younger than 6 months of age should not be vaccinated.

People who are moderately or severely ill with or without fever should usually wait until they recover before getting flu vaccine.

A history of Guillain-Barré syndrome (GBS) within 6 weeks following receipt of influenza vaccine is a precaution for the use of influenza vaccine. Such individuals have a risk of recurrence of GBS with subsequent vaccination, and if not at high risk of severe influenza complications should generally not be vaccinated. However, while data are limited, the established benefits of influenza vaccination might outweigh the risks for many people who have a history of GBS and who also are at high risk for severe complications from influenza.

Vaccination of People with a History of Egg Allergy

Most influenza vaccines are produced by growing influenza virus in embryonated chicken eggs, and therefore contain trace amounts of egg protein.

All vaccines should be administered in settings in which personnel and equipment for rapid recognition and treatment of anaphylaxis are available.

A previous severe allergic reaction to influenza vaccine, regardless of the component suspected to be responsible for the reaction, is a contraindication to future receipt of the vaccine.

Special Consideration Regarding Egg Allergy

People with egg allergies can receive any licensed, recommended age-appropriate influenza vaccine and no longer have to be monitored for 30 minutes after receiving the vaccine. People who have severe egg allergies should be vaccinated in a medical setting and be supervised by a healthcare provider who is able to recognize and manage severe allergic conditions.

Influenza Vaccines and Use of Influenza Antiviral Medications

- Administration of inactivated influenza vaccine to persons receiving influenza antiviral drugs for treatment or chemoprophylaxis is acceptable.

- Live-attenuated influenza vaccine should not be administered until 48 hours after cessation of influenza antiviral therapy.

- If influenza antiviral medications are administered within 2 weeks after receipt of live-attenuated influenza vaccine, the vaccine dose should be repeated 48 or more hours after the last dose of antiviral medication.

Concurrent Administration of Influenza Vaccine with Other Vaccines

- Inactivated vaccines do not interfere with the immune response to other inactivated vaccines or to live vaccines.

- Inactivated or live vaccines can be administered simultaneously with live-attenuated influenza vaccine.

- However, after administration of a live vaccine, at least 4 weeks should pass before another live vaccine is administered.

Chapter 12

Pertussis

Pertussis, also known as **whooping cough**, is a highly contagious respiratory disease. It is caused by the bacterium *Bordetella pertussis.*

Pertussis is known for uncontrollable, violent coughing which often makes it hard to breathe. After fits of many coughs, someone with pertussis often needs to take deep breaths which result in a "whooping" sound. Pertussis can affect people of all ages, but can be very serious, even deadly, for babies less than a year old.

The best way to protect against pertussis is by getting vaccinated.

Causes and Transmission

Causes

Pertussis, a respiratory illness commonly known as whooping cough, is a very contagious disease caused by a type of bacteria called *Bordetella pertussis*. These bacteria attach to the cilia (tiny, hair-like extensions) that line part of the upper respiratory system. The bacteria release toxins (poisons), which damage the cilia and cause airways to swell.

Transmission

Pertussis is a very contagious disease only found in humans. It is spread from person to person. People with pertussis usually spread the

---

This chapter includes text excerpted from "Pertussis (Whooping Cough)," Centers for Disease Control and Prevention (CDC), August 31, 2015.

disease to another person by coughing or sneezing or when spending a lot of time near one another where you share breathing space. Many babies who get pertussis are infected by older siblings, parents, or caregivers who might not even know they have the disease.

Infected people are most contagious up to about 2 weeks after the cough begins. Antibiotics may shorten the amount of time someone is contagious.

While pertussis vaccines are the most effective tool we have to prevent this disease, no vaccine is 100 percent effective. If pertussis is circulating in the community, there is a chance that a fully vaccinated person, of any age, can catch this very contagious disease. If you have been vaccinated but still get sick, the infection is usually not as bad.

Signs and Symptoms

Pertussis (whooping cough) can cause serious illness in babies, children, teens, and adults. Symptoms of pertussis usually develop within 5 to 10 days after being exposed, but sometimes not for as long as 3 weeks.

Early Symptoms

The disease usually starts with cold-like symptoms and maybe a mild cough or fever. In babies, the cough can be minimal or not even there. Babies may have a symptom known as "apnea". Apnea is a pause in the child's breathing pattern. Pertussis is most dangerous for babies. About half of babies younger than 1 year who get the disease need care in the hospital.

Early symptoms can last for 1 to 2 weeks and usually include:

- runny nose
- low-grade fever (generally minimal throughout the course of the disease)
- mild, occasional cough
- apnea—a pause in breathing (in babies)

Because pertussis in its early stages appears to be nothing more than the common cold, it is often not suspected or diagnosed until the more severe symptoms appear.

Later-Stage Symptoms

After 1 to 2 weeks and as the disease progresses, the traditional symptoms of pertussis may appear and include:

- paroxysms (fits) of many, rapid coughs followed by a high-pitched "whoop"
- vomiting (throwing up) during or after coughing fits
- exhaustion (very tired) after coughing fits

Pertussis can cause violent and rapid coughing, over and over, until the air is gone from the lungs and you are forced to inhale with a loud "whooping" sound. This extreme coughing can cause you to throw up and be very tired. Although you are often exhausted after a coughing fit, you usually appear fairly well in-between. Coughing fits generally become more common and bad as the illness continues, and can occur more often at night. The coughing fits can go on for up to 10 weeks or more. In China, pertussis is known as the "100-day cough." However, the "whoop" is often not there for people who have milder (less serious) disease. The infection is generally milder in teens and adults, especially those who have been vaccinated.

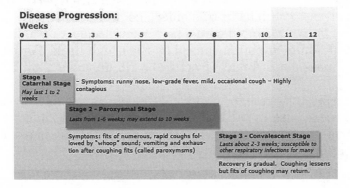

Figure 12.1. *Pertussis Timeline*

Recovery

Recovery from pertussis can happen slowly. The cough becomes milder and less common. However, coughing fits can return with other respiratory infections for many months after the pertussis infection started.

Complications

Babies and Children

Pertussis (whooping cough) can cause serious and sometimes deadly complications in babies and young children, especially those who are not fully vaccinated.

In babies younger than 1 year old who get pertussis, about half need care in the hospital. The younger the baby, the more likely treatment in the hospital will be needed. Of those babies who are treated in the hospital with pertussis about:

- 1 out of 4 (23%) get pneumonia (lung infection)

- 1 out of 100 (1.1%) will have convulsions (violent, uncontrolled shaking)

- 3 out of 5 (61%) will have apnea (slowed or stopped breathing)

- 1 out of 300 (0.3%) will have encephalopathy (disease of the brain)

- 1 out of 100 (1%) will die

Teens and Adults

Teens and adults can also get complications from pertussis. They are usually less serious in this older age group, especially in those who have been vaccinated with a pertussis vaccine. Complications in teens and adults are often caused by the cough itself. For example, you may pass out or break (fracture) a rib during violent coughing fits.

In one study, less than 1 out of 20 (5%) teens and adults with pertussis needed care in the hospital. Pneumonia (lung infection) was diagnosed in 1 out of 50 (2%) of those patients. The most common complications in another study were:

- weight loss in 1 out of 3 (33%) adults

- loss of bladder control in 1 out of 3 (28%) adults

- passing out in 3 out of 50 (6%) adults

- rib fractures from severe coughing in 1 out of 25 (4%) adults

Diagnosis and Treatment

Diagnosis

Pertussis (whooping cough) can be diagnosed by taking into consideration if you have been exposed to pertussis and by doing a:

- history of typical signs and symptoms

- physical examination

- laboratory test which involves taking a sample of mucus (with a swab or syringe filled with saline) from the back of the throat through the nose

- blood test

Treatment

Pertussis is generally treated with antibiotics and early treatment is very important. Treatment may make your infection less serious if it is started early, before coughing fits begin. Treatment can also help prevent spreading the disease to close contacts (people who have spent a lot of time around the infected person). Treatment after three weeks of illness is unlikely to help because the bacteria are gone from your body, even though you usually will still have symptoms. This is because the bacteria have already done damage to your body.

There are several antibiotics (medications that can help treat diseases caused by bacteria) available to treat pertussis. If you or your child is diagnosed with pertussis, your doctor will explain how to treat the infection.

Pertussis can sometimes be very serious, requiring treatment in the hospital. Babies are at greatest risk for serious complications from pertussis.

If Your Child Is Treated for Pertussis at Home

Do not give cough medications unless instructed by your doctor. **Giving cough medicine probably will not** help and is often not recommended for kids younger than 4 years old.

Manage pertussis and reduce the risk of spreading it to others by:

- Following the schedule for giving antibiotics exactly as your child's doctor prescribed.

- Keeping your home free from irritants—as much as possible—that can trigger coughing, such as smoke, dust, and chemical fumes.

- Using a clean, cool mist vaporizer to help loosen mucus and soothe the cough.

- Practicing good handwashing

- Encouraging your child to drink plenty of fluids, including water, juices, and soups, and eating fruits to prevent dehydration (lack of fluids). **Report any signs of dehydration to your doctor immediately.** These include dry, sticky mouth, sleepiness or tiredness, thirst, decreased urination or fewer wet diapers, few or no tears when crying, muscle weakness, headache, dizziness or lightheadedness.

• Encouraging your child to eat small meals every few hours to help prevent vomiting (throwing up) from occurring.

If Your Child Is Treated for Pertussis in the Hospital

Your child may need help keeping breathing passages clear, which may require suctioning (drawing out) of mucus. Breathing is monitored and oxygen will be given, if needed. Intravenous (IV, through the vein) fluids might be required if your child shows signs of dehydration or has difficulty eating. Precautions, like practicing good hand hygiene and keeping surfaces clean, should be taken.

Prevention

Vaccines

The best way to prevent pertussis (whooping cough) among babies, children, teens, and adults is to get vaccinated. Also, keep babies and other people at high risk for pertussis complications away from infected people.

In the United States, the recommended pertussis vaccine for babies and children is called DTaP. This is a combination vaccine that helps protect against three diseases: diphtheria, tetanus and pertussis.

Vaccine protection for these three diseases fades with time. Before 2005, the only booster (called Td) available contained protection against tetanus and diphtheria, and was recommended for teens and adults every 10 years. Today there is a booster (called Tdap) for preteens, teens, and adults that contains protection against tetanus, diphtheria and pertussis.

Infection

If your doctor confirms that you have pertussis, your body will have a natural defense (immunity) to future infections. Some observational studies suggest that pertussis infection can provide immunity for 4 to 20 years. Since this immunity fades and does not offer lifelong protection, vaccination is still recommended.

Antibiotics

If you or a member of your household has been diagnosed with pertussis, your doctor or local health department may recommend preventive antibiotics (medications that can help prevent diseases caused by bacteria) to other members of the household to help prevent the spread of disease. Additionally, some other people outside the household who have been exposed to a person with pertussis may be given preventive antibiotics, including

- people at risk for serious disease
- people who have routine contact with someone that is considered at high risk of serious disease

Babies younger than 1 year old are most at risk for serious complications from pertussis. Although pregnant women are not at increased risk for serious disease, those in their third trimester would be considered at increased risk since they could in turn expose their newborn to pertussis. You should discuss whether or not you need preventative antibiotics with your doctor, especially if there is a baby or pregnant woman in your household or you plan to have contact with a baby or pregnant woman.

Hygiene

Like many respiratory illnesses, pertussis is spread by coughing and sneezing while in close contact with others, who then breathe in the pertussis bacteria. Practicing good hygiene is always recommended to prevent the spread of respiratory illnesses. To practice good hygiene you should:

- cover your mouth and nose with a tissue when you cough or sneeze
- put your used tissue in the waste basket
- cough or sneeze into your upper sleeve or elbow, not your hands, if you don't have a tissue
- wash your hands often with soap and water for at least 20 seconds
- use an alcohol-based hand rub if soap and water are not available

Chapter 13

Pneumonia

What Is Pneumonia?

Pneumonia is an infection in one or both of the lungs. Many germs—such as bacteria, viruses, and fungi—can cause pneumonia.

The infection inflames your lungs air sacs, which are called alveoli. The air sacs may fill up with fluid or pus, causing symptoms such as a cough with phlegm (a slimy substance), fever, chills, and trouble breathing.

Types of Pneumonia

Pneumonia is named for the way in which a person gets the infection or for the germ that causes it.

Community-Acquired Pneumonia

Community-acquired pneumonia (CAP) occurs outside of hospitals and other healthcare settings. Most people get CAP by breathing in germs (especially while sleeping) that live in the mouth, nose, or throat.

CAP is the most common type of pneumonia. Most cases occur during the winter. About 4 million people get this form of pneumonia each year. About 1 out of every 5 people who has CAP needs to be treated in a hospital.

This chapter includes text excerpted from "Pneumonia," PubMed Health, National Center for Biotechnology Information (NCBI), June 11, 2014.

Hospital-Acquired Pneumonia

Some people catch pneumonia during a hospital stay for another illness. This is called hospital-acquired pneumonia (HAP). You're at higher risk of getting HAP if you're on a ventilator (a machine that helps you breathe).

HAP tends to be more serious than CAP because you're already sick. Also, hospitals tend to have more germs that are resistant to antibiotics (medicines used to treat pneumonia).

Healthcare-Associated Pneumonia

Patients also may get pneumonia in other healthcare settings, such as nursing homes, dialysis centers, and outpatient clinics. This type of pneumonia is called healthcare-associated pneumonia.

Other Common Types of Pneumonia

Aspiration Pneumonia

This type of pneumonia can occur if you inhale food, drink, vomit, or saliva from your mouth into your lungs. This may happen if something disturbs your normal gag reflex, such as a brain injury, swallowing problem, or excessive use of alcohol or drugs.

Aspiration pneumonia can cause pus to form in a cavity in the lung. When this happens, it's called a lung abscess.

Atypical Pneumonia

Several types of bacteria—*Legionella pneumophila, mycoplasma pneumonia,* and *Chlamydophila pneumoniae*—cause atypical pneumonia, a type of CAP. Atypical pneumonia is passed from person to person.

Other Names for Pneumonia

- Pneumonitis.

- Bronchopneumonia.

- Nosocomial pneumonia. This is another name for hospital-acquired pneumonia.

- Walking pneumonia. This refers to pneumonia that's mild enough that you're not bedridden.

- Double pneumonia. This refers to pneumonia that affects both lobes of the lungs.

What Causes Pneumonia?

Many germs can cause pneumonia. Examples include different kinds of bacteria, viruses, and, less often, fungi.

Most of the time, the body filters germs out of the air that we breathe to protect the lungs from infection. Your immune system, the shape of your nose and throat, your ability to cough, and fine, hair-like structures called cilia help stop the germs from reaching your lungs.

Sometimes, though, germs manage to enter the lungs and cause infections. This is more likely to occur if:

- your immune system is weak

- a germ is very strong

- your body fails to filter germs out of the air that you breathe

For example, if you can't cough because you've had a stroke or are sedated, germs may remain in your airways. ("Sedated" means you're given medicine to make you sleepy.)

When germs reach your lungs, your immune system goes into action. It sends many kinds of cells to attack the germs. These cells cause the alveoli (air sacs) to become red and inflamed and to fill up with fluid and pus. This causes the symptoms of pneumonia.

Germs That Can Cause Pneumonia

Bacteria

Bacteria are the most common cause of pneumonia in adults. Some people, especially the elderly and those who are disabled, may get bacterial pneumonia after having the flu or even a common cold.

Many types of bacteria can cause pneumonia. Bacterial pneumonia can occur on its own or develop after you've had a cold or the flu. This type of pneumonia often affects one lobe, or area, of a lung. When this happens, the condition is called lobar pneumonia.

The most common cause of pneumonia in the United States is the bacterium *Streptococcus pneumoniae*, or *pneumococcus*.

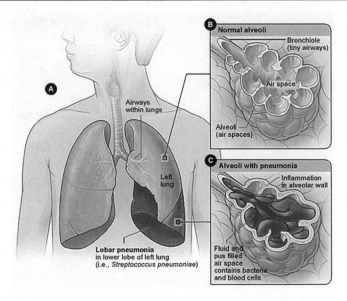

Figure 13.1. *Lobar Pneumonia*

Figure A shows the location of the lungs and airways in the body. This figure also shows pneumonia affecting the lower lobe of the left lung. Figure B shows normal alveoli. Figure C shows infected alveoli.

(Source: "Pneumonia," National Heart, Lung, and Blood Institute (NHLBI), March 1, 2011.)

Another type of bacterial pneumonia is called atypical pneumonia. Atypical pneumonia includes:

- *Legionella pneumophila.* This type of pneumonia sometimes is called Legionnaires' disease, and it has caused serious outbreaks. Outbreaks have been linked to exposure to cooling towers, whirlpool spas, and decorative fountains.

- *Mycoplasma pneumonia.* This is a common type of pneumonia that usually affects people younger than 40 years old. People who live or work in crowded places like schools, homeless shelters, and prisons are at higher risk for this type of pneumonia. It's usually mild and responds well to treatment with antibiotics. However, mycoplasma pneumonia can be very serious. It may be associated with a skin rash and hemolysis (the breakdown of red blood cells).

- *Chlamydophila pneumoniae.* This type of pneumonia can occur all year and often is mild. The infection is most common in people 65 to 79 years old.

Viruses

Respiratory viruses cause up to one-third of the pneumonia cases in the United States each year. These viruses are the most common cause of pneumonia in children younger than 5 years old.

Most cases of viral pneumonia are mild. They get better in about 1 to 3 weeks without treatment. Some cases are more serious and may require treatment in a hospital.

If you have viral pneumonia, you run the risk of getting bacterial pneumonia as well.

The flu virus is the most common cause of viral pneumonia in adults. Other viruses that cause pneumonia include respiratory syncytial virus, rhinovirus, herpes simplex virus, severe acute respiratory syndrome (SARS), and more.

Fungi

Three types of fungi in the soil in some parts of the United States can cause pneumonia. These fungi are:

- **Coccidioidomycosis**. This fungus is found in Southern California and the desert Southwest.

- **Histoplasmosis**. This fungus is found in the Ohio and Mississippi River Valleys.

- **Cryptococcus**. This fungus is found throughout the United States in bird droppings and soil contaminated with bird droppings.

Most people exposed to these fungi don't get sick, but some do and require treatment.

Serious fungal infections are most common in people who have weak immune systems due to the long-term use of medicines to suppress their immune systems or having HIV/AIDS.

Pneumocystis jiroveci, formerly *Pneumocystis carinii*, sometimes is considered a fungal pneumonia. However, it's not treated with the usual antifungal medicines. This type of infection is most common in people who:

- have HIV/AIDS or cancer

- have had an organ transplant and/or blood and marrow stem cell transplant

- take medicines that affect their immune systems

Other kinds of fungal infections also can lead to pneumonia.

Who Is at Risk for Pneumonia?

Pneumonia can affect people of all ages. However, two age groups are at greater risk of developing pneumonia:

- infants who are 2 years old or younger (because their immune systems are still developing during the first few years of life)

- people who are 65 years old or older

Other conditions and factors also raise your risk for pneumonia. You're more likely to get pneumonia if you have a lung disease or other serious disease. Examples include cystic fibrosis, asthma, COPD (chronic obstructive pulmonary disease), bronchiectasis, diabetes, heart failure, and sickle cell anemia.

You're at greater risk for pneumonia if you're in a hospital intensive-care unit, especially if you're on a ventilator (a machine that helps you breathe).

Having a weak or suppressed immune system also raises your risk for pneumonia. A weak immune system may be the result of a disease such as HIV/AIDS. A suppressed immune system may be due to an organ transplant or blood and marrow stem cell transplant, chemotherapy (a treatment for cancer), or long-term steroid use.

Your risk for pneumonia also increases if you have trouble coughing because of a stroke or problems swallowing. You're also at higher risk if you can't move around much or are sedated (given medicine to make you relaxed or sleepy).

Smoking cigarettes, abusing alcohol, or being undernourished also raises your risk for pneumonia. Your risk also goes up if you've recently had a cold or the flu, or if you're exposed to certain chemicals, pollutants, or toxic fumes.

What Are the Signs and Symptoms of Pneumonia?

The signs and symptoms of pneumonia vary from mild to severe. Many factors affect how serious pneumonia is, including the type of germ causing the infection and your age and overall health.

See your doctor promptly if you:

- have a high fever

- have shaking chills

- have a cough with phlegm (a slimy substance), which doesn't improve or worsens

- develop shortness of breath with normal daily activities

- have chest pain when you breathe or cough

- feel suddenly worse after a cold or the flu

People who have pneumonia may have other symptoms, including nausea (feeling sick to the stomach), vomiting, and diarrhea.

Symptoms may vary in certain populations. Newborns and infants may not show any signs of the infection. Or, they may vomit, have a fever and cough, or appear restless, sick, or tired and without energy.

Older adults and people who have serious illnesses or weak immune systems may have fewer and milder symptoms. They may even have a lower than normal temperature. If they already have a lung disease, it may get worse. Older adults who have pneumonia sometimes have sudden changes in mental awareness.

Complications of Pneumonia

Often, people who have pneumonia can be successfully treated and not have complications. But some people, especially those in high-risk groups, may have complications such as:

- **Bacteremia.** This serious complication occurs if the infection moves into your bloodstream. From there, it can quickly spread to other organs, including your brain.

- **Lung abscesses.** An abscess occurs if pus forms in a cavity in the lung. An abscess usually is treated with antibiotics. Sometimes surgery or drainage with a needle is needed to remove the pus.

- **Pleural effusion.** Pneumonia may cause fluid to build up in the pleural space. This is a very thin space between two layers of tissue that line the lungs and the chest cavity. Pneumonia can cause the fluid to become infected—a condition called empyema. If this happens, you may need to have the fluid drained through a chest tube or removed with surgery.

How Is Pneumonia Diagnosed?

Pneumonia can be hard to diagnose because it may seem like a cold or the flu. You may not realize it's more serious until it lasts longer than these other conditions.

Your doctor will diagnose pneumonia based on your medical history, a physical exam, and test results.

Medical History

Your doctor will ask about your signs and symptoms and how and when they began. To find out what type of germ is causing the pneumonia, he or she also may ask about:

- any recent traveling you've done
- your hobbies
- your exposure to animals
- your exposure to sick people at home, school, or work
- your past and current medical conditions, and whether any have gotten worse recently
- any medicines you take
- whether you smoke
- whether you've had flu or pneumonia vaccinations

Physical Exam

Your doctor will listen to your lungs with a stethoscope. If you have pneumonia, your lungs may make crackling, bubbling, and rumbling sounds when you inhale. Your doctor also may hear wheezing.

Your doctor may find it hard to hear sounds of breathing in some areas of your chest.

Diagnostic Tests

If your doctor thinks you have pneumonia, he or she may recommend one or more of the following tests.

Chest X-Ray

A chest X-ray is a painless test that creates pictures of the structures inside your chest, such as your heart, lungs, and blood vessels.

A chest X-ray is the best test for diagnosing pneumonia. However, this test won't tell your doctor what kind of germ is causing the pneumonia.

Blood Tests

Blood tests involve taking a sample of blood from a vein in your body. A complete blood count (CBC) measures many parts of your blood, including the number of white blood cells in the blood sample. The number of white blood cells can show whether you have a bacterial infection.

Your doctor also may recommend a blood culture to find out whether the infection has spread to your bloodstream. This test is used to detect germs in the bloodstream. A blood culture may show which germ caused the infection. If so, your doctor can decide how to treat the infection.

Other Tests

Your doctor may recommend other tests if you're in the hospital, have serious symptoms, are older, or have other health problems.

Sputum test. Your doctor may look at a sample of sputum (spit) collected from you after a deep cough. This may help your doctor find out what germ is causing your pneumonia. Then, he or she can plan treatment.

Chest computed tomography (CT) scan. A chest CT scan is a painless test that creates precise pictures of the structures in your chest, such as your lungs. A chest CT scan is a type of X-ray, but its pictures show more detail than those of a standard chest X-ray.

Pleural fluid culture. For this test, a fluid sample is taken from the pleural space (a thin space between two layers of tissue that line the lungs and chest cavity). Doctors use a procedure called thoracentesis to collect the fluid sample. The fluid is studied for germs that may cause pneumonia.

Pulse oximetry. For this test, a small sensor is attached to your finger or ear. The sensor uses light to estimate how much oxygen is in your blood. Pneumonia can keep your lungs from moving enough oxygen into your bloodstream.

If you're very sick, your doctor may need to measure the level of oxygen in your blood using a blood sample. The sample is taken from an artery, usually in your wrist. This test is called an arterial blood gas test.

Bronchoscopy. Bronchoscopy is a procedure used to look inside the lungs' airways. If you're in the hospital and treatment with antibiotics isn't working well, your doctor may use this procedure.

Your doctor passes a thin, flexible tube through your nose or mouth, down your throat, and into the airways. The tube has a light and small camera that allow your doctor to see your windpipe and airways and take pictures.

Your doctor can see whether something is blocking your airways or whether another factor is contributing to your pneumonia.

How Is Pneumonia Treated?

Treatment for pneumonia depends on the type of pneumonia you have and how severe it is. Most people who have community-acquired pneumonia—the most common type of pneumonia—are treated at home.

The goals of treatment are to cure the infection and prevent complications.

General Treatment

If you have pneumonia, follow your treatment plan, take all medicines as prescribed, and get ongoing medical care. Ask your doctor when you should schedule followup care. Your doctor may want you to have a chest X-ray to make sure the pneumonia is gone.

Although you may start feeling better after a few days or weeks, fatigue (tiredness) can persist for up to a month or more. People who are treated in the hospital may need at least 3 weeks before they can go back to their normal routines.

Bacterial Pneumonia

Bacterial pneumonia is treated with medicines called antibiotics. You should take antibiotics as your doctor prescribes. You may start to feel better before you finish the medicine, but you should continue taking it as prescribed. If you stop too soon, the pneumonia may come back.

Most people begin to improve after 1 to 3 days of antibiotic treatment. This means that they should feel better and have fewer symptoms, such as cough and fever.

Viral Pneumonia

Antibiotics don't work when the cause of pneumonia is a virus. If you have viral pneumonia, your doctor may prescribe an antiviral medicine to treat it.

Viral pneumonia usually improves in 1 to 3 weeks.

Treating Severe Symptoms

You may need to be treated in a hospital if:

- your symptoms are severe

- you're at risk for complications because of other health problems

If the level of oxygen in your bloodstream is low, you may receive oxygen therapy. If you have bacterial pneumonia, your doctor may give you antibiotics through an intravenous (IV) line inserted into a vein.

How Can Pneumonia Be Prevented?

Pneumonia can be very serious and even life threatening. When possible, take steps to prevent the infection, especially if you're in a high-risk group.

Vaccines

Vaccines are available to prevent pneumococcal pneumonia and the flu. Vaccines can't prevent all cases of infection. However, compared to people who don't get vaccinated, those who do and still get pneumonia tend to have:

- milder cases of the infection

- pneumonia that doesn't last as long

- fewer serious complications

Pneumococcal Pneumonia Vaccine

A vaccine is available to prevent pneumococcal pneumonia. In most adults, one shot is good for at least 5 years of protection. This vaccine often is recommended for:

- people who are 65 years old or older

- people who have chronic (ongoing) diseases, serious long-term health problems, or weak immune systems. For example, this may include people who have cancer, HIV/AIDS, asthma, or damaged or removed spleens

- people who smoke

- children who are younger than 5 years old

- children who are 5–18 years of age with certain medical conditions, such as heart or lung diseases or cancer

Influenza Vaccine

The vaccine that helps prevent the flu is good for 1 year. It's usually given in October or November, before peak flu season.

Because many people get pneumonia after having the flu, this vaccine also helps prevent pneumonia.

Hib Vaccine

Haemophilus influenzae type b (Hib) is a type of bacteria that can cause pneumonia and meningitis. (Meningitis is an infection of the covering of the brain and spinal cord.) The Hib vaccine is given to children to help prevent these infections.

The vaccine is recommended for all children in the United States who are younger than 5 years old. The vaccine often is given to infants starting at 2 months of age.

Other Ways to Help Prevent Pneumonia

You also can take the following steps to help prevent pneumonia:

- Wash your hands with soap and water or alcohol-based rubs to kill germs.

- Don't smoke. Smoking damages your lungs' ability to filter out and defend against germs. Although this resource focuses on heart health, it includes general information about how to quit smoking.

- Keep your immune system strong. Get plenty of rest and physical activity and follow a healthy diet.

If you have pneumonia, limit contact with family and friends. Cover your nose and mouth while coughing or sneezing, and get rid of used tissues right away. These actions help keep the infection from spreading.

Chapter 14

Sinusitis (Sinus Infection)

Sinusitis is an inflammation of the membranes lining the paranasal sinuses—small air-filled spaces located within the skull or bones of the head surrounding the nose. Sinusitis can be caused by an infection or other health problem, and symptoms include facial pain and nasal discharge. Nearly 30 million adults in the United States are diagnosed with sinusitis each year, according to the Centers for Disease Control and Prevention (CDC).

The paranasal sinuses comprise four pairs of air-filled spaces:

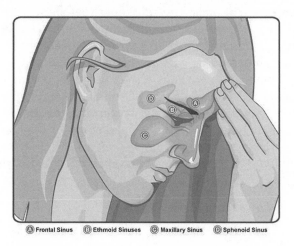

Ⓐ Frontal Sinus   Ⓑ Ethmoid Sinuses   Ⓒ Maxillary Sinus   Ⓓ Sphenoid Sinus

Figure 14.1. *Sinusitis*

This chapter includes text excerpted from "Sinusitis (Sinus Infection)," National Institute of Allergy and Infectious Diseases (NIAID), June 2015.

1. Frontal sinuses—over the eyes in the brow area

2. Ethmoid sinuses—just behind the bridge of the nose, between the eyes

3. Maxillary sinuses—inside each cheekbone

4. Sphenoid sinuses—behind the ethmoids in the upper region of the nose and behind the eyes

There are two basic types of sinusitis:

1. Acute, which lasts up to 4 weeks

2. Chronic, which lasts more than 12 weeks and can continue for months or years

Symptoms

Most people with sinusitis have facial pain or tenderness in several places, and their symptoms usually do not clearly indicate which sinuses are inflamed. The pain of a sinus attack arises because trapped air and mucus put pressure on the membranes of the sinuses and the bony wall behind them. Also, when a swollen membrane at the opening of a paranasal sinus prevents air from entering into the sinuses, it can create a vacuum that causes pain.

People with sinusitis have thick nasal secretions that can be white, yellowish, greenish, or blood-tinged. Sometimes these secretions drain in the back of the throat and are difficult to clear. This is referred to as "postnasal drainage." Chronic postnasal discharge may indicate sinusitis, even in people who do not have facial pain.

However, facial pain without either nasal or postnasal drainage is rarely caused by inflammation of the sinuses. People who experience pain but no nasal discharge often are diagnosed with a pain disorder—such as migraine, cluster headaches, or tension-type headaches—rather than sinusitis.

Less common symptoms of acute or chronic sinusitis include

- tiredness
- decreased sense of smell
- cough that may be worse at night
- sore throat
- bad breath
- fever

On very rare occasions, acute sinusitis can result in brain infection and other serious complications.

Causes

Colds, bacterial infections, allergies, asthma, and other health conditions can cause sinusitis, or inflammation of the paranasal sinuses.

Acute Sinusitis

Acute sinusitis is usually caused by a viral or bacterial infection. The common cold, which is caused by a virus, may lead to swelling of the sinuses, trapping air and mucus behind the narrowed sinus openings. Both the nasal and the sinus symptoms usually go away within two weeks. Sometimes, viral infections are followed by bacterial infections. Many cases of acute sinusitis are caused by bacteria that frequently colonize the nose and throat, such as *Streptococcus pneumoniae, Haemophilus influenzae*, and *Moraxella catarrhalis*. These bacteria typically do not cause problems in healthy people, but in some cases they begin to multiply in the sinuses, causing acute sinusitis. National Institute of Allergy and Infectious Diseases (NIAID) supports studies to better understand what factors put people at risk for bacterial sinusitis. For example, an NIAID-supported clinical trial is investigating relationships between viral respiratory infections, changes in the microbial communities in the nose and throat, and the risk of acute bacterial sinusitis in children.

People who have allergies or other chronic nasal problems are prone to episodes of acute sinusitis. In general, people who have reduced immune function, such as those with HIV infection, are more likely to have sinusitis. Sinusitis also is common in people who have abnormal mucus secretion or mucus movement, such as people with cystic fibrosis, an inherited disease in which thick and sticky mucus clogs the lungs.

Chronic Sinusitis or Rhinosinusitis

In chronic sinusitis, also known as chronic rhinosinusitis, the membranes of both the paranasal sinuses and the nose thicken because they are constantly inflamed. This condition can occur with or without nasal polyps, grape-like growths on the mucous membranes that protrude into the sinuses or nasal passages. The causes of chronic rhinosinusitis are largely unknown. NIAID supports basic research to help explain why people develop this chronic inflammation.

People with asthma and allergies, recurrent acute sinusitis, and other health conditions are at higher risk of developing chronic rhinosinusitis. In fact, some evidence suggests that chronic rhinosinusitis and asthma may be the same disease occurring in the upper and lower parts of the respiratory system, respectively. NIAID supports research to understand the causes of chronic airway inflammation in asthma and its link to chronic rhinosinusitis. For example, NIAID-supported researchers are investigating aspirin-exacerbated respiratory disease (AERD), a condition in which people have asthma and chronic rhinosinusitis with nasal polyps and experience potentially severe respiratory reactions to aspirin and other nonsteroidal anti-inflammatory drugs. Researchers are investigating the basic mechanisms of disease in these people, as well as developing ways to improve treatment. Other groups of NIAID-supported researchers are examining whether viral infections cause worsening of chronic rhinosinusitis and identifying differences in genes and proteins in people with chronic rhinosinusitis and those whose sinuses are healthy.

Diagnosis

Often, healthcare providers can diagnose acute sinusitis by reviewing a person's symptoms and examining the nose and face. Doctors may perform a procedure called rhinoscopy, in which they use a thin, flexible tube-like instrument to examine the inside of the nose.

If symptoms do not clearly indicate sinusitis or if they persist for a long time and do not get better with treatment, the doctor may order a computerized tomography (CT) scan—a form of X-ray that shows some soft-tissue and other structures that cannot be seen in conventional X-rays—to confirm the diagnosis of sinusitis and to evaluate how severe it is.

Laboratory tests that a healthcare professional may use to check for possible causes of chronic rhinosinusitis include

- Allergy testing

- Blood tests to rule out conditions that are associated with sinusitis, such as an immune deficiency disorder

- A sweat test or a blood test to rule out cystic fibrosis

- Tests on the material inside the sinuses to detect a bacterial or fungal infection

- An aspirin challenge to test for aspirin-exacerbated respiratory disease. In an aspirin challenge, a person takes small but gradually increasing doses of aspirin under the careful supervision of a healthcare professional.

Treatment

Acute Sinusitis

Medications can help ease the symptoms of acute sinusitis. Healthcare providers may recommend pain relievers or decongestants—medicines that shrink the swollen membranes in the nose and make it easier to breathe. Decongestant nose drops and sprays should be used for only a few days, as longer term use can lead to even more congestion and swelling of the nasal passages. A doctor may prescribe antibiotics if the sinusitis is caused by a bacterial infection.

Chronic Rhinosinusitis

Chronic rhinosinusitis can be difficult to treat. Medicines may offer some symptom relief. Surgery can be helpful if medication fails.

Medicine

Nasal steroid sprays are helpful for many people, but most still do not get full relief of symptoms with these medicines. Saline (salt water) washes or nasal sprays can be helpful in chronic rhinosinusitis because they remove thick secretions and allow the sinuses to drain. Doctors may prescribe oral steroids, such as prednisone, for severe chronic rhinosinusitis. However, oral steroids are powerful medicines that can cause side effects such as weight gain and high blood pressure if used long-term. Oral steroids typically are prescribed when other medicines have failed. Desensitization to aspirin may be helpful for patients with aspirin-exacerbated respiratory disease. During desensitization, which is performed under close medical supervision, a person is given gradually increasing doses of aspirin over time to induce tolerance to the drug.

Surgery

When medicine fails, surgery may be the only alternative for treating chronic rhinosinusitis. The goal of surgery is to improve sinus drainage and reduce blockage of the nasal passages. Sinus surgery usually is performed to

- enlarge the natural openings of the sinuses

- remove nasal polyps

- correct significant structural problems inside the nose and the sinuses if they contribute to sinus obstruction

Although most people have fewer symptoms and a better quality of life after surgery, problems can recur, sometimes after a short period of time.

In children, problems can sometimes be eliminated by removing the adenoids. These gland-like tissues, located high in the throat behind and above the roof of the mouth, can obstruct the nasal passages.

Prevention

There is little information about the prevention of acute or chronic sinusitis, but the following measures may help:

- Avoid exposure to irritants such as cigarette and cigar smoke or strong chemicals.

- To avoid infections, wash hands frequently during common cold season and try to avoid touching your face.

- If you have allergies, avoid exposure to allergy-inducing substances, or consider asking your healthcare provider for an allergy evaluation or a referral to an allergy specialist.

Chapter 15

Streptococcal Pharyngitis (Strep Throat) and Tonsillitis

Chapter Contents

Section 15.1

Strep Throat

This section includes text excerpted from "Is It Strep Throat?"
Centers for Disease Control and Prevention (CDC), October 19, 2015.

Strep throat is a common type of sore throat in children, but it's not very common in adults. Healthcare professionals can do a quick test to determine if a sore throat is strep throat and decide if antibiotics are needed. Proper treatment can help you feel better faster and prevent spreading it to others!

Many things can cause that unpleasant, scratchy, and sometimes painful condition known as a sore throat. Viruses, bacteria, allergens, environmental irritants (such as cigarette smoke), chronic postnasal drip, and fungi can all cause a sore throat. While many sore throats will get better without treatment, some throat infections—including strep throat—may need antibiotic treatment.

How You Get Strep Throat

Strep throat is an infection in the throat and tonsils caused by group A *Streptococcus* bacteria (called "group A strep"). Group A strep bacteria can also live in a person's nose and throat without causing illness. The bacteria are spread through contact with droplets after an infected person coughs or sneezes. If you touch your mouth, nose, or eyes after touching something that has these droplets on it, you may become ill. If you drink from the same glass or eat from the same plate as the infected person, you could also become ill. It is also possible to get strep throat from contact with sores from group A strep skin infections.

Common Symptoms of Strep Throat

The most common symptoms of strep throat include:

- sore throat, usually starts quickly and can cause severe pain when swallowing

- a fever (101°F or above)

- red and swollen tonsils, sometimes with white patches or streaks of pus

- tiny, red spots (petechiae) on the roof of the mouth (the soft or hard palate)

- headache, nausea, or vomiting

- swollen lymph nodes in the front of the neck

- sandpaper-like rash

A Simple Test Gives Fast Results

Healthcare professionals can test for strep by swabbing the throat to quickly see if group A strep bacteria are causing a sore throat. **A strep test is needed to tell if you have strep throat; just looking at your throat is not enough to make a diagnosis.** If the test is positive, your healthcare professional can prescribe antibiotics. If the strep test is negative, but your clinician still strongly suspects you have this infection, then they can take a throat culture swab to test for the bacteria, but those results will take a little longer to come back.

Antibiotics Get You Well Fast

The strep test results will help your healthcare professional decide if you need antibiotics, which can:

- decrease the length of time you're sick

- reduce your symptoms

- help prevent the spread of infection to friends and family members

- prevent more serious complications, such as tonsil and sinus infections, and acute rheumatic fever (a rare inflammatory disease that can affect the heart, joints, skin, and brain)

You should start feeling better in just a day or two after starting antibiotics. Call your healthcare professional if you don't feel better after taking antibiotics for 48 hours. People with strep throat should stay home from work, school, or daycare until they have taken antibiotics for at least 24 hours so they don't spread the infection to others.

Be sure to finish the entire prescription, even when you start feeling better, unless your healthcare professional tells you to stop taking the medicine. When you stop taking antibiotics early, you risk getting an infection later that is resistant to antibiotic treatment.

More Prevention Tips: Wash Those Hands

The best way to keep from getting strep throat is to wash your hands often and avoid sharing eating utensils, like forks or cups. It is especially important for anyone with a sore throat to wash their hands often and cover their mouth when coughing and sneezing. There is no vaccine to prevent strep throat.

Section 15.2

Tonsillitis

Text in this section is excerpted from "Tonsillitis," © 1995–2016. The Nemours Foundation/KidsHealth®. Reprinted with permission.

What Are Tonsils?

The tonsils' job is to help fight germs that come in through our mouth or nose before they cause infections in the rest of the body. Usually, tonsils do their job well. But sometimes bacteria or viruses get into the tonsils and infect them. When this happens, you have tonsillitis.

How Can I Tell If I Have Tonsillitis?

If you have tonsillitis, your throat usually hurts and it's hard to eat, drink, or even swallow. You also might have a fever. Here are some other signs that bacteria or a virus are infecting your tonsils:

- red (swollen or irritated) tonsils

- a yellow or white coating on the tonsils

- swollen glands in the neck

- fever

- bad breath

What Will the Doctor Do?

The doctor will ask you how you've been feeling and then look at your tonsils. He or she will probably use a wooden stick called a tongue depressor to help hold your tongue down to get a good look at what's going on in there.

The doctor also might look into your nose and ears, listen to your chest, feel your neck, and look for other signs of infection. Bacteria and viruses both can cause tonsillitis. It's important for your doctor to know if it's strep. Strep is short for **streptococci** bacteria. If you have this kind of infection, you need medicine, called an antibiotic, to kill the strep bacteria.

To check for strep, the doctor will use a long cotton swab to swipe the back of your throat. This test, called a throat culture, doesn't hurt, but it might make you gag. Your doctor may use the swab to do a test called a rapid strep test.

Within minutes, this test will tell your doctor if there are any strep bacteria in your throat. But sometimes, the rapid strep test does not show any strep bacteria. Your doctor may send the throat culture to a lab and get results back in 1–2 days.

How Is Tonsillitis Treated?

If the tonsillitis is caused by strep bacteria, the doctor will prescribe antibiotics, a type of medicine that kills bacteria. It's very important to take the antibiotics exactly as you're supposed to and finish the entire prescription to kill all the bacteria. You should finish the medicine even if you start feeling better in the first few days.

If the tonsillitis is caused by a virus, antibiotics won't work and your body will fight off the infection on its own. Sometimes kids get an operation to remove their tonsils, but only if their tonsils get infected a lot during the year or are so big they make it hard for the kid to breathe at night.

If you get tonsillitis, here are some tips that can help you feel better:

- Drink plenty of fluids.

- If you are having trouble swallowing regular food, you can eat smooth foods, including flavored gelatin, soups, ice-pops, and applesauce.

- Take it easy until you feel better.

- Wash your hands often.

Soon your tonsils will be back in action and ready to fight germs again!

Chapter 16

Tuberculosis

Basic TB Facts

Tuberculosis (TB) is caused by a bacterium called *Mycobacterium tuberculosis*. The bacteria usually attack the lungs, but TB bacteria can attack any part of the body such as the kidney, spine, and brain. Not everyone infected with TB bacteria becomes sick. As a result, two TB-related conditions exist: latent TB infection (LTBI) and TB disease. If not treated properly, TB disease can be fatal.

How TB Spreads

TB bacteria are spread through the air from one person to another. The TB bacteria are put into the air when a person with TB disease of the lungs or throat coughs, speaks, or sings. People nearby may breathe in these bacteria and become infected.

TB is NOT spread by

- shaking someone's hand

- sharing food or drink

- touching bed linens or toilet seats

- sharing toothbrushes

- kissing

This chapter includes text excerpted from "Tuberculosis (TB)," Centers for Disease Control and Prevention (CDC), March 20, 2016.

When a person breathes in TB bacteria, the bacteria can settle in the lungs and begin to grow. From there, they can move through the blood to other parts of the body, such as the kidney, spine, and brain.

TB disease in the lungs or throat can be infectious. This means that the bacteria can be spread to other people. TB in other parts of the body, such as the kidney or spine, is usually not infectious.

People with TB disease are most likely to spread it to people they spend time with every day. This includes family members, friends, and coworkers or schoolmates.

Latent TB Infection and TB Disease

Not everyone infected with TB bacteria becomes sick. As a result, two TB-related conditions exist: latent TB infection and TB disease.

Latent TB Infection

TB bacteria can live in the body without making you sick. This is called latent TB infection. In most people who breathe in TB bacteria and become infected, the body is able to fight the bacteria to stop them from growing. People with latent TB infection:

- have no symptoms

- don't feel sick

- can't spread TB bacteria to others

- usually have a positive TB skin test reaction or positive TB blood test

- may develop TB disease if they do not receive treatment for latent TB infection

Many people who have latent TB infection never develop TB disease. In these people, the TB bacteria remain inactive for a lifetime without causing disease. But in other people, especially people who have a weak immune system, the bacteria become active, multiply, and cause TB disease.

TB Disease

TB bacteria become active if the immune system can't stop them from growing. When TB bacteria are active (multiplying in your body), this is called TB disease. People with TB disease are sick. They may also be able to spread the bacteria to people they spend time with every day.

Many people who have latent TB infection never develop TB disease. Some people develop TB disease soon after becoming infected (within weeks) before their immune system can fight the TB bacteria. Other people may get sick years later when their immune system becomes weak for another reason.

For people whose immune systems are weak, especially those with HIV infection, the risk of developing TB disease is much higher than for people with normal immune systems.

The Difference between Latent TB Infection (LTBI) and TB Disease

Table 16.1. Latent TB Infection (LTBI) and TB Disease

A Person with Latent TB Infection	A Person with TB Disease

• Has no symptoms	• Has symptoms that may include
	  • a bad cough that lasts 3 weeks or longer
	  • pain in the chest
	  • coughing up blood or sputum
	  • weakness or fatigue
	  • weight loss
	  • no appetite
	  • chills
	  • fever
	  • sweating at night

• Does not feel sick	• Usually feels sick
• Cannot spread TB bacteria to others	• May spread TB bacteria to others
• Usually has a skin test or blood test result indicating TB infection	• Usually has a skin test or blood test result indicating TB infection
• Has a normal chest X-ray and a negative sputum smear	• May have an abnormal chest X-ray, or positive sputum smear or culture
• Needs treatment for latent TB infection to prevent TB disease	• Needs treatment to treat TB disease

Signs and Symptoms

Symptoms of TB disease depend on where in the body the TB bacteria are growing. TB bacteria usually grow in the lungs (pulmonary TB). TB disease in the lungs may cause symptoms such as

• a bad cough that lasts 3 weeks or longer

- pain in the chest

- coughing up blood or sputum (phlegm from deep inside the lungs)

Other symptoms of TB disease are

- weakness or fatigue

- weight loss

- no appetite

- chills

- fever

- sweating at night

Symptoms of TB disease in other parts of the body depend on the area affected.

People who have latent TB infection do not feel sick, do not have any symptoms, and cannot spread TB to others.

TB Risk Factors

Some people develop TB disease soon after becoming infected (within weeks) before their immune system can fight the TB bacteria. Other people may get sick years later, when their immune system becomes weak for another reason.

Overall, about 5 to 10 percent of infected persons who do not receive treatment for latent TB infection will develop TB disease at some time in their lives. For persons whose immune systems are weak, especially those with HIV infection, the risk of developing TB disease is much higher than for persons with normal immune systems.

Generally, persons at high risk for developing TB disease fall into two categories:

- persons who have been recently infected with TB bacteria

- persons with medical conditions that weaken the immune system

Persons Who Have Been Recently Infected with TB Bacteria

This includes:

- close contacts of a person with infectious TB disease

- persons who have immigrated from areas of the world with high rates of TB

- children less than 5 years of age who have a positive TB test

- groups with high rates of TB transmission, such as homeless persons, injection drug users, and persons with HIV infection

- persons who work or reside with people who are at high risk for TB in facilities or institutions such as hospitals, homeless shelters, correctional facilities, nursing homes, and residential homes for those with HIV

Persons with Medical Conditions That Weaken the Immune System

Babies and young children often have weak immune systems. Other people can have weak immune systems, too, especially people with any of these conditions:

- HIV infection (the virus that causes AIDS)

- substance abuse

- silicosis

- diabetes mellitus

- severe kidney disease

- low body weight

- organ transplants

- head and neck cancer

- medical treatments such as corticosteroids or organ transplant

- specialized treatment for rheumatoid arthritis or Crohn's disease

Exposure to TB

What to Do If You Have Been Exposed to TB

You may have been exposed to TB bacteria if you spent time near someone with TB disease. The TB bacteria are put into the air when a person with active TB disease of the lungs or throat coughs, sneezes, speaks, or sings. You cannot get TB from

- clothes

- drinking glass

- eating utensils

- handshake

- toilet

- other surfaces

If you think you have been exposed to someone with TB disease, you should contact your doctor or local health department about getting a TB skin test or a special TB blood test. Be sure to tell the doctor or nurse when you spent time with the person who has TB disease.

It is important to know that a person who is exposed to TB bacteria is not able to spread the bacteria to other people right away. Only persons with active TB disease can spread TB bacteria to others. Before you would be able to spread TB to others, you would have to breathe in TB bacteria and become infected. Then the active bacteria would have to multiply in your body and cause active TB disease. At this point, you could possibly spread TB bacteria to others. People with TB disease are most likely to spread the bacteria to people they spend time with every day, such as family members, friends, coworkers, or schoolmates.

Some people develop TB disease soon (within weeks) after becoming infected, before their immune system can fight the TB bacteria. Other people may get sick years later, when their immune system becomes weak for another reason. Many people with TB infection never develop TB disease.

TB Prevention

Preventing Latent TB Infection from Progressing to TB Disease

Many people who have latent TB infection never develop TB disease. But some people who have latent TB infection are more likely to develop TB disease than others. Those at high risk for developing TB disease include:

- people with HIV infection

- people who became infected with TB bacteria in the last 2 years

- babies and young children

- people who inject illegal drugs

- people who are sick with other diseases that weaken the immune system

- elderly people

- people who were not treated correctly for TB in the past

If you have latent TB infection and you are in one of these high-risk groups, you should take medicine to keep from developing TB disease. There are several treatment options for latent TB infection. You and your healthcare provider must decide which treatment is best for you. If you take your medicine as instructed, it can keep you from developing TB disease. Because there are less bacteria, treatment for latent TB infection is much easier than treatment for TB disease. A person with TB disease has a large amount of TB bacteria in the body. Several drugs are needed to treat TB disease.

Preventing Exposure to TB Disease While Traveling Abroad

In many countries, TB is much more common than in the United States. Travelers should avoid close contact or prolonged time with known TB patients in crowded, enclosed environments (for example, clinics, hospitals, prisons, or homeless shelters).

Although multidrug-resistant (MDR) and extensively drug-resistant (XDR) TB are occurring globally, they are still rare. HIV-infected travelers are at greatest risk if they come in contact with a person with MDR or XDR TB.

Air travel itself carries a relatively low risk of infection with TB of any kind. Travelers who will be working in clinics, hospitals, or other healthcare settings where TB patients are likely to be encountered should consult infection control or occupational health experts. They should ask about administrative and environmental procedures for preventing exposure to TB. Once those procedures are implemented, additional measures could include using personal respiratory protective devices.

Travelers who anticipate possible prolonged exposure to people with TB (for example, those who expect to come in contact routinely with clinic, hospital, prison, or homeless shelter populations) should have a TB skin test or a TB blood test before leaving the United States. If the test reaction is negative, they should have a repeat test 8 to 10 weeks after returning to the United States. Additionally, annual testing may be recommended for those who anticipate repeated or prolonged exposure or an extended stay over a period of years. Because people with HIV infection are more likely to have an impaired response to TB tests, travelers who are HIV positive should tell their physicians about their HIV infection status.

Vaccines

TB Vaccine (BCG)

Bacille Calmette-Guérin (BCG) is a vaccine for tuberculosis (TB) disease. This vaccine is not widely used in the United States, but it is often given to infants and small children in other countries where TB is common. BCG does not always protect people from getting TB.

BCG Recommendations

In the United States, BCG should be considered for only very select people who meet specific criteria and in consultation with a TB expert. Healthcare providers who are considering BCG vaccination for their patients are encouraged to discuss this intervention with the TB control program in their area.

Children

BCG vaccination should only be considered for children who have a negative TB test and who are continually exposed, and cannot be separated from adults who

- Are untreated or ineffectively treated for TB disease, and the child cannot be given long-term primary preventive treatment for TB infection; or

- Have TB disease caused by strains resistant to isoniazid and rifampin.

Healthcare Workers

BCG vaccination of healthcare workers should be considered on an individual basis in settings in which

- A high percentage of TB patients are infected with TB strains resistant to both isoniazid and rifampin

- There is ongoing transmission of drug-resistant TB strains to healthcare workers and subsequent infection is likely; or

- Comprehensive TB infection-control precautions have been implemented, but have not been successful.

Healthcare workers considered for BCG vaccination should be counseled regarding the risks and benefits associated with both BCG vaccination and treatment of latent TB infection.

Testing for TB in BCG-Vaccinated People

Many people born outside of the United States have been BCG-vaccinated.

People who were previously vaccinated with BCG may receive a TB skin test to test for TB infection. Vaccination with BCG may cause a positive reaction to a TB skin test. A positive reaction to a TB skin test may be due to the BCG vaccine itself or due to infection with TB bacteria.

TB blood tests (IGRAs), unlike the TB skin test, are not affected by prior BCG vaccination and are not expected to give a false-positive result in people who have received BCG.

For children under the age of five, the TB skin test is preferred over TB blood tests.

A positive TB skin test or TB blood test only tells that a person has been infected with TB bacteria. It does not tell whether the person has latent TB infection or has progressed to TB disease. Other tests, such as a chest X-ray and a sample of sputum, are needed to see whether the person has TB disease.

TB and HIV Coinfection

Tuberculosis is a serious health threat, especially for people living with HIV. People living with HIV are more likely than others to become sick with TB. Worldwide, TB is one of the leading causes of death among people living with HIV.

Without treatment, as with other opportunistic infections, HIV and TB can work together to shorten lifespan.

- Someone with untreated latent TB infection and HIV infection is **much more** likely to develop TB disease during his or her lifetime than someone without HIV infection.

- Among people with latent TB infection, HIV infection is the strongest known risk factor for progressing to TB disease.

- A person who has both HIV infection and TB disease has an AIDS-defining condition.

People infected with HIV who also have either latent TB infection or TB disease can be effectively treated. The first step is to ensure that people living with HIV are tested for TB infection. If found to have TB infection, further tests are needed to rule out TB disease. The next step is to start treatment for latent TB infection or TB disease based on test results.

Treatment

Untreated latent TB infection can quickly progress to TB disease in people living with HIV since the immune system is already weakened. And without treatment, TB disease can progress from sickness to death.

Fortunately, there are a number of treatment options for people living with HIV who also have either latent TB infection or TB disease.

Chapter 17

Other Viral Respiratory Infections

Chapter Contents

Section 17.1

Adenovirus

About Adenovirus Infections

Adenoviruses are a group of viruses that can infect the membranes (tissue linings) of the respiratory tract, eyes, intestines, urinary tract, and nervous system. They account for about 10 percent of fever-related illnesses and acute respiratory infections in kids and are a frequent cause of diarrhea.

Adenoviral infections affect babies and young children much more often than adults. Childcare centers and schools sometimes have multiple cases of respiratory infections and diarrhea caused by adenovirus.

Adenoviral infections can occur at any time of the year, but:

- respiratory tract problems caused by adenovirus are more common in late winter, spring, and early summer

- conjunctivitis (pinkeye) and pharyngoconjunctival fever caused by adenovirus tend to affect older kids, mostly in the summer

Adenoviral infections can affect children of any age, but most occur in the first years of life—and most kids have had at least one before age 10. There are many different types of adenoviruses, so some kids can have repeated adenoviral infections.

Signs and Symptoms

Depending on which part of the body is affected, the signs and symptoms of adenoviral infections vary:

Febrile respiratory disease, an infection with fever of the respiratory tract, is the most common result of adenoviral infection in kids. The illness often appears flu-like and can include symptoms of pharyngitis (inflammation of the pharynx, or sore throat), rhinitis (inflammation of nasal membranes, or a congested, runny nose), cough, and swollen lymph nodes (glands). Sometimes the respiratory infection leads to acute otitis media, an infection of the middle ear.

Adenovirus often affects the lower respiratory tract as well, causing bronchiolitis, croup, or viral pneumonia, which is less common but can cause serious illness in infants. Adenovirus can also produce a dry, harsh cough that can resemble whooping cough (pertussis).

Gastroenteritis is an inflammation of the stomach and the small and large intestines. Symptoms include watery diarrhea, vomiting, headache, fever, and abdominal cramps.

Genitourinary infections: Urinary tract infections can cause frequent urination, burning, pain, and blood in the urine. Adenoviruses are also known to cause a condition called **hemorrhagic cystitis**, which is characterized by blood in the urine. Hemorrhagic cystitis usually resolves on its own.

Eye Infections:

- **Pinkeye (conjunctivitis)** is a mild inflammation of the conjunctiva (membranes that cover the eye and inner surfaces of the eyelids). Symptoms include red eyes, discharge, tearing, and the feeling that there's something in the eye.

- **Pharyngoconjunctival fever**, often seen in small outbreaks among school-age kids, occurs when adenovirus affects both the lining of the eye and the respiratory tract. Symptoms include very red eyes and a severe sore throat, sometimes accompanied by low-grade fever, rhinitis, and swollen lymph nodes.

- **Keratoconjunctivitis** is a more severe infection that involves both the conjunctiva and cornea (the transparent front part of the eye) in both eyes. This type of adenoviral infection is extremely contagious and occurs most often in older kids and young adults, causing red eyes, photophobia (discomfort of the eyes upon exposure to light), blurry vision, tearing, and pain.

Nervous System Infections:

- Meningitis and encephalitis (inflammation of the lining of the brain and spinal cord) can sometimes happen due to adenovirus infection. Symptoms can include fever, headache, nausea and vomiting, stiff neck, or skin rash.

Contagiousness

Adenovirus is highly contagious, so multiple cases are common in close-contact settings like childcare centers, schools, hospitals, and summer camps.

The types of adenovirus that cause respiratory and intestinal infections spread from person to person through respiratory secretions (coughs or sneezes) or fecal contamination. Fecal material can spread via contaminated water, eating food contaminated by houseflies, and poor hand washing (such as after using the bathroom, before eating or preparing food, or after handling dirty diapers).

A child might also pick up the virus by holding hands or sharing a toy with an infected person. Adenovirus can survive on surfaces for long periods, so indirect transmission can occur through exposure to the contaminated surfaces of furniture and other objects.

The types of adenovirus causing pinkeye may be transmitted by water (in lakes and swimming pools), by sharing contaminated objects (such as towels or toys), or by touch.

Once a child is exposed to adenovirus, symptoms usually develop from 2 days to 2 weeks later.

Treatment

Adenoviral illnesses often resemble certain bacterial infections, which can be treated with antibiotics. But antibiotics don't work against viruses. To diagnose the true cause of the symptoms so that proper treatment can be prescribed, your doctor may want to test respiratory or conjunctival secretions, a stool specimen, or a blood or urine sample.

The doctor will decide on a course of action based on your child's condition. Adenoviral infections usually don't require hospitalization. However, babies and young children may not be able to drink enough fluids to replace what they lose during vomiting or diarrhea and so might need to be hospitalized to treat or prevent dehydration. Also, young (especially premature) infants with pneumonia usually need to be hospitalized.

In most cases, a child's body, with the help of the immune system, will get rid of the virus over time. Antibiotics cannot treat a viral infection, so it's best to just make your child more comfortable. Children with weakened immune systems, transplants, HIV or AIDS, or congenital immunodeficiencies may have a more difficult time fighting adenovirus, so stronger treatment might be needed. (A congenital immunodeficiency is a condition a baby is born with that causes the immune system to not work properly.)

If your child has a respiratory infection or fever, getting plenty of rest and taking in extra fluids are essential. A cool-mist humidifier (vaporizer) may help loosen congestion and make your child more comfortable. Be sure to clean and dry the humidifier thoroughly each day to prevent bacterial or mold contamination. If your child is under 6 months old, you may need to clear his or her nose with nasal saline drops and a bulb syringe.

Don't give any over-the-counter (OTC) cold remedies or cough medicines without checking with your doctor. You can use acetaminophen to treat a fever (your doctor will tell you the proper dose); however, do **not** give aspirin because of the risk of Reye syndrome, a life-threatening illness.

If your child has diarrhea or is vomiting, increase fluid intake and check with the doctor about giving an oral rehydration solution to prevent dehydration.

To relieve the symptoms of pinkeye, use warm compresses and, if your doctor recommends them, a topical eye ointment or drops.

Duration

Most adenoviral infections last from a few days to a week. However:

- severe respiratory infections may last longer and cause lingering symptoms, such as a cough
- pneumonia can last anywhere from 2–4 weeks
- pinkeye can persist for another several days to a week
- more severe keratoconjunctivitis can last for several weeks
- adenovirus can cause diarrhea that lasts up to 2 weeks (longer than other viral diarrhea episodes)

Prevention

There's no way to completely prevent adenoviral infections in kids. To reduce their spread, parents and other caregivers should encourage frequent hand washing, keep shared surfaces (such as countertops and toys) clean, and remove kids with infections from group settings until symptoms pass.

When to Call the Doctor

Most of these adenoviral conditions and their symptoms are also associated with other causes. Call your doctor if:

- a fever continues more than a few days
- symptoms seem to get worse after a week
- your child has breathing problems
- your child is under 3 months old
- any swelling and redness around the eye becomes more severe or painful
- your child shows signs of dehydration, such as appearing tired or lacking energy, producing less urine or tears, or having a dry mouth or sunken eyes

Section 17.2

Bronchiolitis Obliterans Organizing Pneumonia

This section includes text excerpted from "Bronchiolitis Obliterans Organizing Pneumonia," Genetic and Rare Diseases Information Center (GARD), February 16, 2016.

What Is Bronchiolitis Obliterans Organizing Pneumonia (BOOP)?

Bronchiolitis obliterans organizing pneumonia (BOOP) is a lung disease that causes inflammation in the small air tubes (bronchioles) and air sacs (alveoli). BOOP typically develops in individuals between 40–60 years old; however the disorder may affect individuals of any age. The signs and symptoms of BOOP vary but often include shortness of breath, a dry cough, and fever. BOOP can be caused by viral infections, various drugs, and other medical conditions. If the cause is known, the condition is called secondary BOOP. In many cases, the underlying cause of BOOP is unknown. These cases are called idiopathic BOOP or cryptogenic organizing pneumonia. Treatment often includes corticosteroid medications.

Symptoms

Signs and symptoms of BOOP vary. Some individuals with BOOP may have no apparent symptoms, while others may have severe respiratory distress as in acute, rapidly-progressive BOOP. The most common signs and symptoms of BOOP include shortness of breath (dyspnea), dry cough, and fever. Some people with BOOP develop a flu-like illness with cough, fever, fatigue, and weight loss.

Causes

BOOP may be caused by a variety of factors, including viral infections, inhalation of toxic gases, drugs, connective tissue disorders, radiation therapy, cocaine, inflammatory bowel disease, and HIV infection. In many cases, the underlying cause of BOOP is unknown. These cases are called idiopathic BOOP or cryptogenic organizing pneumonia (COP).

Diagnosis

BOOP is typically diagnosed by lung biopsy, although imaging tests and pulmonary function tests can also provide information for diagnosis.

Treatment

Most cases of BOOP respond well to treatment with corticosteroids. If the condition is caused by a particular drug, stopping the drug can also improve a patient's condition.

Other medications reported in the medical literature to be beneficial for individuals on a case-by-case basis include: cyclophosphamide, erythromycin in the form of azithromycin, and Mycophenolate Mofetil (CellCept). More research is needed to determine the long-term safety and effectiveness of these potential treatment options for individuals with BOOP.

In rare cases, lung transplantation may be necessary for individuals with BOOP who do not respond to standard treatment options.

Section 17.3

Hantavirus Pulmonary Syndrome

This section includes text excerpted from "Hantavirus
Pulmonary Syndrome," Centers for Disease Control and
Prevention (CDC), January 31, 2013.

Hantavirus Pulmonary Syndrome (HPS) is a rare but severe, sometimes fatal, respiratory disease in humans caused by infection with
hantavirus.

What Are the Symptoms of HPS?

Early symptoms include fatigue, fever and muscle aches, especially in the large muscle groups—thighs, hips, back, and sometimes
shoulders. About half of all HPS patients also experience headaches,
dizziness, chills, and abdominal problems, such as nausea, vomiting,
diarrhea, and abdominal pain.

Four to ten days after the initial phase of illness, the late symptoms
of HPS appear. These include coughing and shortness of breath, with
the sensation of, as one survivor put it, a "tight band around my chest
and a pillow over my face" as the lungs fill with fluid.

How Do People Get HPS?

People can get HPS when they are exposed to infected rodents.
Exposures may include:

- Breathing in the virus. This may happen when rodent urine and
  droppings containing hantavirus are stirred up into the air.

- Touching eyes, nose or mouth after touching rodent droppings,
  urine, or nesting materials that contain the virus.

- A bite from an infected rodent.

HPS is not spread from person to person.

Which Rodents Can Cause Humans to Get HPS?

Rodents known to carry hantavirus include:

- deer mouse

- cotton rat

- rice rat

- white-footed mouse

Not all rodents carry hantavirus and there is usually no way to tell when a rodent has the virus. So, it is wise to avoid all contact with rodents when possible.

How Is HPS Diagnosed?

Diagnosing HPS in an individual who has only been infected for a few days is difficult, because early symptoms such as fever, muscle aches, and fatigue are easily confused with influenza.

Experiencing all of the following would strongly suggest HPS infection:

- a history of potential rodent exposure

- fever and fatigue

- shortness of breath

Anyone experiencing these symptoms and having a history of recent rodent exposure should see their physician immediately and mention their potential rodent exposure.

How Is HPS Treated?

There is no specific treatment, cure, or vaccine for HPS.

If infected individuals are recognized early and receive medical care in an intensive care unit, they may do better. In intensive care, patients are intubated and given oxygen therapy to help them through the period of severe respiratory distress.

The earlier the patient is brought in to intensive care, the better. If a patient is experiencing full respiratory distress, it is less likely that the treatment will be effective.

How Can HPS Be Prevented?

When people get HPS, it's usually because they've been exposed to infected rodents or their droppings. So, the best way to help prevent HPS is to eliminate or minimize contact with rodents in your home, workplace, or campsite.

There's an easy way to do this—it's known as **Seal Up! Trap Up! Clean Up!**

- Seal Up!—Seal up holes inside and outside the home to keep rodents out.

- Trap Up!—Trap rodents around the home to help reduce the population.

- Clean Up!—Clean up any food that is easy to get to.

Section 17.4

Laryngitis

Text in this section is excerpted from "Laryngitis," © 1995–2016.
The Nemours Foundation/KidsHealth®. Reprinted with permission.

How Your Voice Works

Open up your mouth and say something. Anything. Answer the question: "What's your favorite flavor of ice cream?"

At the top of your windpipe—also called your **trachea**—is your **larynx**, or voice box. It's the source of your voice. Inside your larynx are two bands of muscles called vocal cords, or vocal folds. When you breathe, your vocal cords are relaxed and open so that you can get air into and out of your lungs.

But when you decide to say something, these cords come together. Now the air from your lungs has to pass through a smaller space. This causes your vocal cords to vibrate. The sound from these vibrations goes up your throat and comes out your mouth as "Chocolate is the best flavor!" (or whatever your favorite flavor of ice cream happens to be).

You can make different sounds by lengthening or shortening, or tensing or relaxing, the vocal cords. Although you don't even think about it, every time you want to talk with a deeper voice you lengthen and relax these vocal muscles. When you talk with a higher pitched voice, you tighten the vocal cords and make them smaller. You can try this right now. Make your voice go from deep to high pitch and back again. Do you feel the vibrations along your throat coming from your vocal cords?

What Causes Laryngitis?

When your cords become inflamed and swollen, they can't work properly. Your voice may sound hoarse. This is called **laryngitis**.

In kids, laryngitis often comes from too much yelling and screaming. You may be hollering at your younger brother or sister. Or you might be cheering on your favorite team, yelling with the crowd during a great play—touchdown! Or you may be in a group of noisy kids and have to talk loudly to be heard. Even a lot of loud singing can irritate your vocal cords and cause laryngitis.

Although it sounds odd, sometimes your stomach can cause laryngitis. Just like you have a tube for air to go into and out of your lungs, you have a tube for food to go into your stomach. Sometimes the stomach acid that helps break down that food comes back up your swallowing tube. The acid can irritate your vocal cords.

Allergies or smoking can also irritate your vocal cords (another good reason not to start messing with cigarettes). Did you ever notice that people who smoke a lot have rough, raspy voices?

Infections from germs are a very common cause of laryngitis—in kids as well as adults. Sometimes bacteria can infect the vocal cords, but most of the time it's viruses—like those that cause runny noses or flu-like illnesses. That's why sometimes when you have a cold or a bad cough, your voice also sounds funny.

Kids who yell and talk loudly can irritate their vocal cords. Over time, people who yell all the time may develop nodules, or little bumps, on their vocal cords. This can make your voice hoarse, rough, and deeper than usual.

How Do I Know If I Have Laryngitis?

A hoarse or raspy voice is the main symptom or sign of laryngitis. You also may have no voice at all or maybe just little squeaks come out when you try to talk. You might need to cough to clear your throat, or you may feel a tickle deep in your throat. These are all signs that you may have laryngitis. You may have this strange voice for a few days, but if you have it longer, you probably will have to go to the doctor.

How Will My Doctor Know I Have It?

Most of the time, doctors can diagnose laryngitis just from the changes in your voice, and knowing that you've had a cold or have been yelling too much.

But sometimes the doctor might think you need to see an **ENT specialist**—a doctor that specializes in diseases of the ears, nose, and throat. This doctor can look into your throat using a special mirror. The mirror is angled so that when it's in your mouth, the doctor can look down into your larynx.

Sometimes doctors use a tiny tube with an even tinier camera that goes through your nose or mouth. This cool camera that goes into your throat is a little uncomfortable. Luckily, it only takes a minute for the doctor to take a good look at your vocal cords.

How Will My Doctor Treat Laryngitis?

How the doctor treats your laryngitis depends on why you have it. If the laryngitis is from a viral infection, the doctor will recommend lots of fluids and resting your voice by talking as little as possible. Being quiet can be hard, but it can be fun, too—especially if you get to show people what you're trying to say by drawing pictures or acting things out.

If your laryngitis is from too much yelling, you will have to be more careful with your voice. Try not to yell at your brother, even if he drives you crazy! It's OK to cheer during the big game, but remember not to yell too loudly for too long.

If stomach acid is causing your laryngitis, the doctor will talk to you about medication. You may have to change your diet and give up some foods that make the problem worse.

Can I Prevent It?

To prevent laryngitis, try not to talk or yell in a way that hurts your voice. A humidifier that puts more water into the air may also help keep your throat from drying out. Also, never smoke and try not to be around people who are smoking.

Section 17.5

Legionella (Legionnaires' Disease)

This section includes text excerpted from "Legionella (Legionnaires' Disease and Pontiac Fever)," Centers for Disease Control and Prevention (CDC), May 31, 2016.

About the Disease

Legionellosis is a respiratory disease caused by *Legionella* bacteria. Sometimes the bacteria cause a serious type of pneumonia (lung infection) called Legionnaires' disease. The bacteria can also cause a less serious infection called Pontiac fever that has symptoms similar to a mild case of the flu.

Causes

Causes and Common Sources of Infection

Legionella is a type of bacterium found naturally in freshwater environments, like lakes and streams. It can become a health concern when it grows and spreads in human-made water systems like

- hot tubs that aren't drained after each use

- hot water tanks and heaters

- large plumbing systems

- cooling towers (air-conditioning units for large buildings)

- decorative fountains

- This bacterium grows best in warm water.

How It Spreads

After *Legionella* grows and multiplies in a building water system, that contaminated water then has to spread in droplets small enough for people to breathe in. People are exposed to *Legionella* when they breathe in mist (small droplets of water in the air) containing the bacteria. One example might be from breathing in droplets sprayed from a hot tub that has not been properly cleaned and disinfected.

Less commonly, *Legionella* can be spread by aspiration of drinking water, which is when water "goes down the wrong pipe," into the trachea (windpipe) and lungs instead of down the digestive tract. People at increased risk of aspiration include those with swallowing difficulties. In general, Legionnaires' disease and Pontiac fever are not spread from one person to another. However, this may be possible in rare cases.

If you have reason to believe you were exposed to the bacteria, talk to your doctor or local health department. Your local health department can determine if an investigation is needed. Be sure to mention if you spent any nights away from home in the last two weeks.

People at Increased Risk

Most healthy people do not get sick after being exposed to *Legionella*. People at increased risk of getting sick are:

- people 50 years or older
- current or former smokers
- people with a chronic lung disease (like chronic obstructive pulmonary disease or emphysema)
- people with a weak immune system from diseases like cancer, diabetes, or kidney failure
- people who take drugs that suppress (weaken) the immune system (like after a transplant operation or chemotherapy)

Signs and Symptoms

People who get sick after being exposed to *Legionella* can develop two different illnesses: Legionnaires' disease and Pontiac fever.

Legionnaires' Disease

Legionnaires' disease is very similar to other types of pneumonia (lung infection), with symptoms that include:

- cough
- shortness of breath
- fever

- muscle aches

- headaches

Legionnaires' disease can also be associated with other symptoms such as diarrhea, nausea, and confusion. Symptoms usually begin 2 to 10 days after being exposed to the bacteria, but it can take longer so people should watch for symptoms for about 2 weeks after exposure.

If you develop pneumonia symptoms, see a doctor right away. Be sure to mention if you may have been exposed to *Legionella*, have used a hot tub, spent any nights away from home, or stayed in a hospital in the last two weeks.

Pontiac Fever

Pontiac fever symptoms are primarily fever and muscle aches; it is a milder infection than Legionnaires' disease. Symptoms begin between a few hours to 3 days after being exposed to the bacteria and usually last less than a week. Pontiac fever is different from Legionnaires' disease because someone with Pontiac fever does not have pneumonia.

Diagnosis, Treatment, and Complications

Diagnosis

People with Legionnaires' disease have pneumonia (lung infection), which can be confirmed by chest X-ray. Clinicians typically use two preferred types of tests to see if a patient's pneumonia is caused by *Legionella*:

- urine test

- laboratory test that involves taking a sample of sputum (phlegm) or washing from the lung

Treatment and Complications

Legionnaires' disease requires treatment with antibiotics (medicines that kill bacteria in the body), and most cases of this illness can be treated successfully. Healthy people usually get better after being sick with Legionnaires' disease, but they often need care in the hospital.

Possible complications of Legionnaires' disease include

- lung failure

- death

About 1 out of every 10 people who get sick with Legionnaires' disease will die due to complications from their illness.

Prevention

There are no vaccines that can prevent legionellosis.

Instead, the key to preventing legionellosis is making sure that the water systems in buildings are maintained in order to reduce the risk of growing and spreading *Legionella*. Examples of water systems that might spread *Legionella* include

- hot tubs
- hot water tanks and heaters
- large plumbing systems
- cooling towers (air-conditioning systems for large buildings)
- decorative fountains

Legionella and Hot Tubs

Legionella grows best in warm water, like the water temperatures used in hot tubs. However, warm temperatures also make it hard to keep disinfectants, such as chlorine, at the levels needed to kill germs like *Legionella*. Disinfectant and other chemical levels in hot tubs should be checked regularly and hot tubs should be cleaned as recommended by the manufacturer.

Section 17.6

Otitis Media

This section includes text excerpted from "Ear Infection," Centers for Disease Control and Prevention (CDC), April 17, 2015.

Otitis Media with Effusion

Otitis media with effusion, or OME, is a buildup of fluid in the middle ear without signs and symptoms of infection (pain, redness of the eardrum, pus, fever). The most common reasons for this fluid buildup include:

- allergies

- changes in air pressure due to travel or elevation changes

- drinking while laying on your back

- irritants such as cigarette smoke

- previous respiratory infections

OME almost always goes away on its own and will not benefit from antibiotics. After a respiratory tract infection has gone away, fluid may remain inside the ear and take a month or longer to go away. Sometimes this fluid can become infected, leading to acute otitis media (AOM). OME is more common than AOM.

Acute Otitis Media

Acute otitis media, or AOM, is the type of ear infection that affects the inside of the ear and can be painful. AOM is often caused by bacteria, but can also be caused by viruses. The bacteria that usually cause AOM are *Streptococcus pneumoniae*, *Haemophilus influenzae*, and *Moraxella catarrhalis*. The viruses that most commonly cause AOM are respiratory syncytial virus (RSV), rhinoviruses, influenza viruses, and adenoviruses.

AOM may improve with antibiotics, but they are not always necessary since not all AOM is caused by bacteria.

Risk Factors

There are many things that can increase your risk for OME or AOM, including:

- age (children younger than 2 years are at higher risk)

- daycare attendance

- drinking from a bottle while laying down

- exposure to air pollution or secondhand smoke

- season (ear infections are more common during fall and winter)

Signs and Symptoms

Children with OME do not act sick and will not have any obvious symptoms, although temporary problems with hearing may be present. Symptoms more commonly associated with AOM include:

- difficulty balancing
- excessive crying
- fever
- fluid draining from ears
- headache
- irritability, especially with infants and toddlers
- problems with hearing
- pulling at ears, especially with children
- sleep disturbances

When to Seek Medical Care

See a healthcare professional if you or your child has any of the following:

- temperature higher than 100.4 °F
- discharge of blood or pus from the ears
- symptoms that have not improved or have gotten worse after being diagnosed with an ear infection

If your child is younger than three months of age and has a fever, it's important to always call your healthcare professional right away.

Diagnosis and Treatment

Ear infections can be diagnosed with a special instrument called an otoscope, which is used to look inside the ear at the eardrum. Your healthcare professional can also perform a special test using the otoscope to see if fluid has collected behind the eardrum. If OME is present, fluid may be visible, but there will be no signs of infection. If there are signs of infection, then AOM may be present.

Your healthcare professional will consider several factors when determining if antibiotics are needed for an ear infection: age, illness severity, certainty a bacterial infection is present, and options for fol-low-up. Since ear infections will often get better on their own without antibiotic treatment, your healthcare professional may decide to wait a few days before prescribing antibiotics. When an ear infection is caused by a virus, antibiotic treatment will not help it get better and may even cause harm in both children and adults.

If symptoms continue to last for more than one month for OME or 2 days for AOM, you should schedule a follow-up appointment with your healthcare professional.

Symptom Relief

Rest, over-the-counter (OTC) medicines and other self-care methods may help you or your child feel better. Remember, always use OTC products as directed. Many OTC products are not recommended for children of certain ages.

Prevention

There are steps you can take to help prevent getting an ear infec-tion, including:

- avoid smoking and exposure to secondhand smoke
- bottle feed your baby in the upright position
- breastfeed your baby for 12 months or more if possible
- keep you and your child up to date with recommended immunizations

Section 17.7

Psittacosis

This section includes text excerpted from "Psittacosis,"
Centers for Disease Control and Prevention (CDC), July 7, 2016.

Clinical Features

In humans, fever, chills, headache, muscle aches, and a dry cough.
Pneumonia is often evident on chest X-ray.

Etiologic Agent

Chlamydia psittaci, a gram-negative bacterium; the bacterium was
previously known as *Chlamydophila psittaci*.

Incidence

Since 2010, fewer than 10 confirmed cases are reported in the
United States each year. More cases may occur that are not correctly
diagnosed or reported.

Sequelae

Endocarditis, hepatitis, and neurologic complications may occasionally occur. Severe pneumonia requiring intensive-care support may
also occur. Fatal cases have been reported but are rare.

Transmission

Birds are the natural reservoirs of *C. psittaci* and infection is usually acquired by inhaling dried secretions from infected birds. The
incubation period is 5 to 19 days. Although all birds are susceptible, pet
birds (parrots, parakeets, macaws, and cockatiels) and poultry (turkeys
and ducks) are most frequently involved in transmission to humans.
Personal protective equipment (PPE), such as gloves and appropriate
masks, should be used when handling birds or cleaning their cages.

Risk Groups

Bird owners, aviary and pet shop employees, poultry workers, and veterinarians. Outbreaks of psittacosis in poultry processing plants have been reported.

Treatment

Tetracyclines are the treatment of choice.

Surveillance

Psittacosis is a reportable condition in most states.

Trends

Annual incidence varies considerably because of periodic outbreaks. A decline in reported cases since 1988 may be the result of improved diagnostic tests that distinguish *C. psittaci* from more common *C. pneumoniae* infections.

Challenges

Diagnosis of psittacosis can be difficult. Serologic tests are often used to confirm a diagnosis, but antibiotic treatment may prevent an antibody response, thus limiting diagnosis by serologic methods. Infected birds are often asymptomatic. Tracebacks of infected birds to distributors and breeders often is not possible because of limited regulation of the pet bird industry.

Chapter 18

Fungal Infections That Cause Respiratory Complications

Chapter Contents

Section 18.1

Aspergillosis

This section includes text excerpted from "Aspergillosis," Centers for Disease Control and Prevention (CDC), November 13, 2015.

What Is Aspergillosis?

Aspergillosis is a disease caused by *Aspergillus*, a common mold (a type of fungus) that lives indoors and outdoors. Most people breathe in *Aspergillus* spores every day without getting sick. However, people with weakened immune systems or lung diseases are at a higher risk of developing health problems due to *Aspergillus*. There are different types of aspergillosis. Some types are mild, but some of them are very serious.

Types of Aspergillosis

- **Allergic bronchopulmonary aspergillosis (ABPA)**: *Aspergillus* causes inflammation in the lungs and allergy symptoms such as coughing and wheezing, but doesn't cause an infection.

- **Allergic *Aspergillus* sinusitis**: *Aspergillus* causes inflammation in the sinuses and symptoms of a sinus infection (drainage, stuffiness, headache) but doesn't cause an infection.

- **Aspergilloma**: also called a "fungus ball." As the name suggests, it is a ball of *Aspergillus* that grows in the lungs or sinuses, but usually does not spread to other parts of the body.

- **Chronic pulmonary aspergillosis**: a long-term (3 months or more) condition in which *Aspergillus* can cause cavities in the lungs. One or more fungal balls (aspergillomas) may also be present in the lungs.

- **Invasive aspergillosis**: a serious infection that usually affects people who have weakened immune systems, such as people who have had an organ transplant or a stem cell transplant. Invasive aspergillosis most commonly affects the lungs, but it can also spread to other parts of the body.

- **Cutaneous (skin) aspergillosis**: *Aspergillus* enters the body through a break in the skin (for example, after surgery or a burn wound) and causes infection, usually in people who have weakened immune systems. Cutaneous aspergillosis can also occur if invasive aspergillosis spreads to the skin from somewhere else in the body, such as the lungs.

Symptoms of Aspergillosis

The different types of aspergillosis can cause different symptoms. The symptoms of **allergic bronchopulmonary aspergillosis (ABPA)** are similar to asthma symptoms, including:

- wheezing
- shortness of breath
- cough
- fever (in rare cases)

Symptoms of **allergic *Aspergillus* sinusitis** include:

- stuffiness
- runny nose
- headache
- reduced ability to smell

Symptoms of an **aspergilloma** ("fungus ball") include:

- cough
- coughing up blood
- shortness of breath

Symptoms of **chronic pulmonary aspergillosis** include:

- weight loss
- cough
- coughing up blood
- fatigue
- shortness of breath

Invasive aspergillosis usually occurs in people who are already sick from other medical conditions, so it can be difficult to know which symptoms are related to an *Aspergillus* infection. However, the symptoms of invasive aspergillosis in the lungs include:

- fever
- chest pain
- cough
- coughing up blood
- shortness of breath
- other symptoms can develop if the infection spreads from the lungs to other parts of the body

Contact your healthcare provider if you have symptoms that you think are related to any form of aspergillosis.

Aspergillosis Risk and Prevention

Who Gets Aspergillosis?

The different types of aspergillosis affect different groups of people.

- **Allergic bronchopulmonary aspergillosis (ABPA)** most often occurs in people who have cystic fibrosis or asthma.
- **Aspergillomas** usually affect people who have other lung diseases like tuberculosis.
- **Chronic pulmonary aspergillosis** typically occurs in people who have other lung diseases, including tuberculosis, chronic obstructive pulmonary disease (COPD), or sarcoidosis.
- **Invasive aspergillosis** affects people who have weakened immune systems, such as people who have had a stem cell transplant or organ transplant, are getting chemotherapy for cancer, or are taking high doses of corticosteroids.

How Does Someone Get Aspergillosis?

People can get aspergillosis by breathing in microscopic *Aspergillus* spores from the environment. Most people breathe in *Aspergillus* spores every day without getting sick. However, people with weakened immune systems or lung diseases are at a higher risk of developing health problems due to *Aspergillus*.

Is Aspergillosis Contagious?

No. Aspergillosis can't spread between people or between people and animals from the lungs.

How Can I Prevent Aspergillosis?

It's difficult to avoid breathing in *Aspergillus* spores because the fungus is common in the environment. For people who have weakened immune systems, there may be some ways to lower the chances of developing a severe *Aspergillus* infection.

- **Protect yourself from the environment.** It's important to note that although these actions are recommended, they haven't been proven to prevent aspergillosis.

  - Try to avoid areas with a lot of dust like construction or excavation sites. If you can't avoid these areas, wear an N95 respirator (a type of face mask) while you're there.

  - Avoid activities that involve close contact to soil or dust, such as yard work or gardening. If this isn't possible,

  - Wear shoes, long pants, and a long-sleeved shirt when doing outdoor activities such as gardening, yard work, or visiting wooded areas.

  - Wear gloves when handling materials such as soil, moss, or manure.

  - To reduce the chances of developing a skin infection, clean skin injuries well with soap and water, especially if they have been exposed to soil or dust.

- **Antifungal medication.** If you are at high risk for developing invasive aspergillosis (for example, if you've had an organ transplant or a stem cell transplant), your healthcare provider may prescribe medication to prevent aspergillosis. Scientists are still learning about which transplant patients are at highest risk and how to best prevent fungal infections.

- **Testing for early infection.** Some high-risk patients may benefit from blood tests to detect invasive aspergillosis. Talk to your doctor to determine if this type of test is right for you.

Sources of Aspergillosis

Aspergillus Lives in the Environment

Aspergillus, the mold (a type of fungus) that causes aspergillosis, is very common both indoors and outdoors, so most people breathe in fungal spores every day. It's probably impossible to completely avoid breathing in some *Aspergillus* spores. For people with healthy immune systems, breathing in *Aspergillus* isn't harmful. However, for people who have weakened immune systems, breathing in *Aspergillus* spores can cause an infection in the lungs or sinuses which can spread to other parts of the body.

I'm Worried That the Mold in My Home Is Aspergillus. Should Someone Test the Mold to Find out What It Is?

No. Generally, it's not necessary to identify the species of mold growing in a home, and Centers for Disease Control and Prevention (CDC) doesn't recommend routine sampling for molds.

Types of Aspergillus

There are approximately 180 species of *Aspergillus*, but fewer than 40 of them are known to cause infections in humans. *Aspergillus fumigatus* is the most common cause of human *Aspergillus* infections. Other common species include *A. flavus*, *A. terreus*, and *A. niger*.

Diagnosis and Testing for Aspergillosis

How Is Aspergillosis Diagnosed?

Healthcare providers consider your medical history, risk factors, symptoms, physical examinations, and lab tests when diagnosing aspergillosis. You may need imaging tests such as a chest X-ray or a CT scan of your lungs or other parts of your body depending on the location of the suspected infection. If your healthcare provider suspects that you have an *Aspergillus* infection in your lungs, he or she might collect a sample of fluid from your respiratory system to send to a laboratory. Healthcare providers may also perform a tissue biopsy, in which a small sample of affected tissue is analyzed in a laboratory for evidence of *Aspergillus* under a microscope or in a fungal culture. A blood test can help diagnose invasive aspergillosis early in people who have severely weakened immune systems.

Treatment for Aspergillosis

Allergic Forms of Aspergillosis

For allergic forms of aspergillosis such as allergic bronchopulmonary aspergillosis (ABPA) or allergic *Aspergillus* sinusitis, the recommended treatment is itraconazole, a prescription antifungal medication. Corticosteroids may also be helpful.

Invasive Aspergillosis

Invasive aspergillosis needs to be treated with prescription antifungal medication, usually voriconazole. There are other medications that can be used to treat invasive aspergillosis in patients who can't take voriconazole or whose infections don't get better after taking voriconazole. These include itraconazole, lipid amphotericin formulations, caspofungin, micafungin, and posaconazole. Whenever possible, immunosuppressive medications should be discontinued or decreased. People who have severe cases of aspergillosis may need surgery.

Section 18.2

Blastomycosis

This section includes text excerpted from "Blastomycosis," Centers for Disease Control and Prevention (CDC), December 28, 2015.

What Is Blastomycosis?

Blastomycosis is an infection caused by the fungus *Blastomyces*. The fungus lives in the environment, particularly in moist soil and in decomposing organic matter such as wood and leaves. In the United States, *Blastomyces* mainly lives in the midwestern, south-central, and southeastern states, particularly in areas surrounding the Ohio and Mississippi River valleys, the Great Lakes, and the Saint Lawrence River. The fungus also lives in Canada, and a few blastomycosis cases have been reported from Africa and India.

People can get blastomycosis after breathing in the microscopic fungal spores from the air, often after participating in activities that disturb the soil. Although most people who breathe in the spores don't get sick, some of those who do may have flu-like symptoms. In some people, such as those who have weakened immune systems, the infection can become severe, especially if it spreads from the lungs to other organs.

Symptoms of Blastomycosis

Approximately half of people who are infected with the fungus *Blastomyces* will show symptoms. The symptoms of blastomycosis are often similar to the symptoms of flu or other lung infections, and can include:

- fever
- cough
- night sweats
- muscle aches or joint pain
- weight loss
- chest pain
- fatigue (extreme tiredness)

How Soon Do the Symptoms of Blastomycosis Appear?

Symptoms of blastomycosis usually appear between 3 weeks and 3 months after a person breathes in the fungal spores.

Severe Blastomycosis

In some people, particularly those who have weakened immune systems, blastomycosis can spread from the lungs to other parts of the body, such as the skin, bones and joints, and the central nervous system (the brain and spinal cord).

Blastomycosis Risk and Prevention

Who Gets Blastomycosis?

Anyone can get blastomycosis if they've been in an area where *Blastomyces* lives in the environment. People who participate in outdoor activities that expose them to wooded areas (such as forestry work, hunting, and camping) in these areas may be at higher risk for getting blastomycosis. People who have weakened immune systems may be more likely to develop severe blastomycosis than people who are otherwise healthy.

Is Blastomycosis Contagious?

No. Blastomycosis can't spread between people or between people and animals.

Can My Pets Get Blastomycosis?

Yes. Pets, particularly dogs, can get blastomycosis, but it is **not** contagious between animals and people.The symptoms of blastomycosis in animals are similar to the symptoms in humans. If you are concerned about your pet's risk of getting blastomycosis or if you think that your pet has blastomycosis, please talk to a veterinarian.

How Can I Prevent Blastomycosis?

There is no vaccine to prevent blastomycosis, and it may not be possible to completely avoid being exposed to the fungus that causes blastomycosis in areas where it is common in the environment. People who have weakened immune systems may want to consider avoiding activities that involve disrupting soil in these areas.

Sources of Blastomycosis

Where Does Blastomyces Live?

Blastomyces lives in the environment, particularly in moist soil and in decomposing organic matter such as wood and leaves. In the United States, the fungus mainly lives in the midwestern, south-central, and southeastern states, particularly in areas surrounding the Ohio and Mississippi River valleys, the Great Lakes, and the Saint Lawrence River. The fungus also lives in Canada, and a small number of blastomycosis cases have been reported from Africa and India.

I'm Worried That Blastomyces Is in the Soil near My Home. Can Someone Test the Environment to Find out If the Fungus Is There?

No, in this situation, testing the environment for *Blastomyces* isn't likely to be useful. When a soil sample tests positive for *Blastomyces,* it isn't necessarily a source of infection, and when a sample tests negative, that doesn't necessarily mean that the fungus isn't in the soil. Also, there are no commercially-available tests to detect *Blastomyces* in the environment. Testing environmental samples for *Blastomyces* is currently only done for scientific research.

Diagnosis and Testing for Blastomycosis

How Is Blastomycosis Diagnosed?

Healthcare providers use your medical and travel history, symptoms, physical examinations, and laboratory tests to diagnose blastomycosis. A doctor will likely test for blastomycosis by taking a blood sample or a urine sample and sending it to a laboratory.

Healthcare providers may do imaging tests such as chest X-rays or CT scans of your lungs. They may also collect a sample of fluid from your respiratory tract or perform a tissue biopsy, in which a small sample of affected tissue is taken from the body and examined under a microscope. Laboratories may also see if *Blastomyces* will grow from body fluids or tissues (this is called a culture).

Where Can I Get Tested for Blastomycosis?

Most healthcare providers can order a test for blastomycosis.

How Long Will It Take to Get My Test Results?

It depends on the type of test. Results from a blood test or a urine test are usually available in a few days. If your healthcare provider sends a sample to a laboratory to be cultured, the results could take a couple of weeks.

Treatment for Blastomycosis

Most people with blastomycosis will need treatment with prescription antifungal medication. Itraconazole is a type of antifungal medication that is typically used to treat mild to moderate blastomycosis. Amphotericin B is usually recommended for severe blastomycosis in the lungs or infections that have spread to other parts of the body. Depending on the severity of the infection and the person's immune status, the course of treatment can range from six months to one year.

Section 18.3

Coccidioidomycosis (Valley Fever)

This section includes text excerpted from "Valley Fever
(Coccidioidomycosis)," Centers for Disease Control and
Prevention (CDC), June 29, 2015.

What Is Valley Fever?

Valley fever is an infection caused by the fungus *Coccidioides*. The
scientific name for Valley fever is "coccidioidomycosis," and it's also
sometimes called "San Joaquin Valley fever" or "desert rheumatism".
The term "Valley fever" usually refers to *Coccidioides* infection in the
lungs, but the infection can spread to other parts of the body in severe
cases (this is called "disseminated coccidioidomycosis").

The fungus is known to live in the soil in the southwestern United
States and parts of Mexico and Central and South America. The fungus
was also recently found in south-central Washington. People can get
Valley fever by breathing in the microscopic fungal spores from the
air in these areas.

Most people who breathe in the spores don't get sick, but some
people do. Usually, people who get sick with Valley fever will get better on their own within weeks to months, but some people will need
antifungal medication. Certain groups of people are at higher risk for
developing the severe forms of the infection, and these people typically
need antifungal treatment. It's difficult to prevent exposure to *Coccidioides* in areas where it's common in the environment, but people who
are at higher risk for severe Valley fever should try to avoid breathing
in large amounts of dust if they're in these areas.

Symptoms of Valley Fever

Many people who are exposed to the fungus *Coccidioides* never have
symptoms. Other people may have flu-like symptoms that go usually
away on their own after weeks to months. If your symptoms last for
more than a week, contact your healthcare provider.

Symptoms of Valley fever include:

- fatigue (tiredness)
- cough
- fever
- shortness of breath
- headache
- night sweats
- muscle aches or joint pain
- rash on upper body or legs

In extremely rare cases, the fungal spores can enter the skin through a cut, wound, or splinter and cause a skin infection.

How Soon Do the Symptoms Appear?

Symptoms of Valley fever may appear between 1 and 3 weeks after a person breathes in the fungal spores.

How Long Do the Symptoms Last?

The symptoms of Valley fever usually last for a few weeks to a few months. However, some patients have symptoms that last longer than this, especially if the infection becomes severe.

Severe Valley Fever

Approximately 5 to 10 percent of people who get Valley fever will develop serious or long-term problems in their lungs. In an even smaller percent of people (about 1%), the infection spreads from the lungs to other parts of the body, such as the central nervous system (brain and spinal cord), skin, or bones and joints.

Valley Fever Risk and Prevention

Who Gets Valley Fever?

Anyone who lives in or travels to the southwestern United States (Arizona, California, Nevada, New Mexico, Texas, or Utah), or parts of Mexico or Central or South America can get Valley fever. Valley fever can affect people of any age, but it's most common in adults aged 60 and older. Certain groups of people may be at higher risk for developing the severe forms of Valley fever, such as:

- people who have weakened immune systems, for example, people who:
  - have HIV/AIDS
  - have had an organ transplant
  - are taking medications such as corticosteroids or tumor necrosis factor (TNF)-inhibitors
- pregnant women
- people who have diabetes
- people who are black or Filipino

Is Valley Fever Contagious?

No. The fungus that causes Valley fever, *Coccidioides*, can't spread from the lungs between people or between people and animals. However, in **extremely** rare instances, a wound infection with *Coccidioides* can spread Valley fever to someone else, or the infection can be spread through an organ transplant with an infected organ.

Traveling to an Endemic Area

The risk of getting Valley fever is low when traveling to an area where *Coccidioides* lives in the environment, such as the southwestern United States, Mexico, or Central or South America. Your risk for infection could increase if you will be in a very dusty setting, but even then the risk is still low. If you have questions about your risk of getting Valley fever while traveling, talk to your healthcare provider.

I've Had It Before; Could I Get It Again?

Usually not. If you've already had Valley fever, your immune system will most likely protect you from getting it again. Some people can have the infection come back again (a relapse) after getting better the first time, but this is very rare.

Can My Pets Get Valley Fever?

Yes. Pets, particularly dogs, can get valley fever, but it is **not** contagious between animals and people. Valley fever in dogs is similar to valley fever in humans. Like humans, many dogs that are exposed to *Coccidioides* never get sick. Dogs that do develop symptoms often have symptoms that include coughing, lack of energy, and weight loss. If you're concerned about your pet's risk of getting Valley fever or if you think that your pet has Valley fever, please talk to a veterinarian.

Coccidioides at My Workplace

If you think you've been exposed to *Coccidioides* at work or in a laboratory, you should contact your Occupational Health, Infection Control, Risk Management, or Safety/Security Department. If your workplace or laboratory doesn't have these services, you should contact your local city, county, or state health department. Recommendations about what to do in the event of a laboratory exposure have been published. There is no evidence showing that antifungal medication (i.e., prophylaxis) prevents people from getting sick with Valley fever after a workplace exposure to *Coccidioides*. If you develop symptoms of Valley fever, contact your healthcare provider.

How Can I Prevent Valley Fever?

It's very difficult to avoid breathing in the fungus *Coccidioides* in areas where it's common in the environment. People who live in these areas can try to avoid spending time in dusty places as much as possible. People who are at risk for severe Valley fever (such as people who have weakened immune systems, pregnant women, people who have diabetes, or people who are Black or Filipino) may be able to lower their chances of developing the infection by trying to avoid breathing in the fungal spores.

The following are some common-sense methods that may be helpful to avoid getting Valley fever. It's important to know that although these steps are recommended, they haven't been proven to prevent Valley fever.

- Try to avoid areas with a lot of dust like construction or excavation sites. If you can't avoid these areas, wear an N95 respirator (a type of face mask) while you're there.

- Stay inside during dust storms and close your windows.

- Avoid activities that involve close contact to dirt or dust, including yard work, gardening, and digging.

- Use air filtration measures indoors.

- Clean skin injuries well with soap and water to reduce the chances of developing a skin infection, especially if the wound was exposed to dirt or dust.

- Take preventive antifungal medication if your healthcare provider says you need it.

Is There a Vaccine for Valley Fever?

No. Currently, there is no vaccine to prevent Valley fever, but scientists have been trying to make one since the 1960s. Because people who've had Valley fever are usually protected from getting it again, a vaccine could make the body's immune system think that it's already had Valley fever, which would likely prevent a person from being able to get the infection.

Scientists have tried several different ways to make a Valley fever vaccine. When one version of the vaccine was tested on humans in the 1980s, it didn't provide good protection, and it also caused people to develop side effects such as swelling at the injection site. Since then, scientists have been looking at ways to make a vaccine with different ingredients that will provide better protection against Valley fever and won't cause side effects. Studies of these vaccines are ongoing, so it's possible that a vaccine to prevent Valley fever could become available in the future.

Sources of Valley Fever

Where Does Coccidioides Live?

Coccidioides lives in dust and soil in some areas in the southwestern United States, Mexico, and South America. In the United States, *Coccidioides* lives in Arizona, California, Nevada, New Mexico, Texas, and Utah. The fungus was also recently found in south-central Washington.

Uncommon Sources of Valley Fever

The most common way for someone to get Valley fever is by inhaling *Coccidioides* spores that are in the air. In **extremely** rare cases, people can get the infection from other sources, such as:

- from an organ transplant if the organ donor had Valley fever

- from inhaling spores from a wound infected with *Coccidioides*

- from contact with objects (such as rocks or shoes) that have been contaminated with *Coccidioides*

Testing Soil

I'm Worried That Coccidioides Is in the Soil near My Home. Can Someone Test the Soil to Find out If the Fungus Is There?

No, in this situation, testing soil for *Coccidioides* isn't likely to be useful because the fungus is thought to be common in the soil in certain areas. A soil sample that tests positive for *Coccidioides* doesn't necessarily mean that the soil will release the fungus into the air and cause infection. Also, there are no commercially-available tests to detect *Coccidioides* in soil. Testing soil for *Coccidioides* is currently only done for scientific research.

Testing Soil for Research

Scientists sometimes test soil or other environmental samples for *Coccidioides* to understand more about its habitat and how weather or climate patterns may affect its growth. The available methods to detect *Coccidioides* in the soil don't always detect *Coccidioides* spores even if they are present. However, new tests are being developed so that researchers can better detect *Coccidioides* in the environment.

Valley Fever and the Weather

Scientists continue to study how weather and climate patterns affect the habitat of the fungus that causes Valley fever. *Coccidioides* is thought to grow best in soil after heavy rainfall and then disperse into the air most effectively during hot, dry conditions. For example, hot and dry weather conditions have been shown to correlate with an increase in the number of Valley fever cases in Arizona and in California (but to a lesser extent). The ways in which climate change may be affecting the number of Valley fever infections, as well as the geographic range of *Coccidioides*, isn't known yet, but is a subject for further research.

Diagnosis and Testing for Valley Fever

How Is Valley Fever Diagnosed?

Healthcare providers rely on your medical and travel history, symptoms, physical examinations, and laboratory tests to diagnose Valley fever. The most common way that healthcare providers test for Valley fever is by taking a blood sample and sending it to a laboratory to look for *Coccidioides* antibodies or antigens.

Healthcare providers may do imaging tests such as chest X-rays or CT scans of your lungs to look for Valley fever pneumonia. They may also perform a tissue biopsy, in which a small sample of tissue is taken from the body and examined under a microscope. Laboratories may also see if *Coccidioides* will grow from body fluids or tissues (this is called a culture).

Where Can I Get Tested for Valley Fever?

Any healthcare provider can order a test for Valley fever.

How Long Will It Take to Get My Test Results?

It depends on the type of test. Results from a blood test will usually be available in a few days. If your healthcare provider sends a sample to a laboratory to be cultured, the results could take a few days to a couple of weeks.

Treatment for Valley Fever

How Is Valley Fever Treated?

For many people, the symptoms of Valley fever will go away within a few months without any treatment. Healthcare providers choose to prescribe antifungal medication for some people to try to reduce the severity of symptoms or prevent the infection from getting worse. Antifungal medication is typically given to people who are at higher risk for developing severe Valley fever. The treatment is usually 3 to 6 months of fluconazole or another type of antifungal medication. There are no over-the-counter medications to treat Valley fever. If you have Valley fever, you should talk to your healthcare provider about whether you need treatment. The healthcare provider who diagnoses you with Valley fever may suggest that you see other healthcare providers who specialize in treating Valley fever.

People who have severe lung infections or infections that have spread to other parts of the body always need antifungal treatment and may need to stay in the hospital. For these types of infections, the course of treatment is usually longer than 6 months. Valley fever that develops into meningitis is fatal if it's not treated, so lifelong antifungal treatment is necessary for those cases.

If I Have Valley Fever, Should I Stay at Home?

Valley fever isn't contagious, so you don't need to stay at home to avoid spreading the infection to other people. However, your healthcare provider may recommend that you rest at home to help your body fight off the infection.

Does Valley Fever Have Any Long-Term Effects?

Most people who have Valley fever will make a full recovery. A small percent of people develop long-term lung infections that can take several years to get better. In very severe cases of Valley fever, the nervous system can be affected and there may be long-term damage, but this is very rare. Most people who have Valley fever will make a full recovery. A small percent of people develop long-term lung infections that can take several years to get better. In very severe cases of Valley fever, the nervous system can be affected and there may be long-term damage, but this is very rare.

Section 18.4

Cryptococcosis

This section includes text excerpted from "*C. neoformans* Infection," Centers for Disease Control and Prevention (CDC), November 28, 2015.

What Is Cryptococcosis?

Cryptococcus neoformans is a fungus that lives in the environment throughout the world. People can become infected with *C. neoformans* after breathing in the microscopic fungus, although most people who are exposed to the fungus never get sick from it.

Infection with the fungus *Cryptococcus* (either *C. neoformans* or *C. gattii*) is called cryptococcosis. Cryptococcosis usually affects the lungs or the central nervous system (the brain and spinal cord), but it can also affect other parts of the body. Brain infections due to the fungus *Cryptococcus* are called cryptococcal meningitis.

C. neoformans infections are extremely rare in people who are otherwise healthy. Most cases of *C. neoformans* infection occur in people

214

who have weakened immune systems, particularly those who have advanced HIV/AIDS.

Symptoms of C. neoformans Infection

C. neoformans usually infects the lungs or the central nervous system (the brain and spinal cord), but it can also affect other parts of the body. The symptoms of the infection depend on the parts of the body that are affected.

In the Lungs

A *C. neoformans* infection in the lungs can cause a pneumonia-like illness. The symptoms are often similar to those of many other illnesses, and can include:

- cough
- shortness of breath
- chest pain
- fever

In the Brain (Cryptococcal Meningitis)

Cryptococcal meningitis is an infection caused by the fungus *Cryptococcus* after it spreads from the lungs to the brain. The symptoms of cryptococcal meningitis include:

- headache
- fever
- neck pain
- nausea and vomiting
- sensitivity to light
- confusion or changes in behavior

If you have symptoms that you think may be due to a *C. neoformans* infection, please contact your healthcare provider.

C. neoformans Infection Risk and Prevention

Who Gets C. neoformans Infections?

C. neoformans infections are extremely rare among people who are otherwise healthy. Most cases of *C. neoformans* infection occur in people who have weakened immune systems, such as people who:

- have advanced HIV/AIDS

- have had an organ transplant, or

- are taking corticosteroids, medications to treat rheumatoid arthritis, or other medications that weaken the immune system

Is C. neoformans *Infection Contagious?*

No. The infection can't spread between people or between people and animals.

Can Pets Get C. neoformans *Infections?*

Yes. Pets can get *C. neoformans* infections, but it is very rare, and the infection **cannot** spread between animals and people. If you're concerned about your pet's risk of getting a *C. neoformans* infection, or if you think that your pet has the infection, please talk to a veterinarian.

How Can I Prevent a C. neoformans *Infection?*

It's difficult to avoid breathing in *C. neoformans* because it's thought to be common in the environment. Most people who breathe in *C. neoformans* never get sick from it. However, in people who have weakened immune systems, *C. neoformans* can stay hidden in the body and cause infection later when the immune system becomes too weak to fight it off. This leaves a window of time when the silent infection can be detected and treated early, before symptoms develop.

Detecting Silent Cryptococcal Infections in People Who Have HIV/AIDS

One approach to prevent cryptococcal meningitis is called "targeted screening." Research suggests that *C. neoformans* is able to live in the body undetected, especially when a person's immune system is weaker than normal. In a targeted screening program, a simple blood test is used to detect cryptococcal antigen (an indicator of cryptococcal infection) in HIV-infected patients before they begin taking antiretroviral treatment (ART). A patient who tests positive for cryptococcal antigen can take fluconazole, an antifungal medication, to fight off the silent fungal infection and prevent it from developing into life-threatening meningitis.

Sources of C. neoformans

Where Does C. neoformans *Live?*

C. neoformans lives in the environment throughout the world. The fungus is typically found in soil, on decaying wood, in tree hollows, or in bird droppings.

How Does Someone Get a C. neoformans *Infection?*

C. neoformans infections are **not** contagious. Humans and animals can get the infection after inhaling the microscopic fungus from the environment. Some research suggests that people may be exposed to *C. neoformans* in the environment when they are children. Most people who breathe in *C. neoformans* never get sick from it. However, in people who have weakened immune systems, *C. neoformans* can stay hidden in the body and cause infection later when the immune system becomes too weak to fight it off.

Diagnosis and Testing for C. neoformans Infection

How Is a C. neoformans *Infection Diagnosed?*

Healthcare providers rely on your medical history, symptoms, physical examinations, and laboratory tests to diagnose a *C. neoformans* infection.

Your healthcare provider will take a sample of tissue or body fluid (such as blood, cerebrospinal fluid, or sputum) and send the sample to a laboratory to be examined under a microscope, tested with an antigen test, or cultured. Your healthcare provider may also perform tests such as a chest X-ray or CT scan of your lungs, brain, or other parts of the body.

Treatment for C. neoformans Infection

How Are C. neoformans *Infections Treated?*

People who have *C. neoformans* infection need to take prescription antifungal medication for at least 6 months, often longer. The type of treatment usually depends on the severity of the infection and the parts of the body that are affected.

- For people who have **asymptomatic infections (e.g., diagnosed via targeted screening) or mild-to-moderate pulmonary infections**, the treatment is usually fluconazole.

- For people who have **severe lung infections or infections in the central nervous system** (brain and spinal cord), the recommended initial treatment is amphotericin B in combination with flucytosine. After that, patients usually need to take fluconazole for an extended time to clear the infection.

The type, dose, and duration of antifungal treatment may differ for certain groups of people, such as pregnant women, children, and people in resource-limited settings. Some people may also need surgery to remove fungal growths (cryptococcomas).

Section 18.5

Histoplasmosis

This section includes text excerpted from "Histoplasmosis," Centers for Disease Control and Prevention (CDC), November 21, 2015.

What Is Histoplasmosis?

Histoplasmosis is an infection caused by the fungus *Histoplasma*. The fungus lives in the environment, particularly in soil that contains large amounts of bird or bat droppings. In the United States, *Histoplasma* mainly lives in soil in the central and eastern states, especially areas around the Ohio and Mississippi River valleys. The fungus also lives in parts of Central and South America, Africa, Asia, and Australia.

People can get histoplasmosis after breathing in the microscopic fungal spores from the air, often after participating in activities that disturb the soil. Although most people who breathe in the spores don't get sick, those who do may have a fever, cough, and fatigue. Many people who get sick will get better on their own without medication. In some people, such as those who have weakened immune systems, the infection can become severe, especially if it spreads from the lungs to other organs.

Symptoms of Histoplasmosis

Most people who are exposed to the fungus *Histoplasma* never have symptoms. Other people may have flu-like symptoms that usually go away on their own.

Symptoms of histoplasmosis include:

- fever
- cough
- fatigue (extreme tiredness)
- chills
- headache
- chest pain
- body aches

How Soon Do the Symptoms of Histoplasmosis Appear?

Symptoms of histoplasmosis may appear between 3 and 17 days after a person breathes in the fungal spores.

How Long Do the Symptoms of Histoplasmosis Last?

For most people, the symptoms of histoplasmosis will go away within a few weeks to a month. However, some people have symptoms that last longer than this, especially if the infection becomes severe.

Severe Histoplasmosis

In some people, usually those who have weakened immune systems, histoplasmosis can develop into a long-term lung infection, or it can spread from the lungs to other parts of the body, such as the central nervous system (the brain and spinal cord).

Histoplasmosis Risk and Prevention

Who Gets Histoplasmosis?

Anyone can get histoplasmosis if they've been in an area where *Histoplasma* lives in the environment. Histoplasmosis is often associated with activities that disturb soil, particularly soil that contains bird or bat droppings. Certain groups of people are at higher risk for developing the severe forms of histoplasmosis:

- people who have weakened immune systems, for example, people who:
  - have HIV/AIDS

- have had an organ transplant
- are taking medications such as corticosteroids or TNF-inhibitors

- infants
- adults aged 55 and older

Is Histoplasmosis Contagious?

No. Histoplasmosis can't spread from the lungs between people or between people and animals. However, in **extremely** rare cases, the infection can be passed through an organ transplant with an infected organ.

If I've Already Had Histoplasmosis, Could I Get It Again?

It's possible for someone who's already had histoplasmosis to get it again, but the body's immune system usually provides some partial protection so that the infection is less severe the second time. In people who have weakened immune systems, histoplasmosis can remain hidden in the body for months or years and then cause symptoms later (also called a relapse of infection).

Can My Pets Get Histoplasmosis?

Yes. Pets, particularly cats, can get histoplasmosis, but it is **not** contagious between animals and people. Histoplasmosis in cats and dogs is similar to histoplasmosis in humans. Like humans, many cats and dogs that are exposed to *Histoplasma* never get sick. Cats and dogs that do develop symptoms often have symptoms that include coughing, lack of energy, and weight loss. The fungus that causes histoplasmosis grows well in soil that contains bird droppings, but birds don't appear to be able to get histoplasmosis. If you're concerned about your pet's risk of getting histoplasmosis or if you think that your pet has histoplasmosis, please talk to a veterinarian.

How Can I Prevent Histoplasmosis?

It can be difficult to avoid breathing in *Histoplasma* in areas where it's common in the environment. In areas where *Histoplasma* is known to live, people who have weakened immune systems (for example, by HIV/AIDS, an organ transplant, or medications such as corticosteroids or TNF-inhibitors) should avoid doing activities that are known to be associated with getting histoplasmosis, including:

- disturbing material (for example, digging in soil or chopping wood) where there are bird or bat droppings

- cleaning chicken coops

- exploring caves

- cleaning, remodeling, or tearing down old buildings

Large amounts of bird or bat droppings should be cleaned up by professional companies that specialize in the removal of hazardous waste.

What Are Public Health Agencies Doing about Histoplasmosis?

- **Surveillance.** In some states, healthcare providers and laboratories are required to report histoplasmosis cases to public health authorities. Disease reporting helps government officials and healthcare providers understand how and why outbreaks occur and allows them to monitor trends in the number of histoplasmosis cases.

- **Developing better diagnostic tools.** The symptoms of histoplasmosis can be similar to those of other respiratory diseases. Faster, more reliable methods to diagnosis histoplasmosis are in development, which could help minimize delays in treatment, save money and resources looking for other diagnoses, and reduce unnecessary treatment for other suspected illnesses.

- **Building laboratory capacity**. Equipping laboratories in Latin America to be able to diagnose histoplasmosis and perform laboratory-based surveillance will help reduce the burden of HIV-associated histoplasmosis in these areas.

Sources of Histoplasmosis

Where Does Histoplasma Live?

Histoplasma, the fungus that causes histoplasmosis, lives throughout the world, but it's most common in North America and Central America. In the United States, *Histoplasma* mainly lives in soil in the central and eastern states, particularly areas around the Ohio and Mississippi River Valleys, but it can likely live in other parts of the

United States as well. The fungus also lives in parts of Central and South America, Africa, Asia, and Australia.

Histoplasma grows best in soil that contains bird or bat droppings. Bats can get histoplasmosis and spread the fungus in their droppings.

I'm Worried That **Histoplasma** *Is in the Soil or in Bird / Bat Droppings near My Home. Can Someone Test the Environment to Find out If the Fungus Is There?*

No, in this situation, testing the environment for *Histoplasma* isn't likely to be useful because the fungus is thought to be common in the environment in certain areas. A soil sample that tests positive for *Histoplasma* doesn't necessarily mean that it's a source of infection, and a sample that tests negative doesn't necessarily mean that the fungus isn't there. Also, there are no commercially-available tests to detect *Histoplasma* in the environment. Testing environmental samples for *Histoplasma* is currently only done for scientific research. If there are bird or bat droppings near your home, you should have it cleaned up, if possible. If it's not possible to clean up, try not to disturb it.

Diagnosis and Testing for Histoplasmosis

How Is Histoplasmosis Diagnosed?

Healthcare providers rely on your medical and travel history, symptoms, physical examinations, and laboratory tests to diagnose histoplasmosis. The most common way that healthcare providers test for histoplasmosis is by taking a blood sample or a urine sample and sending it to a laboratory.

Healthcare providers may do imaging tests such as chest X-rays or CT scans of your lungs. They may also collect a sample of fluid from your respiratory tract or perform a tissue biopsy, in which a small sample of affected tissue is taken from the body and examined under a microscope. Laboratories may also see if *Histoplasma* will grow from body fluids or tissues (this is called a culture).

Where Can I Get Tested for Histoplasmosis?

Most healthcare providers can order a test for histoplasmosis.

How Long Will It Take to Get My Test Results?

It depends on the type of test. Results from a blood test or a urine test will usually be available in a few days. If your healthcare provider sends a sample to a laboratory to be cultured, the results could take a couple of weeks.

Treatment for Histoplasmosis

How Is Histoplasmosis Treated?

For some people, the symptoms of histoplasmosis will go away without treatment. However, prescription antifungal medication is needed to treat severe histoplasmosis in the lungs, chronic histoplasmosis, and infections that have spread from the lungs to other parts of the body (disseminated histoplasmosis). Itraconazole is one type of antifungal medication that's commonly used to treat histoplasmosis. Depending on the severity of the infection and the person's immune status, the course of treatment can range from 3 months to 1 year.

Chapter 19

Inhalation Anthrax

What Is Anthrax?

Anthrax is the disease caused by the bacterium *Bacillus anthracis*, which lives in soil. The bacterial cell lives as a hardy spore to survive harsh conditions. The spores germinate into thriving colonies of bacteria once inside an animal or person. Anthrax usually affects livestock far more than humans, but—as we know from the 2001 anthrax attacks in the United States—anthrax is feared as a modern biological weapon.

Anthrax occurs in three forms:

1. Cutaneous (affecting the skin)

2. Inhalational (in the lungs)

3. Gastrointestinal (in the digestive tract)

Cutaneous Anthrax

Cutaneous anthrax is the most common form of the disease. People with cuts or open sores can get cutaneous anthrax if they come in direct contact with the bacteria or its spores, usually through contaminated animal products. The skin will redden and swell, much like an insect bite, and then develop a painless blackened lesion or ulcer that may form a brown or black scab, which is actually dead tissue. Cutaneous

---

This chapter includes text excerpted from "Anthrax," National Institute of Allergy and Infectious Diseases (NIAID), September 30, 2013.

anthrax responds well to antibiotics but may spread throughout the body if untreated. People who work with certain animals or animal carcasses are at risk of getting this form of the disease. Cutaneous anthrax is rare in the United States.

Inhalational Anthrax

When a person inhales the spores of *Bacillus anthracis*, they germinate and the bacteria infect the lungs, spreading to the lymph nodes in the chest. As the bacteria grow, they produce two kinds of deadly toxins.

Symptoms usually appear 1 to 7 days after exposure, but they may first appear more than a month later. Fever, nausea, vomiting, aches, and fatigue are among the early symptoms of inhalational anthrax; it progresses to labored breathing, shock, and often death.

Historically, the mortality rate for naturally occurring inhalational anthrax has been 75 percent, even with appropriate treatment. But inhalational anthrax is rare. In the 2001 anthrax attacks, 11 people were infected with inhalational anthrax and 6 survived. Prior to 2001, the last known U.S. case was in 1976, when a California craftsman died after getting the infection from imported yarn contaminated with anthrax spores.

Gastrointestinal Anthrax

People can get gastrointestinal anthrax from eating meat contaminated with anthrax bacteria or their spores. Symptoms are stomach pain, loss of appetite, diarrhea, and fever. Antibiotic treatment can cure this form of anthrax, but left untreated, it may kill half of those who get it.

Gastrointestinal anthrax occurs naturally in warm and tropical regions of Asia, Africa, and the Middle East. It is the least common form of anthrax in the United States.

Causes

Bacillus anthracis is a bacterium that lives in soil and has developed a survival tactic that allows it to endure for decades under the harshest conditions. An anthrax bacterial cell can transform itself into a spore, a very hardy resting phase which can withstand extreme heat, cold, and drought, without nutrients or air. When environmental conditions are favorable, the spores will germinate into thriving colonies of bacteria. For example, a grazing animal may ingest spores that begin to grow, spread, and eventually kill the animal. The bacteria will form spores in the carcass and then return to the soil to infect other animals in the future.

While its spore form allows the bacteria to survive in any environment, the ability to produce toxins is what makes the bacteria such a potent killer. Together, the hardiness and toxicity of *B. anthracis* make it a formidable bioterror agent. Its toxin is made of three proteins: protective antigen, edema factor, and lethal factor.

Protective antigen binds to select cells of an infected person or animal and forms a channel that permits edema factor and lethal factor to enter those cells.

Edema factor, once inside the cell, causes fluid to accumulate at the site of infection. Edema factor can contribute to a fatal build-up of fluid in the cavity surrounding the lungs. It also can inhibit some of the body's immune functions.

Lethal factor also works inside the cell, disrupting a key molecular switch that regulates the cell's functions. Lethal factor can kill infected cells or prevent them from working properly.

Treatment

If diagnosed early, anthrax is easily treated with antibiotics. Unfortunately, infected people often confuse early symptoms with more common infections and do not seek medical help until severe symptoms appear. By that time, the destructive anthrax toxins have already risen to high levels, making treatment difficult. Antibiotics can kill the bacteria, but antibiotics have no effect on anthrax toxins.

Prevention

In 1970, the U.S. Food and Drug Administration (FDA) approved an anthrax vaccine for humans which is licensed for limited use. The vaccine is currently used to protect members of the military and people most at risk for occupational exposure to the bacteria, such as slaughterhouse workers, veterinarians, laboratory workers, and livestock handlers. The vaccine does not contain the whole bacterium. Rather, it is made mostly of the anthrax protective antigen protein, so people cannot get anthrax infection from the vaccine.

Health experts currently do not recommend the vaccine for general use by the public because anthrax illness is rare and the vaccine potentially can cause adverse side effects in some people. Researchers have not determined the safety and efficacy of the vaccine in children, the elderly, and people with weakened immune systems. Although the vaccine trials indicate that three to four doses of anthrax vaccine can generate significant protective immunity, the recommended vaccination schedule is five doses given over an 18-month period and efforts are underway to reduce the number of doses further. Nonetheless, to enhance public protection in the event of an anthrax bioterror attack, scientists are seeking to develop an improved anthrax vaccine.

Part Three

Inflammatory Respiratory Disorders

Chapter 20

Asthma

Chapter Contents

Section 20.1

Facts about Asthma

This section includes text excerpted from "Asthma," National Heart, Lung, and Blood Institute (NHLBI), August 4, 2014.

What Is Asthma?

Asthma is a chronic (long-term) lung disease that inflames and narrows the airways. Asthma causes recurring periods of wheezing (a whistling sound when you breathe), chest tightness, shortness of breath, and coughing. The coughing often occurs at night or early in the morning.

Asthma affects people of all ages, but it most often starts during childhood.

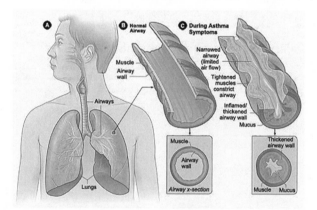

Figure 20.1. *Asthma*

Figure A shows the location of the lungs and airways in the body. Figure B shows a cross-section of a normal airway. Figure C shows a cross-section of an airway during asthma symptoms.

What Causes Asthma?

The exact cause of asthma isn't known. Researchers think some genetic and environmental factors interact to cause asthma, most often early in life. These factors include:

- An inherited tendency to develop allergies, called atopy.

- Parents who have asthma.

- Certain respiratory infections during childhood.

- Contact with some airborne allergens or exposure to some viral infections in infancy or in early childhood when the immune system is developing.

If asthma or atopy runs in your family, exposure to irritants (for example, tobacco smoke) may make your airways more reactive to substances in the air.

Some factors may be more likely to cause asthma in some people than in others. Researchers continue to explore what causes asthma.

The "Hygiene Hypothesis"

One theory researchers have for what causes asthma is the "hygiene hypothesis." They believe that our Western lifestyle—with its emphasis on hygiene and sanitation—has resulted in changes in our living conditions and an overall decline in infections in early childhood.

Many young children no longer have the same types of environmental exposures and infections as children did in the past. This affects the way that young children's immune systems develop during very early childhood, and it may increase their risk for atopy and asthma. This is especially true for children who have close family members with one or both of these conditions.

Who Is at Risk for Asthma?

Asthma affects people of all ages, but it most often starts during childhood. In the United States, more than 22 million people are known to have asthma. Nearly 6 million of these people are children.

Young children who often wheeze and have respiratory infections—as well as certain other risk factors—are at highest risk of developing asthma that continues beyond 6 years of age. The other risk factors include having allergies, eczema (an allergic skin condition), or parents who have asthma.

Among children, more boys have asthma than girls. But among adults, more women have the disease than men. It's not clear whether or how sex and sex hormones play a role in causing asthma.

Most, but not all, people who have asthma have allergies.

Some people develop asthma because of contact with certain chemical irritants or industrial dusts in the workplace. This type of asthma is called occupational asthma.

What Are the Signs and Symptoms of Asthma?

Common signs and symptoms of asthma include:

- Coughing. Coughing from asthma often is worse at night or early in the morning, making it hard to sleep.

- Wheezing. Wheezing is a whistling or squeaky sound that occurs when you breathe.

- Chest tightness. This may feel like something is squeezing or sitting on your chest.

- Shortness of breath. Some people who have asthma say they can't catch their breath or they feel out of breath. You may feel like you can't get air out of your lungs.

Not all people who have asthma have these symptoms. Likewise, having these symptoms doesn't always mean that you have asthma. The best way to diagnose asthma for certain is to use a lung function test, a medical history (including type and frequency of symptoms), and a physical exam.

The types of asthma symptoms you have, how often they occur, and how severe they are may vary over time. Sometimes your symptoms may just annoy you. Other times, they may be troublesome enough to limit your daily routine.

Severe symptoms can be fatal. It's important to treat symptoms when you first notice them so they don't become severe.

With proper treatment, most people who have asthma can expect to have few, if any, symptoms either during the day or at night.

What Causes Asthma Symptoms to Occur?

Many things can trigger or worsen asthma symptoms. Your doctor will help you find out which things (sometimes called triggers) may cause your asthma to flare up if you come in contact with them. Triggers may include:

- Allergens from dust, animal fur, cockroaches, mold, and pollens from trees, grasses, and flowers.

- Irritants such as cigarette smoke, air pollution, chemicals or dust in the workplace, compounds in home décor products, and sprays (such as hairspray).

- Medicines such as aspirin or other nonsteroidal anti-inflammatory drugs and nonselective beta blockers.

- Sulfites in foods and drinks.

- Viral upper respiratory infections, such as colds.

- Physical activity, including exercise.

Other health conditions can make asthma harder to manage. Examples of these conditions include a runny nose, sinus infections, reflux disease, psychological stress, and sleep apnea. These conditions need treatment as part of an overall asthma care plan.

Asthma is different for each person. Some of the triggers listed above may not affect you. Other triggers that do affect you may not be on the list. Talk with your doctor about the things that seem to make your asthma worse.

How Is Asthma Diagnosed?

Your primary care doctor will diagnose asthma based on your medical and family histories, a physical exam, and test results.

Your doctor also will figure out the severity of your asthma—that is, whether it's intermittent, mild, moderate, or severe. The level of severity will determine what treatment you'll start on.

You may need to see an asthma specialist if:

- You need special tests to help diagnose asthma

- You've had a life-threatening asthma attack

- You need more than one kind of medicine or higher doses of medicine to control your asthma, or if you have overall problems getting your asthma well controlled

- You're thinking about getting allergy treatments

Medical and Family Histories

Your doctor may ask about your family history of asthma and allergies. He or she also may ask whether you have asthma symptoms and when and how often they occur.

Let your doctor know whether your symptoms seem to happen only during certain times of the year or in certain places, or if they get worse at night.

Your doctor also may want to know what factors seem to trigger your symptoms or worsen them.

Your doctor may ask you about related health conditions that can interfere with asthma management. These conditions include a runny nose, sinus infections, reflux disease, psychological stress, and sleep apnea.

Physical Exam

Your doctor will listen to your breathing and look for signs of asthma or allergies. These signs include wheezing, a runny nose or swollen nasal passages, and allergic skin conditions (such as eczema).

Keep in mind that you can still have asthma even if you don't have these signs on the day that your doctor examines you.

Diagnostic Tests

Lung Function Test

Your doctor will use a test called spirometry to check how your lungs are working. This test measures how much air you can breathe in and out. It also measures how fast you can blow air out.

Your doctor also may give you medicine and then test you again to see whether the results have improved.

If the starting results are lower than normal and improve with the medicine, and if your medical history shows a pattern of asthma symptoms, your diagnosis will likely be asthma.

Other Tests

Your doctor may recommend other tests if he or she needs more information to make a diagnosis. Other tests may include:

- Allergy testing to find out which allergens affect you, if any.

- A test to measure how sensitive your airways are. This is called a bronchoprovocation test. Using spirometry, this test repeatedly measures your lung function during physical activity or after you receive increasing doses of cold air or a special chemical to breathe in.

- A test to show whether you have another condition with the same symptoms as asthma, such as reflux disease, vocal cord dysfunction, or sleep apnea.

- A chest X-ray or an EKG (electrocardiogram). These tests will help find out whether a foreign object or other disease may be causing your symptoms.

Diagnosing Asthma in Young Children

Most children who have asthma develop their first symptoms before 5 years of age. However, asthma in young children (aged 0 to 5 years) can be hard to diagnose.

Sometimes it's hard to tell whether a child has asthma or another childhood condition. This is because the symptoms of asthma also occur with other conditions.

Also, many young children who wheeze when they get colds or respiratory infections don't go on to have asthma after they're 6 years old.

A child may wheeze because he or she has small airways that become even narrower during colds or respiratory infections. The airways grow as the child grows older, so wheezing no longer occurs when the child gets colds.

A young child who has frequent wheezing with colds or respiratory infections is more likely to have asthma if:

- one or both parents have asthma

- the child has signs of allergies, including the allergic skin condition eczema

- the child has allergic reactions to pollens or other airborne allergens

- the child wheezes even when he or she doesn't have a cold or other infection

The most certain way to diagnose asthma is with a lung function test, a medical history, and a physical exam. However, it's hard to do lung function tests in children younger than 5 years. Thus, doctors must rely on children's medical histories, signs and symptoms, and physical exams to make a diagnosis.

Doctors also may use a 4–6 week trial of asthma medicines to see how well a child responds.

How Is Asthma Treated and Controlled?

Asthma is a long-term disease that has no cure. The goal of asthma treatment is to control the disease. Good asthma control will:

- prevent chronic and troublesome symptoms, such as coughing and shortness of breath

- reduce your need for quick-relief medicines

- help you maintain good lung function

- let you maintain your normal activity level and sleep through the night

- prevent asthma attacks that could result in an emergency room visit or hospital stay

To control asthma, partner with your doctor to manage your asthma or your child's asthma. Children aged 10 or older—and younger children who are able—should take an active role in their asthma care. Taking an active role to control your asthma involves:

- Working with your doctor to treat other conditions that can interfere with asthma management.

- Avoiding things that worsen your asthma (asthma triggers). However, one trigger you should not avoid is physical activity. Physical activity is an important part of a healthy lifestyle. Talk with your doctor about medicines that can help you stay active.

- Working with your doctor and other healthcare providers to create and follow an asthma action plan.

An asthma action plan gives guidance on taking your medicines properly, avoiding asthma triggers (except physical activity), tracking your level of asthma control, responding to worsening symptoms, and seeking emergency care when needed.

Asthma is treated with two types of medicines: long-term control and quick-relief medicines. Long-term control medicines help reduce airway inflammation and prevent asthma symptoms. Quick-relief, or "rescue," medicines relieve asthma symptoms that may flare up.

Your initial treatment will depend on the severity of your asthma. Followup asthma treatment will depend on how well your asthma action plan is controlling your symptoms and preventing asthma attacks.

Your level of asthma control can vary over time and with changes in your home, school, or work environments. These changes can alter how often you're exposed to the factors that can worsen your asthma.

Your doctor may need to increase your medicine if your asthma doesn't stay under control. On the other hand, if your asthma is well controlled for several months, your doctor may decrease your medicine. These adjustments to your medicine will help you maintain the best control possible with the least amount of medicine necessary.

Asthma treatment for certain groups of people—such as children, pregnant women, or those for whom exercise brings on asthma symptoms—will be adjusted to meet their special needs.

Follow an Asthma Action Plan

You can work with your doctor to create a personal asthma action plan. The plan will describe your daily treatments, such as which medicines to take and when to take them. The plan also will explain when to call your doctor or go to the emergency room.

If your child has asthma, all of the people who care for him or her should know about the child's asthma action plan. This includes babysitters and workers at daycare centers, schools, and camps. These caretakers can help your child follow his or her action plan.

Avoid Things That Can Worsen Your Asthma

Many common things (called asthma triggers) can set off or worsen your asthma symptoms. Once you know what these things are, you can take steps to control many of them.

For example, exposure to pollens or air pollution might make your asthma worse. If so, try to limit time outdoors when the levels of these substances in the outdoor air are high. If animal fur triggers your asthma symptoms, keep pets with fur out of your home or bedroom.

One possible asthma trigger you shouldn't avoid is physical activity. Physical activity is an important part of a healthy lifestyle. Talk with your doctor about medicines that can help you stay active.

If your asthma symptoms are clearly related to allergens, and you can't avoid exposure to those allergens, your doctor may advise you to get allergy shots.

You may need to see a specialist if you're thinking about getting allergy shots. These shots can lessen or prevent your asthma symptoms, but they can't cure your asthma.

Several health conditions can make asthma harder to manage. These conditions include runny nose, sinus infections, reflux disease, psychological stress, and sleep apnea. Your doctor will treat these conditions as well.

Medicines

Your doctor will consider many things when deciding which asthma medicines are best for you. He or she will check to see how well a medicine works for you. Then, he or she will adjust the dose or medicine as needed.

Asthma medicines can be taken in pill form, but most are taken using a device called an inhaler. An inhaler allows the medicine to go directly to your lungs.

Not all inhalers are used the same way. Ask your doctor or another healthcare provider to show you the right way to use your inhaler. Review the way you use your inhaler at every medical visit.

Long-Term Control Medicines

Most people who have asthma need to take long-term control medicines daily to help prevent symptoms. The most effective long-term medicines reduce airway inflammation, which helps prevent symptoms from starting. These medicines don't give you quick relief from symptoms.

Inhaled corticosteroids. Inhaled corticosteroids are the preferred medicine for long-term control of asthma. They're the most effective option for long-term relief of the inflammation and swelling that makes your airways sensitive to certain inhaled substances.

Reducing inflammation helps prevent the chain reaction that causes asthma symptoms. Most people who take these medicines daily find they greatly reduce the severity of symptoms and how often they occur.

Inhaled corticosteroids generally are safe when taken as prescribed. These medicines are different from the illegal anabolic steroids taken by some athletes. Inhaled corticosteroids aren't habit-forming, even if you take them every day for many years.

Like many other medicines, though, inhaled corticosteroids can have side effects. Most doctors agree that the benefits of taking inhaled corticosteroids and preventing asthma attacks far outweigh the risk of side effects.

One common side effect from inhaled corticosteroids is a mouth infection called thrush. You might be able to use a spacer or holding chamber on your inhaler to avoid thrush. These devices attach to your inhaler. They help prevent the medicine from landing in your mouth or on the back of your throat.

Check with your doctor to see whether a spacer or holding chamber should be used with the inhaler you have. Also, work with your healthcare team if you have any questions about how to use a spacer or holding chamber. Rinsing your mouth out with water after taking inhaled corticosteroids also can lower your risk for thrush.

If you have severe asthma, you may have to take corticosteroid pills or liquid for short periods to get your asthma under control.

If taken for long periods, these medicines raise your risk for cataracts and osteoporosis. A cataract is the clouding of the lens in your eye. Osteoporosis is a disorder that makes your bones weak and more likely to break.

Your doctor may have you add another long-term asthma control medicine so he or she can lower your dose of corticosteroids. Or, your doctor may suggest you take calcium and vitamin D pills to protect your bones.

Other long-term control medicines. Other long-term control medicines include:

- Cromolyn. This medicine is taken using a device called a nebulizer. As you breathe in, the nebulizer sends a fine mist of medicine to your lungs. Cromolyn helps prevent airway inflammation.

- Omalizumab (anti-IgE). This medicine is given as a shot (injection) one or two times a month. It helps prevent your body from reacting to asthma triggers, such as pollen and dust mites. Anti-IgE might be used if other asthma medicines have not worked well.

A rare, but possibly life-threatening allergic reaction called anaphylaxis might occur when the Omalizumab injection is given. If you take this medication, work with your doctor to make sure you understand the signs and symptoms of anaphylaxis and what actions you should take.

- Inhaled long-acting beta$_2$-agonists. These medicines open the airways. They might be added to inhaled corticosteroids to improve asthma control. Inhaled long-acting beta$_2$-agonists should never be used on their own for long-term asthma control. They must used with inhaled corticosteroids.

- Leukotriene modifiers. These medicines are taken by mouth. They help block the chain reaction that increases inflammation in your airways.

- Theophylline. This medicine is taken by mouth. Theophylline helps open the airways.

If your doctor prescribes a long-term control medicine, take it every day to control your asthma. Your asthma symptoms will likely return or get worse if you stop taking your medicine.

Long-term control medicines can have side effects. Talk with your doctor about these side effects and ways to reduce or avoid them.

With some medicines, like theophylline, your doctor will check the level of medicine in your blood. This helps ensure that you're getting enough medicine to relieve your asthma symptoms, but not so much that it causes dangerous side effects.

Quick-Relief Medicines

All people who have asthma need quick-relief medicines to help relieve asthma symptoms that may flare up. Inhaled short-acting beta$_2$-agonists are the first choice for quick relief.

These medicines act quickly to relax tight muscles around your airways when you're having a flareup. This allows the airways to open up so air can flow through them.

You should take your quick-relief medicine when you first notice asthma symptoms. If you use this medicine more than 2 days a week, talk with your doctor about your asthma control. You may need to make changes to your asthma action plan.

Carry your quick-relief inhaler with you at all times in case you need it. If your child has asthma, make sure that anyone caring for him or her has the child's quick-relief medicines, including staff at the child's school. They should understand when and how to use these medicines and when to seek medical care for your child.

You shouldn't use quick-relief medicines in place of prescribed long-term control medicines. Quick-relief medicines don't reduce inflammation.

Track Your Asthma

To track your asthma, keep records of your symptoms, check your peak flow number using a peak flow meter, and get regular asthma checkups.

Record Your Symptoms

You can record your asthma symptoms in a diary to see how well your treatments are controlling your asthma.

Asthma is well controlled if:

- You have symptoms no more than 2 days a week, and these symptoms don't wake you from sleep more than 1 or 2 nights a month.

- You can do all your normal activities.

- You take quick-relief medicines no more than 2 days a week.

- You have no more than one asthma attack a year that requires you to take corticosteroids by mouth.

- Your peak flow doesn't drop below 80 percent of your personal best number.

If your asthma isn't well controlled, contact your doctor. He or she may need to change your asthma action plan.

Use a Peak Flow Meter

This small, hand-held device shows how well air moves out of your lungs. You blow into the device and it gives you a score, or peak flow number. Your score shows how well your lungs are working at the time of the test.

Your doctor will tell you how and when to use your peak flow meter. He or she also will teach you how to take your medicines based on your score.

Your doctor and other healthcare providers may ask you to use your peak flow meter each morning and keep a record of your results. You may find it very useful to record peak flow scores for a couple of weeks before each medical visit and take the results with you.

When you're first diagnosed with asthma, it's important to find your "personal best" peak flow number. To do this, you record your score each day for a 2- to 3-week period when your asthma is well-controlled. The highest number you get during that time is your personal best. You can compare this number to future numbers to make sure your asthma is controlled.

Your peak flow meter can help warn you of an asthma attack, even before you notice symptoms. If your score shows that your breathing is getting worse, you should take your quick-relief medicines the way your asthma action plan directs. Then you can use the peak flow meter to check how well the medicine worked.

Get Asthma Checkups

When you first begin treatment, you'll see your doctor about every 2 to 6 weeks. Once your asthma is controlled, your doctor may want to see you from once a month to twice a year.

During these checkups, your doctor may ask whether you've had an asthma attack since the last visit or any changes in symptoms or peak flow measurements. He or she also may ask about your daily activities. This information will help your doctor assess your level of asthma control.

Your doctor also may ask whether you have any problems or concerns with taking your medicines or following your asthma action plan. Based on your answers to these questions, your doctor may change the dose of your medicine or give you a new medicine.

If your control is very good, you might be able to take less medicine. The goal is to use the least amount of medicine needed to control your asthma.

Emergency Care

Most people who have asthma, including many children, can safely manage their symptoms by following their asthma action plans. However, you might need medical attention at times.

Call your doctor for advice if:

- Your medicines don't relieve an asthma attack.

- Your peak flow is less than half of your personal best peak flow number.

Call 9–1–1 for emergency care if:

- You have trouble walking and talking because you're out of breath.

- You have blue lips or fingernails.

At the hospital, you'll be closely watched and given oxygen and more medicines, as well as medicines at higher doses than you take at home. Such treatment can save your life.

Asthma Treatment for Special Groups

The treatments described above generally apply to all people who have asthma. However, some aspects of treatment differ for people in certain age groups and those who have special needs.

Children

It's hard to diagnose asthma in children younger than 5 years. Thus, it's hard to know whether young children who wheeze or have other asthma symptoms will benefit from long-term control medicines. (Quick-relief medicines tend to relieve wheezing in young children whether they have asthma or not.)

Doctors will treat infants and young children who have asthma symptoms with long-term control medicines if, after assessing a child, they feel that the symptoms are persistent and likely to continue after 6 years of age.

Inhaled corticosteroids are the preferred treatment for young children. Montelukast and cromolyn are other options. Treatment might be given for a trial period of 1 month to 6 weeks. Treatment usually is stopped if benefits aren't seen during that time and the doctor and parents are confident the medicine was used properly.

Inhaled corticosteroids can possibly slow the growth of children of all ages. Slowed growth usually is apparent in the first several months of treatment, is generally small, and doesn't get worse over time. Poorly controlled asthma also may reduce a child's growth rate.

Many experts think the benefits of inhaled corticosteroids for children who need them to control their asthma far outweigh the risk of slowed growth.

Older Adults

Doctors may need to adjust asthma treatment for older adults who take certain other medicines, such as beta blockers, aspirin and other pain relievers, and anti-inflammatory medicines. These medicines can prevent asthma medicines from working well and may worsen asthma symptoms.

Be sure to tell your doctor about all of the medicines you take, including over-the-counter medicines.

Older adults may develop weak bones from using inhaled corticosteroids, especially at high doses. Talk with your doctor about taking calcium and vitamin D pills, as well as other ways to help keep your bones strong.

Pregnant Women

Pregnant women who have asthma need to control the disease to ensure a good supply of oxygen to their babies. Poor asthma control increases the risk of preeclampsia, a condition in which a pregnant woman develops high blood pressure and protein in the urine. Poor asthma control also increases the risk that a baby will be born early and have a low birth weight.

Studies show that it's safer to take asthma medicines while pregnant than to risk having an asthma attack.

Talk with your doctor if you have asthma and are pregnant or planning a pregnancy. Your level of asthma control may get better or it may get worse while you're pregnant. Your healthcare team will check your asthma control often and adjust your treatment as needed.

People Whose Asthma Symptoms Occur with Physical Activity

Physical activity is an important part of a healthy lifestyle. Adults need physical activity to maintain good health. Children need it for growth and development.

In some people, however, physical activity can trigger asthma symptoms. If this happens to you or your child, talk with your doctor about the best ways to control asthma so you can stay active.

The following medicines may help prevent asthma symptoms caused by physical activity:

- Short-acting beta$_2$-agonists (quick-relief medicine) taken shortly before physical activity can last 2 to 3 hours and prevent exercise-related symptoms in most people who take them.

- Long-acting beta$_2$-agonists can be protective for up to 12 hours. However, with daily use, they'll no longer give up to 12 hours of protection. Also, frequent use of these medicines for physical activity might be a sign that asthma is poorly controlled.

- Leukotriene modifiers. These pills are taken several hours before physical activity. They can help relieve asthma symptoms brought on by physical activity.

- Long-term control medicines. Frequent or severe symptoms due to physical activity may suggest poorly controlled asthma and the need to either start or increase long-term control medicines that reduce inflammation. This will help prevent exercise-related symptoms.

Easing into physical activity with a warmup period may be helpful. You also may want to wear a mask or scarf over your mouth when exercising in cold weather.

If you use your asthma medicines as your doctor directs, you should be able to take part in any physical activity or sport you choose.

People Having Surgery

Asthma may add to the risk of having problems during and after surgery. For instance, having a tube put into your throat may cause an asthma attack.

Tell your surgeon about your asthma when you first talk with him or her. The surgeon can take steps to lower your risk, such as giving you asthma medicines before or during surgery.

How Can Asthma Be Prevented?

You can't prevent asthma. However, you can take steps to control the disease and prevent its symptoms. For example:

- Learn about your asthma and ways to control it.
- Follow your written asthma action plan.
- Use medicines as your doctor prescribes.
- Identify and try to avoid things that make your asthma worse (asthma triggers). However, one trigger you should not avoid is physical activity. Physical activity is an important part of a healthy lifestyle. Talk with your doctor about medicines that can help you stay active.
- Keep track of your asthma symptoms and level of control.
- Get regular checkups for your asthma.

Section 20.2

Allergic Asthma

This section includes text excerpted from "Allergic Asthma,"
Genetics Home Reference (GHR), National Institute of
Health (NIH), December 2015.

What Is Allergic Asthma

Asthma is a breathing disorder characterized by inflammation of the airways and recurrent episodes of breathing difficulty. These episodes, sometimes referred to as asthma attacks, are triggered by irritation of the inflamed airways. In allergic/extrinsic asthma, the attacks occur when substances known as allergens are inhaled, causing an allergic reaction. Allergens are harmless substances that the body's immune system mistakenly reacts to as though they are harmful. Common allergens include pollen, dust, animal dander, and mold. The immune response leads to the symptoms of asthma. Allergic asthma is the most common form of the disorder.

A hallmark of asthma is bronchial hyperresponsiveness, which means the airways are especially sensitive to irritants and respond excessively. Because of this hyperresponsiveness, attacks can be triggered by irritants other than allergens, such as physical activity, respiratory infections, or exposure to tobacco smoke, in people with allergic asthma.

An asthma attack is characterized by tightening of the muscles around the airways (bronchoconstriction), which narrows the airway and makes breathing difficult. Additionally, the immune reaction can lead to swelling of the airways and overproduction of mucus. During an attack, an affected individual can experience chest tightness, wheezing, shortness of breath, and coughing. Over time, the muscles around the airways can become enlarged (hypertrophied), further narrowing the airways.

Some people with allergic asthma have another allergic disorder, such as hay fever (allergic rhinitis) or food allergies. Asthma is sometimes part of a series of allergic disorders, referred to as the atopic march. Development of these conditions typically follows a pattern, beginning with eczema (atopic dermatitis), followed by food allergies, then hay fever, and finally asthma. However, not all individuals with asthma have progressed through the atopic march, and not all individuals with one allergic disease will develop others.

Frequency

Approximately 235 million people worldwide have asthma. In the United States, the condition affects an estimated 8 percent of the population. In nearly 90 percent of children and 50 percent of adults with asthma, the condition is classified as allergic asthma.

Genetic Changes

The cause of allergic asthma is complex. It is likely that a combination of multiple genetic and environmental factors contribute to development of the condition. Doctors believe genes are involved because having a family member with allergic asthma or another allergic disorder increases a person's risk of developing asthma.

Studies suggest that more than 100 genes may be associated with allergic asthma, but each seems to be a factor in only one or a few populations. Many of the associated genes are involved in the body's immune response. Others play a role in lung and airway function.

There is evidence that an unbalanced immune response underlies allergic asthma. While there is normally a balance between type 1 (or Th1) and type 2 (or Th2) immune reactions in the body, many individuals with allergic asthma predominantly have type 2 reactions. Type 2 reactions lead to the production of immune proteins called IgE antibodies and the generation of other factors that predispose to bronchial hyperresponsiveness. Normally, the body produces IgE antibodies in response to foreign invaders, particularly parasitic worms. For unknown reasons, in susceptible individuals, the body reacts to an allergen as if it is harmful, producing IgE antibodies specific to it. Upon later encounters with the allergen, IgE antibodies recognize it, which stimulates an immune response, causing bronchoconstriction, airway swelling, and mucus production.

Not everyone with a variation in one of the allergic asthma-associated genes develops the condition; exposure to certain environmental factors also contributes to its development. Studies suggest that these exposures trigger epigenetic changes to the DNA. Epigenetic changes modify DNA without changing the DNA sequence. They can affect gene activity and regulate the production of proteins, which may influence the development of allergies in susceptible individuals.

Inheritance Pattern

Allergic asthma can be passed through generations in families, but the inheritance pattern is unknown. People with mutations in one or more of the associated genes inherit an increased risk of allergic asthma, not the condition itself. Because allergic asthma is a complex condition influenced by genetic and environmental factors, not all people with a mutation in an asthma-associated gene will develop the disorder.

Section 20.3

Acetaminophen Use and the Risk of Developing Asthma

This section includes text excerpted from "Acetaminophen May Increase the Risk of Developing Asthma," National Institute of Environmental Health Sciences (NIEHS), September, 2008. Reviewed September 2016.

There are plausible biological and associative links between acetaminophen and asthma. Acetaminophen became the drug of choice for pain and fever relief in the 1980s after several studies reported a link between Reye syndrome and aspirin use. In 1986, the U.S. Food and Drug Administration (FDA) placed warning labels regarding the Reyes Syndrome link on acetaminophen bottles. Shortly afterwards, pediatricians nationwide started noticing a rise in asthma incidence. Acetaminophen, unlike aspirin and ibuprofen, decreases the level of the antioxidant glutathione in the lungs and other tissues.

In the work funded by National Institute of Environmental Health Sciences (NIEHS), women were recruited during their first trimester of pregnancy. Use of acetaminophen during pregnancy was determined by a questionnaire and related to respiratory outcomes in their newborns during their first year of life. Use of acetaminophen in the second and third trimesters was significantly related to wheezing in the first year. While wheezing is a known symptom of asthma in young children, it alone does not constitute a diagnosis of asthma.

The findings in this report are consistent with previous literature showing increases in asthma symptoms after exposure to acetaminophen. The researchers point out that this is only the second study suggesting that exposure to acetaminophen late in pregnancy may affect the subsequent development of allergic symptoms in the child. Confirmation of these finding in larger cohorts could have substantial public health implications in defining factors attributable to the development of asthma.

Chapter 21

Bronchiectasis

What Is Bronchiectasis?

Bronchiectasis is a condition in which damage to the airways causes them to widen and become flabby and scarred. The airways are tubes that carry air in and out of your lungs.

Bronchiectasis usually is the result of an infection or other condition that injures the walls of your airways or prevents the airways from clearing mucus. Mucus is a slimy substance that the airways produce to help remove inhaled dust, bacteria, and other small particles.

In bronchiectasis, your airways slowly lose their ability to clear out mucus. When mucus can't be cleared, it builds up and creates an environment in which bacteria can grow. This leads to repeated, serious lung infections.

Each infection causes more damage to your airways. Over time, the airways lose their ability to move air in and out. This can prevent enough oxygen from reaching your vital organs.

Bronchiectasis can lead to serious health problems, such as respiratory failure, atelectasis, and heart failure.

This chapter includes text excerpted from "Bronchiectasis," National Heart, Lung, and Blood Institute (NHLBI), June 2, 2014.

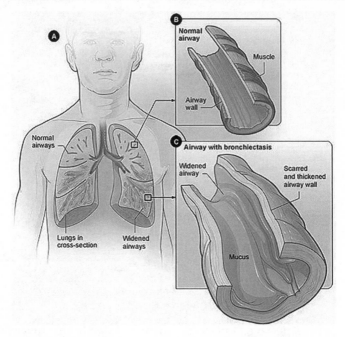

Figure 21.1. *Bronchiectasis*

Figure A shows a cross-section of the lungs with normal airways and with widened airways. Figure B shows a cross-section of a normal airway. Figure C shows a cross-section of an airway with bronchiectasis.

Other Names for Bronchiectasis

- Acquired bronchiectasis
- Congenital bronchiectasis

What Causes Bronchiectasis?

Damage to the walls of the airways usually is the cause of bronchiectasis. A lung infection may cause this damage. Examples of lung infections that can lead to bronchiectasis include:

- Severe pneumonia
- Whooping cough or measles (uncommon in the united states due to vaccination)
- Tuberculosis
- Fungal infections

Conditions that damage the airways and raise the risk of lung infections also can lead to bronchiectasis. Examples of such conditions include:

- Cystic fibrosis. This disease leads to almost half of the cases of bronchiectasis in the United States.

- Immunodeficiency disorders, such as common variable immunodeficiency and, less often, HIV and AIDS.

- Allergic bronchopulmonary aspergillosis. This is an allergic reaction to a fungus called aspergillus. The reaction causes swelling in the airways.

- Disorders that affect cilia function, such as primary ciliary dyskinesia. Cilia are small, hair-like structures that line your airways. They help clear mucus (a slimy substance) out of your airways.

- Chronic (ongoing) pulmonary aspiration. This is a condition in which you inhale food, liquids, saliva, or vomited stomach contents into your lungs. Aspiration can inflame the airways, which can lead to bronchiectasis.

- Connective tissue diseases, such as rheumatoid arthritis, Sjögren syndrome, and Crohn disease.

Other conditions, such as an airway blockage, also can lead to bronchiectasis. Many things can cause a blockage, such as a growth or a noncancerous tumor. An inhaled object, such as a piece of a toy or a peanut that you inhaled as a child, also can cause an airway blockage.

A problem with how the lungs form in a fetus may cause congenital bronchiectasis. This condition affects infants and children.

Who Is at Risk for Bronchiectasis?

People who have conditions that damage the lungs or increase the risk of lung infections are at risk for bronchiectasis. Such conditions include:

- Cystic fibrosis.

- Immunodeficiency disorders

- Allergic bronchopulmonary aspergillosis

- Disorders that affect cilia function

Bronchiectasis can develop at any age. Overall, two-thirds of people who have the condition are women. However, in children, the condition is more common in boys than in girls.

What Are the Signs and Symptoms of Bronchiectasis?

The initial airway damage that leads to bronchiectasis often begins in childhood. However, signs and symptoms may not appear until months or even years after you start having repeated lung infections. The most common signs and symptoms of bronchiectasis are:

- A daily cough that occurs over months or years.

- Daily production of large amounts of sputum (spit). Sputum, which you cough up and spit out, may contain mucus (a slimy substance), trapped particles, and pus.

- Shortness of breath and wheezing (a whistling sound when you breathe).

- Chest pain

- Clubbing (the flesh under your fingernails and toenails gets thicker).

If your doctor listens to your lungs with a stethoscope, he or she may hear abnormal lung sounds.

Over time, you may have more serious symptoms. You may cough up blood or bloody mucus and feel very tired. Children may lose weight or not grow at a normal rate.

Complications of Bronchiectasis

Severe bronchiectasis can lead to other serious health conditions, such as respiratory failure and atelectasis.

Respiratory failure is a condition in which not enough oxygen passes from your lungs into your blood. The condition also can occur if your lungs can't properly remove carbon dioxide (a waste gas) from your blood.

Respiratory failure can cause shortness of breath, rapid breathing, and air hunger (feeling like you can't breathe in enough air). In severe cases, signs and symptoms may include a bluish color on your skin, lips, and fingernails; confusion; and sleepiness.

Atelectasis is a condition in which one or more areas of your lungs collapse or don't inflate properly. As a result, you may feel short of breath. Your heart rate and breathing rate may increase, and your skin and lips may turn blue.

If bronchiectasis is so advanced that it affects all parts of your airways, it may cause heart failure. Heart failure is a condition in which the heart can't pump enough blood to meet the body's needs.

The most common signs and symptoms of heart failure are shortness of breath or trouble breathing, tiredness, and swelling in the ankles, feet, legs, abdomen, and veins in the neck.

How Is Bronchiectasis Diagnosed?

Your doctor may suspect bronchiectasis if you have a daily cough that produces large amounts of sputum (spit).

To find out whether you have bronchiectasis, your doctor may recommend tests to:

- identify any underlying causes that require treatment

- rule out other causes of your symptoms

- find out how much your airways are damaged

Diagnostic Tests and Procedures

Chest CT Scan

A chest computed tomography scan, or chest CT scan, is the most common test for diagnosing bronchiectasis.

This painless test creates precise pictures of your airways and other structures in your chest. A chest CT scan can show the extent and location of lung damage. This test gives more detailed pictures than a standard chest X-ray.

Chest X-Ray

This painless test creates pictures of the structures in your chest, such as your heart and lungs. A chest X-ray can show areas of abnormal lung and thickened, irregular airway walls.

Other Tests

Your doctor may recommend other tests, such as:

- Blood tests. These tests can show whether you have an underlying condition that can lead to bronchiectasis. Blood tests also

257

can show whether you have an infection or low levels of certain infection-fighting blood cells.

- A sputum culture. Lab tests can show whether a sample of your sputum contains bacteria (such as the bacteria that cause tuberculosis) or fungi.

- Lung function tests. These tests measure how much air you can breathe in and out, how fast you can breathe air out, and how well your lungs deliver oxygen to your blood. Lung function tests help show how much lung damage you have.

- A sweat test or other tests for cystic fibrosis.

Bronchoscopy

If your bronchiectasis doesn't respond to treatment, your doctor may recommend bronchoscopy. Doctors use this procedure to look inside the airways.

During bronchoscopy, a flexible tube with a light on the end is inserted through your nose or mouth into your airways. The tube is called a bronchoscope. It provides a video image of your airways. You'll be given medicine to numb your upper airway and help you relax during the procedure.

Bronchoscopy can show whether you have a blockage in your airways. The procedure also can show the source of any bleeding in your airways.

How Is Bronchiectasis Treated?

Bronchiectasis often is treated with medicines, hydration, and chest physical therapy (CPT). Your doctor may recommend surgery if the bronchiectasis is isolated to a section of lung or you have a lot of bleeding.

If the bronchiectasis is widespread and causing respiratory failure, your doctor may recommend oxygen therapy.

The goals of treatment are to:

- treat any underlying conditions and lung infections.

- remove mucus (a slimy substance) from your lungs. Maintaining good hydration helps with mucus removal.

- prevent complications.

Early diagnosis and treatment of the underlying cause of bronchiectasis may help prevent further lung damage.

In addition, any disease associated with the bronchiectasis, such as cystic fibrosis or immunodeficiency, also should be treated.

Medicines

Your doctor may prescribe antibiotics, bronchodilators, expectorants, or mucus-thinning medicines to treat bronchiectasis.

Antibiotics

Antibiotics are the main treatment for the repeated lung infections that bronchiectasis causes. Oral antibiotics often are used to treat these infections.

For hard-to-treat infections, your doctor may prescribe intravenous (IV) antibiotics. These medicines are given through an IV line inserted into your arm. Your doctor may help you arrange for a home care provider to give you IV antibiotics at home.

Expectorants and Mucus-Thinning Medicines

Your doctor may prescribe expectorants and mucus thinners to help you cough up mucus.

Expectorants help loosen the mucus in your lungs. They often are combined with decongestants, which may provide extra relief. Mucus thinners, such as acetylcysteine, loosen the mucus to make it easier to cough up.

For some of these treatments, little information is available to show how well they work.

Hydration

Drinking plenty of fluid, especially water, helps prevent airway mucus from becoming thick and sticky. Good hydration helps keep airway mucus moist and slippery, which makes it easier to cough up.

Chest Physical Therapy

CPT also is called physiotherapy or chest clapping or percussion. This technique is generally performed by a respiratory therapist but can be done by a trained member of the family. It involves the therapist pounding your chest and back over and over with his or her hands or a device. Doing this helps loosen the mucus from your lungs so you can cough it up.

You can sit with your head tilted down or lie on your stomach with your head down while you do CPT. Gravity and force help drain the mucus from your lungs.

Some people find CPT hard or uncomfortable to do. Several devices can help with CPT, such as:

- An electric chest clapper, known as a mechanical percussor.

- An inflatable therapy vest that uses high-frequency air waves to force mucus toward your upper airways so you can cough it up.

- A small handheld device that you breathe out through. It causes vibrations that dislodge the mucus.

- A mask that creates vibrations to help break loose mucus from your airway walls.

Some of these methods and devices are popular with patients and doctors, but little information is available on how well they actually work. Choice usually is based on convenience and cost.

Several breathing techniques also are used to help move mucus to the upper airway so it can be coughed up. These techniques include forced expiration technique (FET) and active cycle breathing (ACB).

FET involves forcing out a couple of breaths and then doing relaxed breathing. ACB is FET that involves deep breathing exercises.

Other Treatments

Depending on your condition, your doctor also may recommend bronchodilators, inhaled corticosteroids, oxygen therapy, or surgery.

Bronchodilators

Bronchodilators relax the muscles around your airways. This helps open your airways and makes breathing easier. Most bronchodilators are inhaled medicines. You will use an inhaler or a nebulizer to breathe in a fine mist of medicine.

Inhaled bronchodilators work quickly because the medicine goes straight to your lungs. Your doctor may recommend that you use a bronchodilator right before you do CPT.

Inhaled Corticosteroids

If you also have wheezing or asthma with your bronchiectasis, your doctor may prescribe inhaled corticosteroids (used to treat inflammation in the airways).

Oxygen Therapy

Oxygen therapy can help raise low blood oxygen levels. For this treatment, you'll receive oxygen through nasal prongs or a mask. Oxygen therapy can be done at home, in a hospital, or in another health facility.

Surgery

Your doctor may recommend surgery if no other treatments have helped and only one part of your airway is affected. If you have major bleeding in your airway, your doctor may recommend surgery to remove part of your airway or a procedure to control the bleeding.

In very rare instances of severe bronchiectasis, your doctor may recommend that you receive a lung transplant replacing your diseased lungs with a healthy set of lungs.

How Can Bronchiectasis Be Prevented?

To prevent bronchiectasis, it's important to prevent the lung infections and lung damage that can cause it.

Childhood vaccines for measles and whooping cough prevent infections related to these illnesses. These vaccines also reduce complications from these infections, such as bronchiectasis.

Avoiding toxic fumes, gases, smoke, and other harmful substances also can help protect your lungs.

Proper treatment of lung infections in children also may help preserve lung function and prevent lung damage that can lead to bronchiectasis.

Stay alert to keep children (and adults) from inhaling small objects (such as pieces of toys and food that might stick in a small airway). If you think you, your child, or someone else has inhaled a small object, seek prompt medical care.

In some cases, treating the underlying cause of bronchiectasis can slow or prevent its progression.

Living with Bronchiectasis

Early diagnosis and treatment of bronchiectasis can prevent further damage to your lungs. People who have bronchiectasis should have ongoing care and try to follow a healthy lifestyle.

Ongoing Care

If you have bronchiectasis, work closely with your doctor to learn how to improve your quality of life. This involves learning as much as you can about bronchiectasis and any underlying conditions that you have.

Take steps to avoid lung infections. Ask your doctor about getting flu and pneumonia vaccines. Wash your hands often to lower your risk of getting viruses and bacterial infections.

Healthy Lifestyle

Following a healthy lifestyle is important for overall health and well-being. For example, if you smoke, try to quit. Smoking harms nearly every organ in your body, including your lungs.

Talk with your doctor about programs and products that can help you quit smoking. Also, try to avoid secondhand smoke.

If you have trouble quitting smoking on your own, consider joining a support group. Many hospitals, workplaces, and community groups offer classes to help people quit smoking.

You also can protect your airways by avoiding toxic fumes, gases, and other harmful substances.

A healthy lifestyle also involves following a healthy diet. A healthy diet includes a variety of vegetables and fruits. It also includes whole grains, fat-free or low-fat dairy products, and protein foods, such as lean meats, poultry without skin, seafood, processed soy products, nuts, seeds, beans, and peas.

A healthy diet is low in sodium (salt), added sugars, solid fats, and refined grains. Solid fats are saturated fat and *trans* fatty acids. Refined grains come from processing whole grains, which results in a loss of nutrients (such as dietary fiber).

Staying hydrated also is important. Drinking plenty of fluids, especially water, helps prevent airway mucus from becoming thick and sticky.

Try to be as physically active as you can. Physical activity, such as walking and swimming, can help loosen mucus. Ask your doctor what types and amounts of activity are safe for you.

Emotional Support

People who have chronic lung diseases are more prone to depression, anxiety, and other emotional problems. Talk about how you feel with your healthcare team. Talking to a professional counselor also can help. If you're very depressed, your doctor may recommend medicines or other treatments that can improve your quality of life.

Joining a patient support group may help you adjust to living with bronchiectasis. You can see how other people who have the same symptoms have coped with them. Talk with your doctor about local support groups or check with an area medical center.

Support from family and friends also can help relieve stress and anxiety. Let your loved ones know how you feel and what they can do to help you.

Chapter 22

Chronic Obstructive Pulmonary Disease (COPD)

Chapter Contents

Section 22.1

What Is COPD (Emphysema/Chronic Bronchitis)?

This section includes text excerpted from "COPD," National Heart, Lung, and Blood Institute (NHLBI), July 31, 2013.

What Is COPD?

COPD, or chronic obstructive pulmonary disease, is a progressive disease that makes it hard to breathe. "Progressive" means the disease gets worse over time.

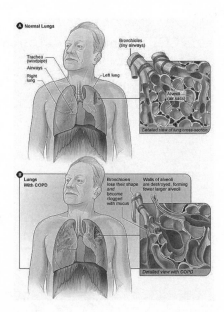

Figure 22.1. *Normal Lungs and Lungs with COPD*

Figure A shows the location of the lungs and airways in the body. The inset image shows a detailed cross-section of the bronchioles and alveoli. Figure B shows lungs damaged by COPD. The inset image shows a detailed cross-section of the damaged bronchioles and alveolar walls.

COPD can cause coughing that produces large amounts of mucus (a slimy substance), wheezing, shortness of breath, chest tightness, and other symptoms.

Cigarette smoking is the leading cause of COPD. Most people who have COPD smoke or used to smoke. Long-term exposure to other lung irritants—such as air pollution, chemical fumes, or dust—also may contribute to COPD.

Other Names for COPD

- Chronic bronchitis

- Chronic obstructive airway disease

- Chronic obstructive lung disease

- Emphysema

What Causes COPD?

Long-term exposure to lung irritants that damage the lungs and the airways usually is the cause of COPD.

In the United States, the most common irritant that causes COPD is cigarette smoke. Pipe, cigar, and other types of tobacco smoke also can cause COPD, especially if the smoke is inhaled.

Breathing in secondhand smoke, air pollution, or chemical fumes or dust from the environment or workplace also can contribute to COPD. (Secondhand smoke is smoke in the air from other people smoking.)

Rarely, a genetic condition called alpha-1 antitrypsin deficiency may play a role in causing COPD. People who have this condition have low levels of alpha-1 antitrypsin (AAT)—a protein made in the liver.

Having a low level of the AAT protein can lead to lung damage and COPD if you're exposed to smoke or other lung irritants. If you have this condition and smoke, COPD can worsen very quickly.

Although uncommon, some people who have asthma can develop COPD. Asthma is a chronic (long-term) lung disease that inflames and narrows the airways. Treatment usually can reverse the inflammation and narrowing. However, if not, COPD can develop.

Who Is at Risk for COPD?

The main risk factor for COPD is smoking. Most people who have COPD smoke or used to smoke. People who have a family history of COPD are more likely to develop the disease if they smoke.

Long-term exposure to other lung irritants also is a risk factor for COPD. Examples of other lung irritants include secondhand smoke, air pollution, and chemical fumes and dust from the environment or workplace. (Secondhand smoke is smoke in the air from other people smoking.)

Most people who have COPD are at least 40 years old when symptoms begin. Although uncommon, people younger than 40 can have COPD. For example, this may happen if a person has alpha-1 antitrypsin deficiency, a genetic condition.

What Are the Signs and Symptoms of COPD?

At first, COPD may cause no symptoms or only mild symptoms. As the disease gets worse, symptoms usually become more severe. Common signs and symptoms of COPD include:

- An ongoing cough or a cough that produces a lot of mucus (often called "smoker's cough")
- Shortness of breath, especially with physical activity
- Wheezing (a whistling or squeaky sound when you breathe)
- Chest tightness

If you have COPD, you also may have colds or the flu (influenza) often.

Not everyone who has the symptoms above has COPD. Likewise, not everyone who has COPD has these symptoms. Some of the symptoms of COPD are similar to the symptoms of other diseases and conditions. Your doctor can find out whether you have COPD.

If your symptoms are mild, you may not notice them, or you may adjust your lifestyle to make breathing easier. For example, you may take the elevator instead of the stairs.

Over time, symptoms may become severe enough to see a doctor. For example, you may get short of breath during physical exertion.

The severity of your symptoms will depend on how much lung damage you have. If you keep smoking, the damage will occur faster than if you stop smoking.

Severe COPD can cause other symptoms, such as swelling in your ankles, feet, or legs; weight loss; and lower muscle endurance.

Some severe symptoms may require treatment in a hospital. You—with the help of family members or friends, if you're unable—should seek emergency care if:

- You're having a hard time catching your breath or talking.

- Your lips or fingernails turn blue or gray. (This is a sign of a low oxygen level in your blood.)

- You're not mentally alert.

- Your heartbeat is very fast.

- The recommended treatment for symptoms that are getting worse isn't working.

How Is COPD Diagnosed?

Your doctor will diagnose COPD based on your signs and symptoms, your medical and family histories, and test results.

Your doctor may ask whether you smoke or have had contact with lung irritants, such as secondhand smoke, air pollution, chemical fumes, or dust.

If you have an ongoing cough, let your doctor know how long you've had it, how much you cough, and how much mucus comes up when you cough. Also, let your doctor know whether you have a family history of COPD.

Your doctor will examine you and use a stethoscope to listen for wheezing or other abnormal chest sounds. He or she also may recommend one or more tests to diagnose COPD.

Lung Function Tests

Lung function tests measure how much air you can breathe in and out, how fast you can breathe air out, and how well your lungs deliver oxygen to your blood.

The main test for COPD is spirometry. Other lung function tests, such as a lung diffusion capacity test, also might be used.

Spirometry

During this painless test, a technician will ask you to take a deep breath in. Then, you'll blow as hard as you can into a tube connected to a small machine. The machine is called a spirometer.

The machine measures how much air you breathe out. It also measures how fast you can blow air out.

Your doctor may have you inhale medicine that helps open your airways and then blow into the tube again. He or she can then compare your test results before and after taking the medicine.

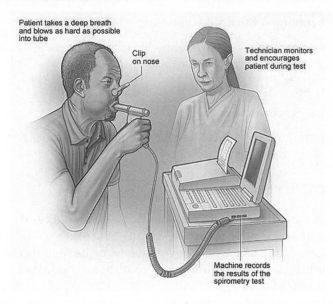

Patient takes a deep breath
and blows as hard as possible
into tube

Clip
on nose

Technician monitors
and encourages
patient during test

Machine records
the results of the
spirometry test

Figure 22.2. *Spirometry*

The image shows how spirometry is done. The patient takes a deep breath and blows as hard as possible into a tube connected to a spirometer. The spirometer measures the amount of air breathed out. It also measures how fast the air was blown out.

Spirometry can detect COPD before symptoms develop. Your doctor also might use the test results to find out how severe your COPD is and to help set your treatment goals.

The test results also may help find out whether another condition, such as asthma or heart failure, is causing your symptoms.

Other Tests

Your doctor may recommend other tests, such as:

- A chest X-ray or chest CT scan. These tests create pictures of the structures inside your chest, such as your heart, lungs, and blood vessels. The pictures can show signs of COPD. They also may show whether another condition, such as heart failure, is causing your symptoms.

- An arterial blood gas test. This blood test measures the oxygen level in your blood using a sample of blood taken from an artery. The results from this test can show how severe your COPD is and whether you need oxygen therapy.

How Is COPD Treated?

COPD has no cure yet. However, lifestyle changes and treatments can help you feel better, stay more active, and slow the progress of the disease.

The goals of COPD treatment include:

- relieving your symptoms
- slowing the progress of the disease
- improving your exercise tolerance (your ability to stay active)
- preventing and treating complications
- improving your overall health

To assist with your treatment, your family doctor may advise you to see a pulmonologist. This is a doctor who specializes in treating lung disorders.

Lifestyle Changes

Quit Smoking and Avoid Lung Irritants

Quitting smoking is the most important step you can take to treat COPD. Talk with your doctor about programs and products that can help you quit.

If you have trouble quitting smoking on your own, consider joining a support group. Many hospitals, workplaces, and community groups offer classes to help people quit smoking. Ask your family members and friends to support you in your efforts to quit.

Also, try to avoid secondhand smoke and places with dust, fumes, or other toxic substances that you may inhale.

Other Lifestyle Changes

If you have COPD, you may have trouble eating enough because of your symptoms, such as shortness of breath and fatigue. (This issue is more common with severe disease.)

As a result, you may not get all of the calories and nutrients you need, which can worsen your symptoms and raise your risk for infections.

Talk with your doctor about following an eating plan that will meet your nutritional needs. Your doctor may suggest eating smaller, more frequent meals; resting before eating; and taking vitamins or nutritional supplements.

Also, talk with your doctor about what types of activity are safe for you. You may find it hard to be active with your symptoms. However, physical activity can strengthen the muscles that help you breathe and improve your overall wellness.

Medicines

Bronchodilators

Bronchodilators relax the muscles around your airways. This helps open your airways and makes breathing easier.

Depending on the severity of your COPD, your doctor may prescribe short-acting or long-acting bronchodilators. Short-acting bronchodilators last about 4–6 hours and should be used only when needed. Long-acting bronchodilators last about 12 hours or more and are used every day.

Most bronchodilators are taken using a device called an inhaler. This device allows the medicine to go straight to your lungs. Not all inhalers are used the same way. Ask your healthcare team to show you the correct way to use your inhaler.

If your COPD is mild, your doctor may only prescribe a short-acting inhaled bronchodilator. In this case, you may use the medicine only when symptoms occur.

If your COPD is moderate or severe, your doctor may prescribe regular treatment with short- and long-acting bronchodilators.

Combination Bronchodilators Plus Inhaled Glucocorticosteroids (Steroids)

If your COPD is more severe, or if your symptoms flare up often, your doctor may prescribe a combination of medicines that includes a bronchodilator and an inhaled steroid. Steroids help reduce airway inflammation.

In general, using inhaled steroids alone is not a preferred treatment.

Your doctor may ask you to try inhaled steroids with the bronchodilator for a trial period of 6 weeks to 3 months to see whether the addition of the steroid helps relieve your breathing problems.

Vaccines

Flu Shots

The flu (influenza) can cause serious problems for people who have COPD. Flu shots can reduce your risk of getting the flu. Talk with your doctor about getting a yearly flu shot.

Pneumococcal Vaccine

This vaccine lowers your risk for pneumococcal pneumonia and its complications. People who have COPD are at higher risk for pneumonia than people who don't have COPD. Talk with your doctor about whether you should get this vaccine.

Pulmonary Rehabilitation

Pulmonary rehabilitation (rehab) is a broad program that helps improve the well-being of people who have chronic (ongoing) breathing problems.

Rehab may include an exercise program, disease management training, and nutritional and psychological counseling. The program's goal is to help you stay active and carry out your daily activities.

Your rehab team may include doctors, nurses, physical therapists, respiratory therapists, exercise specialists, and dietitians. These health professionals will create a program that meets your needs.

Oxygen Therapy

If you have severe COPD and low levels of oxygen in your blood, oxygen therapy can help you breathe better. For this treatment, you're given oxygen through nasal prongs or a mask.

You may need extra oxygen all the time or only at certain times. For some people who have severe COPD, using extra oxygen for most of the day can help them:

- do tasks or activities, while having fewer symptoms

- protect their hearts and other organs from damage

- sleep more during the night and improve alertness during the day

- live longer

Surgery

Surgery may benefit some people who have COPD. Surgery usually is a last resort for people who have severe symptoms that have not improved from taking medicines.

Surgeries for people who have COPD that's mainly related to emphysema include bullectomy and lung volume reduction surgery (LVRS). A lung transplant might be an option for people who have very severe COPD.

Bullectomy

When the walls of the air sacs are destroyed, larger air spaces called bullae form. These air spaces can become so large that they interfere with breathing. In a bullectomy, doctors remove one or more very large bullae from the lungs.

Lung Volume Reduction Surgery

In LVRS, surgeons remove damaged tissue from the lungs. This helps the lungs work better. In carefully selected patients, LVRS can improve breathing and quality of life.

Lung Transplant

During a lung transplant, your damaged lung is removed and replaced with a healthy lung from a deceased donor.

A lung transplant can improve your lung function and quality of life. However, lung transplants have many risks, such as infections. The surgery can cause death if the body rejects the transplanted lung.

If you have very severe COPD, talk with your doctor about whether a lung transplant is an option. Ask your doctor about the benefits and risks of this type of surgery.

Managing Complications

COPD symptoms usually worsen slowly over time. However, they can worsen suddenly. For instance, a cold, the flu, or a lung infection may cause your symptoms to quickly worsen. You may have a much harder time catching your breath. You also may have chest tightness, more coughing, changes in the color or amount of your sputum (spit), and a fever.

Call your doctor right away if your symptoms worsen suddenly. He or she may prescribe antibiotics to treat the infection and other medicines, such as bronchodilators and inhaled steroids, to help you breathe.

Some severe symptoms may require treatment in a hospital.

How Can COPD Be Prevented?

You can take steps to prevent COPD before it starts. If you already have COPD, you can take steps to prevent complications and slow the progress of the disease.

Prevent COPD before It Starts

The best way to prevent COPD is to not start smoking or to quit smoking. Smoking is the leading cause of COPD. If you smoke, talk with your doctor about programs and products that can help you quit.

If you have trouble quitting smoking on your own, consider joining a support group. Many hospitals, workplaces, and community groups offer classes to help people quit smoking. Ask your family members and friends to support you in your efforts to quit.

Also, try to avoid lung irritants that can contribute to COPD. Examples include secondhand smoke, air pollution, chemical fumes, and dust. (Secondhand smoke is smoke in the air from other people smoking.)

Prevent Complications and Slow the Progress of COPD

If you have COPD, the most important step you can take is to quit smoking. Quitting can help prevent complications and slow the progress of the disease. You also should avoid exposure to the lung irritants mentioned above.

Follow your treatments for COPD exactly as your doctor prescribes. They can help you breathe easier, stay more active, and avoid or manage severe symptoms.

Talk with your doctor about whether and when you should get flu (influenza) and pneumonia vaccines. These vaccines can lower your chances of getting these illnesses, which are major health risks for people who have COPD.

Living with COPD

COPD has no cure yet. However, you can take steps to manage your symptoms and slow the progress of the disease. You can:

- avoid lung irritants
- get ongoing care
- manage the disease and its symptoms
- prepare for emergencies

Avoid Lung Irritants

If you smoke, quit. Smoking is the leading cause of COPD. Talk with your doctor about programs and products that can help you quit.

If you have trouble quitting smoking on your own, consider joining a support group. Many hospitals, workplaces, and community groups offer classes to help people quit smoking. Ask your family members and friends to support you in your efforts to quit.

Also, try to avoid lung irritants that can contribute to COPD. Examples include secondhand smoke, air pollution, chemical fumes, and dust. (Secondhand smoke is smoke in the air from other people smoking.)

Keep these irritants out of your home. If your home is painted or sprayed for insects, have it done when you can stay away for a while.

Keep your windows closed and stay at home (if possible) when there's a lot of air pollution or dust outside.

Get Ongoing Care

If you have COPD, it's important to get ongoing medical care. Take all of your medicines as your doctor prescribes. Make sure to refill your prescriptions before they run out. Bring a list of all the medicines you're taking when you have medical checkups.

Talk with your doctor about whether and when you should get flu (influenza) and pneumonia vaccines. Also, ask him or her about other diseases for which COPD may increase your risk, such as heart disease, lung cancer, and pneumonia.

Manage COPD and Its Symptoms

You can do things to help manage COPD and its symptoms. For example:

- Do activities slowly.

- Put items that you need often in one place that's easy to reach.

- Find very simple ways to cook, clean, and do other chores.
  For example, you might want to use a small table or cart with wheels to move things around and a pole or tongs with long handles to reach things.

- Ask for help moving things around in your house so that you won't need to climb stairs as often.

- Keep your clothes loose, and wear clothes and shoes that are easy to put on and take off.

Depending on how severe your disease is, you may want to ask your family and friends for help with daily tasks.

Prepare for Emergencies

If you have COPD, know when and where to seek help for your symptoms. You should get emergency care if you have severe symptoms, such as trouble catching your breath or talking.

Call your doctor if you notice that your symptoms are worsening or if you have signs of an infection, such as a fever. Your doctor may change or adjust your treatments to relieve and treat symptoms.

Keep phone numbers handy for your doctor, hospital, and someone who can take you for medical care. You also should have on hand directions to the doctor's office and hospital and a list of all the medicines you're taking.

Emotional Issues and Support

Living with COPD may cause fear, anxiety, depression, and stress. Talk about how you feel with your healthcare team. Talking to a professional counselor also might help. If you're very depressed, your doctor may recommend medicines or other treatments that can improve your quality of life.

Joining a patient support group may help you adjust to living with COPD. You can see how other people who have the same symptoms have coped with them. Talk with your doctor about local support groups or check with an area medical center.

Support from family and friends also can help relieve stress and anxiety. Let your loved ones know how you feel and what they can do to help you.

Section 22.2

Alpha-1 Antitrypsin Deficiency: Inherited COPD

This section includes text excerpted from "Alpha-1
Antitrypsin Deficiency," Genetic and Rare Diseases
Information Center (GARD), April 8, 2016.

What Is Alpha-1 Antitrypsin Deficiency?

Alpha-1 antitrypsin deficiency (AATD) is a disorder that causes
a deficiency or absence of the alpha-1 antitrypsin (AAT) protein in the
blood. AAT is made in the liver and sent through the bloodstream to
the lungs, to protect the lungs from damage. Having low levels of ATT
(or no ATT) can allow the lungs to become damaged, making breathing
hard. Age of onset and severity of AATD can vary based on how much
ATT an affected person is missing. In adults, symptoms may include
shortness of breath; reduced ability to exercise; wheezing; respiratory infections; fatigue; vision problems; and weight loss. Some people
have chronic obstructive pulmonary disease (COPD) or asthma. Liver
disease (cirrhosis) may occur in affected children or adults. Rarely,
AATD can cause a skin condition called panniculitis. AATD is caused
by mutations in the *SERPINA1* gene and is inherited in a codomi-
nant manner. Treatment is based on each person's symptoms and
may include bronchodilators; antibiotics for upper respiratory tract
infections; intravenous therapy of AAT; and/or lung transplantation
in severe cases.

Symptoms

- Emphysema

- Hepatic failure

- Hepatomegaly

- Nephrotic syndrome

- Cirrhosis

- Autosomal recessive inheritance

- Chronic obstructive pulmonary disease

- Elevated hepatic transaminases

- Hepatocellular carcinoma

Cause

Alpha-1 antitrypsin deficiency (AATD) is caused by mutations in the *SERPINA1* gene. This gene gives the body instructions to make a protein called alpha-1 antitrypsin (AAT), which protects the body from an enzyme called neutrophil elastase. Neutrophil elastase helps the body fight infections, but it can also attack healthy tissues (especially the lungs) if not controlled by AAT.

Mutations that cause AAT can cause a deficiency or absence of AAT, or a form of AAT that does not work well. This allows neutrophil elastase to destroy lung tissue, causing lung disease. In addition, abnormal AAT can build up in the liver and cause damage to the liver.

The severity of AATD may also be worsened by environmental factors such as exposure to tobacco smoke, dust, and chemicals.

Diagnosis

Alpha-1 antitrypsin deficiency (AATD) may first be suspected in people with evidence of liver disease at any age, or lung disease (such as emphysema), especially when there is no obvious cause or it is diagnosed at a younger age.

Confirming the diagnosis involves a blood test showing a low serum concentration of the alpha-1 antitrypsin (AAT) protein, and either:

- Detecting a functionally deficient AAT protein variant by isoelectric focusing (a method for detecting mutations); or

- Detecting *SERPINA1* gene mutations on both copies of the gene with molecular genetic testing. (This confirms the diagnosis when the above-mentioned tests are not performed or their results are not in agreement.)

Specialists involved in the diagnosis may include primary care doctors, pulmonologists (lung specialists), and/or hepatologists (liver specialists).

Treatment

Treatment of alpha-1 antitrypsin deficiency (AATD) depends on the symptoms and severity in each person. COPD and other related lung diseases are typically treated with standard therapy. Bronchodilators and inhaled steroids can help open the airways and make breathing easier.

Intravenous augmentation therapy (regular infusion of purified, human AAT to increase AAT concentrations) has been recommended for people with established fixed airflow obstruction (determined by a specific lung function test). This therapy raises the level of the AAT protein in the blood and lungs.

Lung transplantation may be an appropriate option for people with end-stage lung disease. Liver transplantation is the definitive treatment for advanced liver disease.

When present, panniculitis may resolve on its own or after dapsone or doxycycline therapy. When this therapy does not help, it has responded to intravenous augmentation therapy in higher than usual doses.

All people with severe AATD should have pulmonary function tests every 6 to 12 months. Those with ATT serum concentrations 10 percent to 20 percent of normal should have periodic evaluation of liver function to detect liver disease. People with established liver disease should have periodic ultrasounds of the liver to monitor for fibrotic changes and liver cancer (hepatocellular carcinoma).

Yearly vaccinations against influenza and pneumococcus are recommended to lessen the progression of lung disease. Vaccination against hepatitis A and B is recommended to lessen the risk of liver disease. People with AATD should avoid smoking and occupations with exposure to environmental pollutants.

Parents, older and younger siblings, and children of a person with severe AATD should be evaluated to identify as early as possible those who would benefit from treatment and preventive measures.

Chapter 23

Idiopathic Pulmonary Fibrosis

What Is Idiopathic Pulmonary Fibrosis?

Idiopathic pulmonary fibrosis is a chronic, progressive lung disease. This condition causes scar tissue (fibrosis) to build up in the lungs, which makes the lungs unable to transport oxygen into the bloodstream effectively. The disease usually affects people between the ages of 50 and 70.

The most common signs and symptoms of idiopathic pulmonary fibrosis are shortness of breath and a persistent dry, hacking cough. Many affected individuals also experience a loss of appetite and gradual weight loss. Some people with idiopathic pulmonary fibrosis develop widened and rounded tips of the fingers and toes (clubbing) resulting from a shortage of oxygen. These features are relatively nonspecific; not everyone with these health problems has idiopathic pulmonary fibrosis. Other respiratory diseases, some of which are less serious, can cause similar signs and symptoms.

In people with idiopathic pulmonary fibrosis, scarring of the lungs increases over time until the lungs can no longer provide enough oxygen to the body's organs and tissues. Some people with idiopathic pulmonary fibrosis develop other serious lung conditions, including

---

This chapter includes text excerpted from "Idiopathic Pulmonary Fibrosis," Genetic Home Reference (GHR), National Institutes of Health (NIH), April 2015.

lung cancer, blood clots in the lungs (pulmonary emboli), pneumonia, or high blood pressure in the blood vessels that supply the lungs (pulmonary hypertension). Most affected individuals survive 3 to 5 years after their diagnosis. However, the course of the disease is highly variable; some affected people become seriously ill within a few months, while others may live with the disease for a decade or longer.

In most cases, idiopathic pulmonary fibrosis occurs in only one person in a family. These cases are described as sporadic. However, a small percentage of people with this disease have at least one other affected family member. When idiopathic pulmonary fibrosis occurs in multiple members of the same family, it is known as familial pulmonary fibrosis.

Frequency

Idiopathic pulmonary fibrosis has an estimated prevalence of 13 to 20 per 100,000 people worldwide. About 100,000 people are affected in the United States, and 30,000 to 40,000 new cases are diagnosed each year.

Familial pulmonary fibrosis is less common than the sporadic form of the disease. Only a small percentage of cases of idiopathic pulmonary fibrosis appear to run in families.

Genetic Changes

The cause of idiopathic pulmonary fibrosis is unknown, although the disease probably results from a combination of genetic and environmental factors. It is likely that genetic changes increase a person's risk of developing idiopathic pulmonary fibrosis, and then exposure to certain environmental factors triggers the disease.

Changes in several genes have been suggested as risk factors for idiopathic pulmonary fibrosis. Most of these genetic changes account for only a small proportion of cases. However, mutations in genes known as *TERC* and *TERT* have been found in about 15 percent of all cases of familial pulmonary fibrosis and a smaller percentage of cases of sporadic idiopathic pulmonary fibrosis. The *TERC* and *TERT* genes provide instructions for making components of an enzyme called telomerase, which maintains structures at the ends of chromosomes known as telomeres. It is not well understood how defects in telomerase are associated with the lung damage characteristic of idiopathic pulmonary fibrosis.

Researchers have also examined environmental risk factors that could contribute to idiopathic pulmonary fibrosis. These factors include exposure to wood or metal dust, viral infections, certain medications, and cigarette smoking. Some research suggests that gastroesophageal reflux disease (GERD) may also be a risk factor for idiopathic pulmonary fibrosis; affected individuals may breathe in (aspirate) stomach contents, which over time could damage the lungs.

Inheritance Pattern

Most cases of idiopathic pulmonary fibrosis are sporadic; they occur in people with no history of the disorder in their family.

Familial pulmonary fibrosis appears to have an autosomal dominant pattern of inheritance. Autosomal dominant inheritance means one copy of an altered gene in each cell is sufficient to cause the disorder. However, some people who inherit the altered gene never develop features of familial pulmonary fibrosis. (This situation is known as reduced penetrance.) It is unclear why some people with a mutated gene develop the disease and other people with the mutated gene do not.

Other Names for This Condition

- Cryptogenic fibrosing alveolitis
- Idiopathic fibrosing alveolitis, chronic form
- IPF
- Usual interstitial pneumonia

Chapter 24

Occupational Lung Disorders

Chapter Contents

Section 24.1

Asbestos Related Disease

This section includes text excerpted from
"Asbestos Exposure and Cancer Risk," National Cancer
Institute (NCI), May 1, 2009. Reviewed September 2016.

What Is Asbestos?

Asbestos is the name given to a group of minerals that occur naturally in the environment as bundles of fibers that can be separated into thin, durable threads. These fibers are resistant to heat, fire, and chemicals and do not conduct electricity. For these reasons, asbestos has been used widely in many industries.

Chemically, asbestos minerals are silicate compounds, meaning they contain atoms of silicon and oxygen in their molecular structure.

Asbestos minerals are divided into two major groups: Serpentine asbestos and amphibole asbestos. Serpentine asbestos includes the mineral chrysotile, which has long, curly fibers that can be woven. Chrysotile asbestos is the form that has been used most widely in commercial applications. Amphibole asbestos includes the minerals actinolite, tremolite, anthophyllite, crocidolite, and amosite. Amphibole asbestos has straight, needle-like fibers that are more brittle than those of serpentine asbestos and are more limited in their ability to be fabricated.

What Are the Health Hazards of Exposure to Asbestos?

People may be exposed to asbestos in their workplace, their communities, or their homes. If products containing asbestos are disturbed, tiny asbestos fibers are released into the air. When asbestos fibers are breathed in, they may get trapped in the lungs and remain there for a long time. Over time, these fibers can accumulate and cause scarring and inflammation, which can affect breathing and lead to serious health problems.

Asbestos has been classified as a known human carcinogen (a substance that causes cancer) by the U.S. Department of Health and Human Services (HHS), the U.S. Environmental Protection Agency (EPA), and the International Agency for Research on Cancer (IARC). Studies have shown that exposure to asbestos may increase the risk of lung cancer and mesothelioma (a relatively rare cancer of the thin membranes that line the chest and abdomen). Although rare, mesothelioma is the most common form of cancer associated with asbestos exposure. In addition to lung cancer and mesothelioma, some studies have suggested an association between asbestos exposure and gastrointestinal and colorectal cancers, as well as an elevated risk for cancers of the throat, kidney, esophagus, and gallbladder. However, the evidence is inconclusive.

Asbestos exposure may also increase the risk of asbestosis (an inflammatory condition affecting the lungs that can cause shortness of breath, coughing, and permanent lung damage) and other nonmalignant lung and pleural disorders, including pleural plaques (changes in the membranes surrounding the lung), pleural thickening, and benign pleural effusions (abnormal collections of fluid between the thin layers of tissue lining the lungs and the wall of the chest cavity). Although pleural plaques are not precursors to lung cancer, evidence suggests that people with pleural disease caused by exposure to asbestos may be at increased risk for lung cancer.

Who Is at Risk for an Asbestos-Related Disease?

Everyone is exposed to asbestos at some time during their life. Low levels of asbestos are present in the air, water, and soil. However, most people do not become ill from their exposure. People who become ill from asbestos are usually those who are exposed to it on a regular basis, most often in a job where they work directly with the material or through substantial environmental contact.

Since the early 1940s, millions of American workers have been exposed to asbestos. Health hazards from asbestos fibers have been recognized in workers exposed in the shipbuilding trades, asbestos mining and milling, manufacturing of asbestos textiles and other asbestos products, insulation work in the construction and building trades, and a variety of other trades. Demolition workers, drywall removers, asbestos removal workers, firefighters, and automobile workers also may be exposed to asbestos fibers. Studies evaluating the cancer risk experienced by automobile mechanics exposed to asbestos through brake repair are limited, but the overall evidence suggests there is no safe level of asbestos exposure. As a result of Government regulations and improved work practices, today's workers (those without previous exposure) are likely to face smaller risks than did those exposed in the past.

Individuals involved in the rescue, recovery, and cleanup at the site of the September 11, 2001, attacks on the World Trade Center (WTC) in New York City are another group at risk of developing an asbestos-related disease. Because asbestos was used in the construction of the North Tower of the WTC, when the building was attacked, hundreds of tons of asbestos were released into the atmosphere. Those at greatest risk include firefighters, police officers, paramedics, construction workers, and volunteers who worked in the rubble at Ground Zero. Others at risk include residents in close proximity to the WTC towers and those who attended schools nearby. These individuals will need to be followed to determine the long-term health consequences of their exposure.

Although it is clear that the health risks from asbestos exposure increase with heavier exposure and longer exposure time, investigators have found asbestos-related diseases in individuals with only brief exposures. Generally, those who develop asbestos-related diseases show no signs of illness for a long time after their first exposure. It can take from 10 to 40 years or more for symptoms of an asbestos-related condition to appear.

There is some evidence that family members of workers heavily exposed to asbestos face an increased risk of developing mesothelioma. This risk is thought to result from exposure to asbestos fibers brought into the home on the shoes, clothing, skin, and hair of workers. To decrease these exposures, Federal law regulates workplace practices to limit the possibility of asbestos being brought home in this way. Some employees may be required to shower and change their clothes before they leave work, store their street clothes in a separate area of the workplace, or wash their work clothes at home separately from other clothes.

Cases of mesothelioma have also been seen in individuals without occupational asbestos exposure who live close to asbestos mines.

What Factors Affect the Risk of Developing an Asbestos-Related Disease?

Several factors can help to determine how asbestos exposure affects an individual, including:

- dose (how much asbestos an individual was exposed to)

- duration (how long an individual was exposed)
- size, shape, and chemical makeup of the asbestos fibers
- source of the exposure
- individual risk factors, such as smoking and pre-existing lung disease

Although all forms of asbestos are considered hazardous, different types of asbestos fibers may be associated with different health risks. For example, the results of several studies suggest that amphibole forms of asbestos may be more harmful than chrysotile, particularly for mesothelioma risk, because they tend to stay in the lungs for a longer period of time.

How Does Smoking Affect Risk?

Many studies have shown that the combination of smoking and asbestos exposure is particularly hazardous. Smokers who are also exposed to asbestos have a risk of developing lung cancer that is greater than the individual risks from asbestos and smoking added together. There is evidence that quitting smoking will reduce the risk of lung cancer among asbestos-exposed workers. Smoking combined with asbestos exposure does not appear to increase the risk of mesothelioma. However, people who were exposed to asbestos on the job at any time during their life or who suspect they may have been exposed should not smoke.

How Are Asbestos-Related Diseases Detected?

Individuals who have been exposed (or suspect they have been exposed) to asbestos fibers on the job, through the environment, or at home via a family contact should inform their doctor about their exposure history and whether or not they experience any symptoms. The symptoms of asbestos-related diseases may not become apparent for many decades after the exposure. It is particularly important to check with a doctor if any of the following symptoms develop:

- shortness of breath, wheezing, or hoarseness
- a persistent cough that gets worse over time
- blood in the sputum (fluid) coughed up from the lungs
- pain or tightening in the chest

- difficulty swallowing

- swelling of the neck or face

- loss of appetite

- weight loss

- fatigue or anemia

A thorough physical examination, including a chest X-ray and lung function tests, may be recommended. The chest X-ray is currently the most common tool used to detect asbestos-related diseases. However, it is important to note that chest X-rays cannot detect asbestos fibers in the lungs, but they can help identify any early signs of lung disease resulting from asbestos exposure.

Studies have shown that computed tomography (CT) (a series of detailed pictures of areas inside the body taken from different angles; the pictures are created by a computer linked to an X-ray machine) may be more effective than conventional chest X-rays at detecting asbestos-related lung abnormalities in individuals who have been exposed to asbestos.

A lung biopsy, which detects microscopic asbestos fibers in pieces of lung tissue removed by surgery, is the most reliable test to confirm the presence of asbestos-related abnormalities. A bronchoscopy is a less invasive test than a biopsy and detects asbestos fibers in material that is rinsed out of the lungs. It is important to note that these tests cannot determine how much asbestos an individual may have been exposed to or whether disease will develop. Asbestos fibers can also be detected in urine, mucus, or feces, but these tests are not reliable for determining how much asbestos may be in an individual's lungs.

How Can Workers Protect Themselves from Asbestos Exposure?

The **Occupational Safety and Health Administration (OSHA)** is a component of the U.S. Department of Labor (DOL) and is the Federal agency responsible for health and safety regulations in maritime, construction, manufacturing, and service workplaces. OSHA established regulations dealing with asbestos exposure on the job, specifically in construction work, shipyards, and general industry, that employers are required to follow. In addition, the **Mine Safety and Health Administration (MSHA)**, another component of the DOL, enforces regulations related to mine safety. Workers should use all protective equipment provided by their employers and follow recommended workplace practices and safety procedures. For example, National Institute for Occupational Safety and Health (NIOSH)-approved respirators that fit properly should be worn by workers when required.

Section 24.2

Mold in the Workplace

This section includes text excerpted from "A Brief Guide to Mold in the Workplace," Occupational Safety and Health Administration (OSHA), November 8, 2013.

Mold Basics

Molds are part of the natural environment. Molds are fungi that can be found anywhere—inside or outside—throughout the year. About 1,000 species of mold can be found in the United States, with more than 100,000 known species worldwide.

Outdoors, molds play an important role in nature by breaking down organic matter such as toppled trees, fallen leaves, and dead animals. We would not have food and medicines, like cheese and penicillin, without mold.

Indoors, mold growth should be avoided. Problems may arise when mold starts eating away at materials, affecting the look, smell, and possibly, with the respect to wood-framed buildings, affecting the structural integrity of the buildings.

Molds can grow on virtually any substance, as long as moisture or water, oxygen, and an organic source are present. Molds reproduce by creating tiny spores (viable seeds) that usually cannot be seen without magnification. Mold spores continually float through the indoor and outdoor air.

Molds are usually not a problem unless mold spores land on a damp spot and begin growing. They digest whatever they land on in order to survive. There are molds that grow on wood, paper, carpet, foods and insulation, while other molds feast on the everyday dust and dirt that gather in the moist regions of a building.

When excessive moisture or water accumulates indoors, mold growth often will occur, particularly if the moisture problem remains uncorrected. While it is impossible to eliminate all molds and mold spores, controlling moisture can control indoor mold growth.

All molds share the characteristic of being able to grow without sunlight; mold needs only a viable seed (spore), a nutrient source, moisture, and the right temperature to proliferate. This explains why mold infestation is often found in damp, dark, hidden spaces; light and air circulation dry areas out, making them less hospitable for mold.

Molds gradually damage building materials and furnishings. If left unchecked, mold can eventually cause structural damage to a wood framed building, weakening floors and walls as it feeds on moist wooden structural members. If you suspect that mold has damaged building integrity, consult a structural engineer or other professional with the appropriate expertise.

Since mold requires water to grow, it is important to prevent excessive moisture in buildings. Some moisture problems in buildings have been linked to changes in building construction practices since the 1970s, which resulted in tightly sealed buildings with diminished ventilation, contributing to moisture vapor buildup. Other moisture problems may result from roof leaks, landscaping or gutters that direct water into or under a building, or unvented combustion appliance. Delayed or insufficient maintenance may contribute to moisture problems in buildings. Improper maintenance and design of building heating/ventilating/air-conditioning (HVAC) systems, such as insufficient cooling capacity for an air conditioning system, can result in elevated humidity levels in a building.

Health Effects

Currently, there are no federal standards or recommendations, (e.g., OSHA, NIOSH, EPA) for airborne concentrations of mold or mold spores. Scientific research on the relationship between mold exposures and health effects is ongoing. This section provides a brief overview, but does not describe all potential health effects related to mold exposure.

There are many types of mold. Most typical indoor air exposures to mold do not present a risk of adverse health effects. Molds can cause adverse effects by producing allergens (substances that can cause allergic reactions). Potential health concerns are important reasons to prevent mold growth and to remediate existing problem areas.

The onset of allergic reactions to mold can be either immediate or delayed. Allergic responses include hay fever-type symptoms such as runny nose and red eyes.

Molds may cause localized skin or mucosal infections but, in general, do not cause systemic infections in humans, except for persons with impaired immunity, AIDS, uncontrolled diabetes, or those taking immune suppressive drugs.

Molds can also cause asthma attacks in some individuals who are allergic to mold. In addition, exposure to mold can irritate the eyes, skin, nose and throat in certain individuals. Symptoms other than allergic and irritant types are not commonly reported as a result of inhaling mold in the indoor environment.

Some specific species of mold produce mycotoxins under certain environmental conditions. Potential health effects from mycotoxins are the subject of ongoing scientific research and are beyond the scope of this document.

Eating, drinking, and using tobacco products and cosmetics where mold remediation is taking place should be avoided. This will prevent unnecessary contamination of food, beverage, cosmetics, and tobacco products by mold and other harmful substances within the work area.

Prevention

Moisture control is the key to mold control. When water leaks or spills occur indoors—act promptly. Any initial water infiltration should be stopped and cleaned promptly. A prompt response (within 24–48 hours) and thorough clean-up, drying, and/or removal of water-damaged materials will prevent or limit mold growth.

Mold prevention tips include:

- Repairing plumbing leaks and leaks in the building structure as soon as possible.

- Looking for condensation and wet spots. Fix source(s) of moisture incursion problem(s) as soon as possible.

- Preventing moisture from condensing by increasing surface temperature or reducing the moisture level in the air (humidity). To increase surface temperature, insulate or increase air circulation. To reduce the moisture level in the air, repair leaks, increase ventilation (if outside air is cold and dry), or dehumidify (if outdoor air is warm and humid).

- Keeping HVAC drip pans clean, flowing properly, and unobstructed.

- Performing regularly scheduled building/ HVAC inspections and maintenance, including filter changes.

- Maintaining indoor relative humidity below 70% (25–60%, if possible).

- Venting moisture-generating appliances, such as dryers, to the outside where possible.

- Venting kitchens (cooking areas) and bathrooms according to local code requirements.

- Cleaning and drying wet or damp spots as soon as possible, but no more than 48 hours after discovery.

- Providing adequate drainage around buildings and sloping the ground away from building foundations. Follow all local building codes.

- Pinpointing areas where leaks have occurred, identifying the causes, and taking preventive action to ensure that they do not reoccur.

Section 24.3

Occupational Asthma

This section includes text excerpted from "Do You Have Work-Related Asthma?" Occupational Safety and Health Administration (OSHA), March 2014.

Occupational or work-related asthma is a lung disease caused or made worse by exposures to substances in the workplace. Common exposures include chemicals, dust, mold, animals, and plants. Exposure can occur from both inhalation (breathing) and skin contact. Asthma symptoms may start at work or within several hours after leaving work and may occur with no clear pattern. People who never had asthma can develop asthma due to workplace exposures. People who have had asthma for years may find that their condition worsens due to workplace exposures. Both of these situations are considered work-related asthma.

A group of chemicals called isocyanates are one of the most common chemical causes of work-related asthma. OSHA is working to reduce exposures to isocyanates and has identified their use in numerous workplaces.

Why You Should Care about Work-Related Asthma

Work-related asthma may result in long-term lung damage, loss of work days, disability, or even death. The good news is that early diagnosis and treatment of work-related asthma can lead to a better health outcome.

What to Do If You Think You Have Work-Related Asthma

If you think that you may have work-related asthma, see your doctor as soon as possible.

Work-Related Asthma Quick Facts

- Work-related asthma can develop over ANY period of time (days to years).

- Work-related asthma may occur with changes in work exposures, jobs, or processes.

- It is possible to develop work-related asthma even if your workplace has protective equipment, such as exhaust ventilation or respirators.

- Work-related asthma can continue to cause symptoms even when the exposure stops.

- Before working with isocyanates or any other asthma-causing substances, ask your employer for training, as required under OSHA's Hazard Communication standard.

Chapter 25

Pleural Effusion and Pleurisy (Pleuritis)

What Are Pleurisy and Other Pleural Disorders?

Pleurisy is a condition in which the pleura is inflamed. The pleura is a membrane that consists of two large, thin layers of tissue. One layer wraps around the outside of your lungs. The other layer lines the inside of your chest cavity.

Between the layers of tissue is a very thin space called the pleural space. Normally this space is filled with a small amount of fluid—about 4 teaspoons full. The fluid helps the two layers of the pleura glide smoothly past each other as you breathe in and out.

Pleurisy occurs if the two layers of the pleura become irritated and inflamed. Instead of gliding smoothly past each other, they rub together every time you breathe in. The rubbing can cause sharp pain.

Many conditions can cause pleurisy, including viral infections.

This chapter includes text excerpted from "Pleurisy and Other Pleural Disorders," National Heart, Lung, and Blood Institute (NHLBI), September 21, 2011. Reviewed September 2016.

Other Pleural Disorders

Pneumothorax

Air or gas can build up in the pleural space. When this happens, it's called a pneumothorax. A lung disease or acute lung injury can cause a pneumothorax.

Some lung procedures also can cause a pneumothorax. Examples include lung surgery, drainage of fluid with a needle, bronchoscopy, and mechanical ventilation.

Sometimes the cause of a pneumothorax isn't known.

The most common symptoms of a pneumothorax are sudden pain in one side of the lung and shortness of breath. The air or gas in the pleural space also can put pressure on the lung and cause it to collapse.

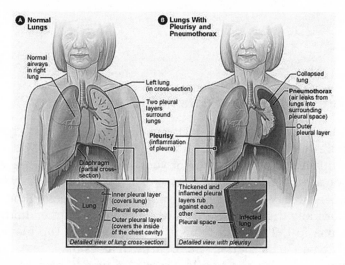

Figure 25.1. *Pleurisy and Pneumothorax*

Figure A shows the location of the lungs, airways, pleura, and diaphragm (a muscle that helps you breathe). The inset image shows a detailed view of the two pleural layers and pleural space. Figure B shows lungs with pleurisy and a pneumothorax. The inset image shows a detailed view of an infected lung with thickened and inflamed pleural layers.

A small pneumothorax may go away without treatment. A large pneumothorax may require a procedure to remove air or gas from the pleural space.

A very large pneumothorax can interfere with blood flow through your chest and cause your blood pressure to drop. This is called a tension pneumothorax.

Pleural Effusion

In some cases of pleurisy, excess fluid builds up in the pleural space. This is called a pleural effusion. A lot of extra fluid can push the pleura against your lung until the lung, or part of it, collapses. This can make it hard for you to breathe.

Sometimes the extra fluid gets infected and turns into an abscess. When this happens, it's called an empyema.

You can develop a pleural effusion even if you don't have pleurisy. For example, pneumonia, heart failure, cancer, or pulmonary embolism can lead to a pleural effusion.

Hemothorax

Blood also can build up in the pleural space. This condition is called a hemothorax. An injury to your chest, chest or heart surgery, or lung or pleural cancer can cause a hemothorax.

A hemothorax can put pressure on the lung and cause it to collapse. A hemothorax also can cause shock. In shock, not enough blood and oxygen reach your body's vital organs.

Other Names for Pleurisy and Other Pleural Disorders

- Pleurisy also is called pleuritis and pleuritic chest pain.

- Pleural effusion also is called fluid in the chest and pleural fluid.

- Pneumothorax also is called air around the lung and air outside the lung.

What Causes Pleurisy and Other Pleural Disorders?

Pleurisy

Many conditions can cause pleurisy. Viral infections are likely the most common cause. Other causes of pleurisy include:

- Bacterial infections, such as pneumonia and tuberculosis, and infections from fungi or parasites

- Pulmonary embolism, a blood clot that travels through the blood vessels to the lungs

- Autoimmune disorders, such as lupus and rheumatoid arthritis

- Cancer, such as lung cancer, lymphoma, and mesothelioma

- Chest and heart surgery, especially coronary artery bypass grafting

- Lung diseases, such as LAM (lymphangioleiomyomatosis) or asbestosis

- Inflammatory bowel disease

- Familial Mediterranean fever, an inherited condition that often causes fever and swelling in the abdomen or lungs

Other causes of pleurisy include chest injuries, pancreatitis (an inflamed pancreas), and reactions to certain medicines. Reactions to certain medicines can cause a condition similar to lupus. These medicines include procainamide, hydralazine, and isoniazid.

Sometimes doctors can't find the cause of pleurisy.

Pneumothorax

Lung diseases or acute lung injury can make it more likely that you will develop a pneumothorax (a buildup of air or gas in the pleural space). Such lung diseases may include COPD (chronic obstructive pulmonary disease), tuberculosis, and LAM.

Surgery or a chest injury also may cause a pneumothorax.

You can develop a pneumothorax without having a recognized lung disease or chest injury. This is called a spontaneous pneumothorax. Smoking increases your risk of spontaneous pneumothorax. Having a family history of the condition also increases your risk.

Pleural Effusion

The most common cause of a pleural effusion (a buildup of fluid in the pleural space) is heart failure. Lung cancer, LAM, pneumonia, tuberculosis, and other lung infections also can lead to a pleural effusion.

Sometimes kidney or liver disease can cause fluid to build up in the pleural space. Asbestosis, sarcoidosis, and reactions to some medicines also can lead to a pleural effusion.

Hemothorax

An injury to the chest, chest or heart surgery, or lung or pleural cancer can cause a hemothorax (buildup of blood in the pleural space).

A hemothorax also can be a complication of an infection (for example, pneumonia), tuberculosis, or a spontaneous pneumothorax.

What Are the Signs and Symptoms of Pleurisy and Other Pleural Disorders

Pleurisy

The main symptom of pleurisy is a sharp or stabbing pain in your chest that gets worse when you breathe in deeply or cough or sneeze.

The pain may stay in one place or it may spread to your shoulders or back. Sometimes the pain becomes a fairly constant dull ache.

Depending on what's causing the pleurisy, you may have other symptoms, such as:

- shortness of breath or rapid, shallow breathing

- coughing

- fever and chills

- unexplained weight loss

Pneumothorax

The symptoms of pneumothorax include:

- sudden, sharp chest pain that gets worse when you breathe in deeply or cough

- shortness of breath

- chest tightness

- easy fatigue (tiredness)

- a rapid heart rate

- a bluish tint to the skin caused by lack of oxygen

Other symptoms of pneumothorax include flaring of the nostrils; anxiety, stress, and tension; and hypotension (low blood pressure).

Pleural Effusion

Pleural effusion often has no symptoms.

Hemothorax

The symptoms of hemothorax often are similar to those of pneumothorax. They include:

- chest pain

- shortness of breath
- respiratory failure
- a rapid heart rate
- anxiety
- restlessness

How Are Pleurisy and Other Pleural Disorders Diagnosed?

Your doctor will diagnose pleurisy or another pleural disorder based on your medical history, a physical exam, and test results.

Your doctor will want to rule out other causes of your symptoms. He or she also will want to find the underlying cause of the pleurisy or other pleural disorder so it can be treated.

Medical History

Your doctor may ask detailed questions about your medical history. He or she likely will ask you to describe any pain, especially:

- what it feels like
- where it's located and whether you can feel it in your arms, jaw, or shoulders
- when it started and whether it goes away and then comes back
- what makes it better or worse

Your doctor also may ask whether you have other symptoms, such as shortness of breath, coughing, or palpitations. Palpitations are feelings that your heart is skipping a beat, fluttering, or beating too hard or fast.

Your doctor also may ask whether you've ever:

- had heart disease
- smoked
- traveled to places where you may have been exposed to tuberculosis
- had a job that exposed you to asbestos. Asbestos is a mineral that, at one time, was widely used in many industries

Your doctor also may ask about medicines you take or have taken. Reactions to some medicines can cause pleurisy or other pleural disorders.

Physical Exam

Your doctor will listen to your breathing with a stethoscope to find out whether your lungs are making any abnormal sounds.

If you have pleurisy, the inflamed layers of the pleura make a rough, scratchy sound as they rub against each other when you breathe. Doctors call this a pleural friction rub. If your doctor hears the friction rub, he or she will know that you have pleurisy.

If you have a pleural effusion, fluid buildup in the pleural space will prevent a friction rub. But if you have a lot of fluid, your doctor may hear a dull sound when he or she taps on your chest. Or, he or she may have trouble hearing any breathing sounds.

Muffled or dull breathing sounds also can be a sign of a pneumothorax (a buildup of air or gas in the pleural space).

Diagnostic Tests

Depending on the results of your physical exam, your doctor may recommend tests.

Chest X-Ray

A chest X-ray is a painless test that creates a picture of the structures in your chest, such as your heart, lungs, and blood vessels. This test may show air or fluid in the pleural space.

A chest X-ray also may show what's causing a pleural disorder—for example, pneumonia, a fractured rib, or a lung tumor.

Sometimes a chest X-ray is taken while you lie on your side. This position can show fluid that didn't appear on an X-ray taken while you were standing.

Chest CT Scan

A chest computed tomography scan, or chest CT scan, is a painless test that creates precise pictures of the structures in your chest.

This test provides a computer-generated picture of your lungs that can show pockets of fluid. A chest CT scan also may show signs of pneumonia, a lung abscess, a tumor, or other possible causes of pleural disorders.

Ultrasound

This test uses sound waves to create pictures of your lungs. An ultrasound may show where fluid is located in your chest. The test also can show some tumors.

Chest MRI

A chest magnetic resonance imaging scan, or chest MRI, uses radio waves, magnets, and a computer to created detailed pictures of the structures in your chest. This test can show pleural effusions and tumors.

This test also is called a magnetic resonance (MR) scan or a nuclear magnetic resonance (NMR) scan.

Blood Tests

Blood tests can show whether you have an illness that increases your risk of pleurisy or another pleural disorder. Such illnesses include bacterial or viral infections, pneumonia, pancreatitis (an inflamed pancreas), kidney disease, or lupus.

Arterial Blood Gas Test

For this test, a blood sample is taken from an artery, usually in your wrist. The blood's oxygen and carbon dioxide levels are checked. This test shows how well your lungs are taking in oxygen.

Thoracentesis

Once your doctor knows whether fluid has built up in the pleural space and where it is, he or she can remove a sample for testing. This is done using a procedure called thoracentesis.

During the procedure, your doctor inserts a thin needle or plastic tube into the pleural space and draws out the excess fluid. After the fluid is removed from your chest, it's sent for testing.

The risks of thoracentesis—such as pain, bleeding, and infection—usually are minor. They get better on their own, or they're easily treated. Your doctor may do a chest X-ray after the procedure to check for complications.

Fluid Analysis

The fluid removed during thoracentesis is examined under a microscope. It's checked for signs of infection, cancer, or other conditions that can cause fluid or blood to build up in the pleural space.

Biopsy

Your doctor may suspect that tuberculosis or cancer has caused fluid to build up in your pleural space. If so, he or she may want to look at a small piece of the pleura under a microscope.

To take a tissue sample, your doctor may do one of the following procedures:

- Insert a needle into your chest to remove a small sample of the pleura's outer layer.

- Insert a tube with a light on the end (endoscope) into tiny cuts in your chest wall so that he or she can see the pleura. Your doctor can then snip out small pieces of tissue. This procedure must be done in a hospital. You'll be given medicine to make you sleep during the procedure.

- Snip out a sample of the pleura through a small cut in your chest wall. This is called an open pleural biopsy. It's usually done if the sample from the needle biopsy is too small for an accurate diagnosis. This procedure must be done in a hospital. You'll be given medicine to make you sleep during the procedure.

How Are Pleurisy and Other Pleural Disorders Treated?

Pleurisy and other pleural disorders are treated with procedures, medicines, and other methods. The goals of treatment include:

- relieving symptoms
- removing the fluid, air, or blood from the pleural space (if a large amount is present)
- treating the underlying condition

Relieving Symptoms

To relieve pleurisy symptoms, your doctor may recommend:

- Acetaminophen or anti-inflammatory medicines (such as ibuprofen) to control pain.
- Codeine-based cough syrups to control coughing.
- Lying on your painful side. This might make you more comfortable.
- Breathing deeply and coughing to clear mucus as the pain eases. Otherwise, you may develop pneumonia.
- Getting plenty of rest.

Removing Fluid, Air, or Blood from the Pleural Space

Your doctor may recommend removing fluid, air, or blood from your pleural space to prevent a lung collapse.

The procedures used to drain fluid, air, or blood from the pleural space are similar.

- During thoracentesis, your doctor will insert a thin needle or plastic tube into the pleural space. An attached syringe will draw fluid out of your chest. This procedure can remove more than 6 cups of fluid at a time.

- If your doctor needs to remove a lot of fluid, he or she may use a chest tube. Your doctor will inject a painkiller into the area of your chest wall where the fluid is. He or she will then insert a plastic tube into your chest between two ribs. The tube will be connected to a box that suctions out the fluid. Your doctor will use a chest X-ray to check the tube's position.

- Your doctor also can use a chest tube to drain blood and air from the pleural space. This process can take several days. The tube will be left in place, and you'll likely stay in the hospital during this time.

Sometimes the fluid in the pleural space contains thick pus or blood clots. It may form a hard skin or peel, which makes the fluid harder to drain. To help break up the pus or blood clots, your doctor may use a chest tube to deliver medicines called fibrinolytics to the pleural space. If the fluid still won't drain, you may need surgery.

If you have a small, persistent air leak into the pleural space, your doctor may attach a one-way valve to the chest tube. The valve allows air to exit the pleural space, but not reenter. Using this type of valve may allow you to continue your treatment from home.

Treat the Underlying Condition

The fluid sample that was removed during thoracentesis will be checked under a microscope. This can tell your doctor what's causing the fluid buildup, and he or she can decide the best way to treat it.

If the fluid is infected, treatment will involve antibiotics and drainage. If you have tuberculosis or a fungal infection, treatment will involve long-term use of antibiotics or antifungal medicines.

Chapter 26

Pneumoconioses

The pneumoconioses are a group of interstitial lung diseases caused by the inhalation of certain dusts and the lung tissue's reaction to the dust. The principal cause of the pneumoconioses is work-place exposure; environmental exposures have rarely given rise to these diseases.

The primary pneumoconioses are asbestosis, silicosis, and coal workers' pneumoconiosis. As their names imply, they are caused by inhalation of asbestos fibers, silica dust, and coal mine dust. Typically, these three diseases take many years to develop and be manifested, although in some cases—silicosis, particularly—rapidly progressive forms can occur after only short periods of intense exposure. When severe, the diseases often lead to lung impairment, disability, and premature death. From a public health perspective, these conditions are entirely man-made, and can be avoided through appropriate dust control.

Other forms of pneumoconioses can be caused by inhaling dusts containing aluminum, antimony, barium, graphite, iron, kaolin, mica, talc, among other dusts. There is also a form called mixed-dust

This chapter contains text excerpted from the following sources: Text in this chapter begins with excerpts from "Pneumoconioses," Centers for Disease Control and Prevention (CDC), October 13, 2011. Reviewed September 2016; Text beginning with the heading "What Is the Health and Safety Problem?" is excerpted from "Mining Topic: Respiratory Diseases," Centers for Disease Control and Prevention (CDC), January 21, 2016; Text beginning with the heading "Silicosis" is excerpted from "Protect Yourself," Occupational Safety and Health Administration (OSHA), September 22, 2005. Reviewed September 2016.

pneumoconiosis. Overall, most physicians do not encounter these diseases very frequently. Byssinosis, caused by exposure to cotton dust, is sometimes included among the pneumoconioses, although its pattern of lung abnormality is different from the pneumoconioses listed above.

What Is the Health and Safety Problem?

Miners are at risk of developing lung diseases called pneumoconioses because of their regular exposure to airborne dust, and miners who are exposed to exhaust from diesel engines have an increased risk of dying from lung cancer.

The two main pneumoconioses (meaning dusty lung) that affect miners are:

- coal workers' pneumoconiosis (CWP) commonly called black lung; and

- silicosis

CWP is associated with coal mining, but silicosis can affect workers in many types of mines and quarries, including coal mines.

Other respiratory diseases, such as chronic obstructive pulmonary disease (COPD), may also occur in miners separately from, or in addition to pneumoconiosis.

What Is the Extent of the Problem?

A newly published report shows that 2 percent of examined surface coal mine workers—most of whom had never worked in underground mines—had CWP.

The recently published Diesel Exhaust in Miners Study of over 12,000 miners showed a significant increased risk of dying from lung cancer among miners who had ever worked underground. This risk increased as the miners' exposure to respirable elemental carbon—representing diesel exhaust—increased.

How Is the NIOSH Mining Program Addressing This Problem?

OMSHR (the NIOSH Office of Mine Safety and Health Research) conducts research to identify sources of respirable dust and diesel exhaust exposure in mining, and develops exposure control technologies.

Reducing miners' exposure to airborne dust directly reduces their risk of developing dust-related respiratory disease.

OMSHR has active programs working to reduce dust exposure to coal miners operating longwall and continuous mining equipment. OMSHR is also investigating how to reduce dust exposure to miners in all commodities who are mobile workers (they don't have a fixed work position), or who perform work:

- with exploratory and blasthole drills

- with other surface mining equipment

- with mills and processing equipment, or

- in operating cabs and rooms

OMSHR is also assessing the application and performance of engineering controls to reduce diesel exhaust 'at the tail pipe' and in areas where miners perform their work.

Finally, OMSHR is continuing work to develop and improve monitors that will provide on-shift information about concentrations of airborne agents so that operators and miners can take steps to quickly correct conditions that could lead to excessive exposures.

What Are the Significant Findings

OMSHR research has produced a continuous personal dust monitor that can provide an accurate measurement of airborne respirable dust at the end of a mine workers' work shift, and provides on-shift information that the worker can use to reduce his or her exposure. This instrument has been approved for use as a coal mine dust personal sampler. Mine Safety and Health Administration (MSHA) rulemaking specifies this instrument be used to measure dust exposure in certain coal mining operations.

OMSHR has also developed a mobile video exposure monitoring method and software application (Helmet-Cam) that combines real-time exposure data with concurrently recorded point-of-view video to identify exposure sources for mobile workers.

Factors affecting the protection from airborne dust by enclosed equipment operator cabs have been identified by OMSHR researchers, and a method to quantify air leakage into cabs has been published.

An instrument to monitor personal exposure to diesel exhaust particulate has been developed and demonstrated by OMSHR researchers. This instrument is commercially available.

What Are the next Steps?

OMSHR is currently evaluating potential dust control technologies such as tailgate spray manifolds on the longwall shearer, improved water sprays on longwall shields, stand-alone dust collectors on continuous mining sections, maintaining the dust control effectiveness of equipment cabs, and the application of optical remote sensing technology to monitor the source and movement of dust over extended areas.

OMSHR has also undertaken development of a methodology that would provide information about a worker's exposure to respirable silica (quartz) at the end of the work shift. If this approach is validated, the delay in receipt of laboratory results would be eliminated. Removing this delay would allow the employer to more rapidly implement enhanced exposure controls, reducing the risk of silicosis among the exposed miners.

Silicosis

Silicosis is caused by exposure to respirable crystalline silica dust. Crystalline silica is a basic component of soil, sand, granite, and most other types of rock, and it is used as an abrasive blasting agent. Silicosis is a progressive, disabling, and often fatal lung disease. Cigarette smoking adds to the lung damage caused by silica.

Effects of Silicosis

- Lung cancer—Silica has been classified as a human lung carcinogen.
- Bronchitis/Chronic Obstructive Pulmonary Disorder.
- Tuberculosis—Silicosis makes an individual more susceptible to TB.
- Scleroderma—a disease affecting skin, blood vessels, joints and skeletal muscles.
- Possible renal disease.

Symptoms of Silicosis

- Shortness of breath; possible fever.
- Fatigue; loss of appetite.
- Chest pain; dry, nonproductive cough.
- Respiratory failure, which may eventually lead to death.

Sources of Exposure

- Sandblasting for surface preparation.

- Crushing and drilling rock and concrete.

- Masonry and concrete work (e.g., building and road construction and repair).

- Mining/tunneling; demolition work.

- Cement and asphalt pavement manufacturing.

Preventing Silicosis

- Use all available engineering controls such as blasting cabinets and local exhaust ventilation. Avoid using compressed air for cleaning surfaces.

- Use water sprays, wet methods for cutting, chipping, drilling, sawing, grinding, etc.

- Substitute non-crystalline silica blasting material.

- Use respirators approved for protection against silica; if sand-blasting, use abrasive blasting respirators.

- Do not eat, drink or smoke near crystalline silica dust.

- Wash hands and face before eating, drinking or smoking away from exposure area.

Chapter 27

Sarcoidosis

What Is Sarcoidosis?

Sarcoidosis is a disease of unknown cause that leads to inflammation. This disease affects your body's organs.

Normally, your immune system defends your body against foreign or harmful substances. For example, it sends special cells to protect organs that are in danger.

These cells release chemicals that recruit other cells to isolate and destroy the harmful substance. Inflammation occurs during this process. Once the harmful substance is gone, the cells and the inflammation go away.

In people who have sarcoidosis, the inflammation doesn't go away. Instead, some of the immune system cells cluster to form lumps called granulomas in various organs in your body.

What Causes Sarcoidosis?

The cause of sarcoidosis isn't known. More than one factor may play a role in causing the disease.

Some researchers think that sarcoidosis develops if your immune system responds to a trigger, such as bacteria, viruses, dust, or chemicals.

This chapter includes text excerpted from "Sarcoidosis," National Heart, Lung, and Blood Institute (NHLBI), June 14, 2013.

Normally, your immune system defends your body against foreign or harmful substances. For example, it sends special cells to protect organs that are in danger.

These cells release chemicals that recruit other cells to isolate and destroy the harmful substance. Inflammation occurs during this process. Once the harmful substance is gone, the cells and the inflammation go away.

In people who have sarcoidosis, the inflammation doesn't go away. Instead, some of the immune system cells cluster to form lumps called granulomas in various organs in your body.

Genetics also may play a role in sarcoidosis. Researchers believe that sarcoidosis occurs if:

- you have a certain gene or genes that raise your risk for the disease

- you're exposed to something that triggers your immune system

Triggers may vary depending on your genetic makeup. Certain genes may influence which organs are affected and the severity of your symptoms.

Who Is at Risk for Sarcoidosis?

Sarcoidosis affects people of all ages and races. However, it's more common among African Americans and Northern Europeans. In the United States, the disease affects African Americans somewhat more often and more severely than Whites.

Studies have shown that sarcoidosis tends to vary amongst ethnic groups. For example, eye problems related to the disease are more common in Japanese people.

Lofgren syndrome, a type of sarcoidosis, is more common in people of European descent. Lofgren syndrome may involve fever, enlarged lymph nodes, arthritis (usually in the ankles), and/or erythema nodosum. Erythema nodosum is a rash of red or reddish-purple bumps on your ankles and shins. The rash may be warm and tender to the touch.

Sarcoidosis is somewhat more common in women than in men. The disease usually develops between the ages of 20 and 50. People who have a family history of sarcoidosis also are at higher risk for the disease.

What Are the Signs and Symptoms of Sarcoidosis?

Many people who have sarcoidosis have no signs or symptoms or mild ones. Often, the disease is found when a chest X-ray is done for another reason (for example, to diagnose pneumonia).

314

The signs and symptoms of sarcoidosis vary depending on which organs are affected. Signs and symptoms also may vary depending on your gender, age, and ethnic background.

Common Signs and Symptoms

In both adults and children, sarcoidosis most often affects the lungs. If granulomas (inflamed lumps) form in your lungs, you may wheeze, cough, feel short of breath, or have chest pain. Or, you may have no symptoms at all.

Some people who have sarcoidosis feel very tired, uneasy, or depressed. Night sweats and weight loss are common symptoms of the disease.

Common signs and symptoms in children are fatigue (tiredness), loss of appetite, weight loss, bone and joint pain, and anemia.

Children who are younger than 4 years old may have a distinct form of sarcoidosis. It may cause enlarged lymph nodes in the chest (which can be seen on chest X-ray pictures), skin lesions, and eye swelling or redness.

Other Signs and Symptoms

Sarcoidosis may affect your lymph nodes. The disease can cause enlarged lymph nodes that feel tender. Sarcoidosis usually affects the lymph nodes in your neck and chest. However, the disease also may affect the lymph nodes under your chin, in your armpits, or in your groin.

Sarcoidosis can cause lumps, ulcers (sores), or areas of discolored skin. These areas may itch, but they don't hurt. These signs tend to appear on your back, arms, legs, and scalp. Sometimes they appear near your nose or eyes. These signs usually last a long time.

Sarcoidosis may cause a more serious skin condition called lupus pernio. Disfiguring skin sores may affect your nose, nasal passages, cheeks, ears, eyelids, and fingers. These sores tend to be ongoing. They can return after treatment is over.

Sarcoidosis also can cause eye problems. If you have sarcoidosis, having an annual eye exam is important. If you have changes in your vision and can't see as clearly or can't see color, call 9–1–1 or have someone drive you to the emergency room.

You should call your doctor if you have any new eye symptoms, such as burning, itching, tearing, pain, or sensitivity to light.

Signs and symptoms of sarcoidosis also may include an enlarged liver, spleen, or salivary glands.

Although less common, sarcoidosis can affect the heart and brain. This can cause many symptoms, such as abnormal heartbeats, shortness of breath, headaches, and vision problems. If sarcoidosis affects the heart or brain, serious complications can occur.

Lofgren Syndrome

Lofgren syndrome is a classic set of signs and symptoms that occur in some people when they first have sarcoidosis. Signs and symptoms may include:

- Fever. This symptom only occurs in some people.

- Enlarged lymph nodes (which can be seen on a chest X-ray).

- Arthritis, usually in the ankles. This symptom is more common in men than women.

- Erythema nodosum. This is a rash of red or reddish-purple bumps on your ankles and shins. The rash may be warm and tender to the touch. This symptom is more common in women than men.

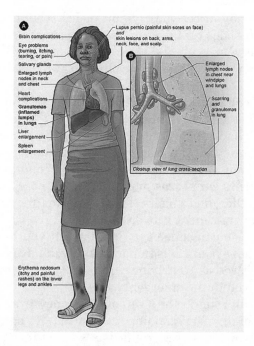

Figure 27.1. *Sarcoidosis: Signs and Symptoms*

How Is Sarcoidosis Diagnosed?

Your doctor will diagnose sarcoidosis based on your medical history, a physical exam, and test results. He or she will look for granulomas (inflamed lumps) in your organs. Your doctor also will try to rule out other possible causes of your symptoms.

Medical History

Your doctor may ask you detailed questions about your medical history. For example, he or she may ask whether you:

- Have a family history of sarcoidosis.
- Have had any jobs that may have raised your risk for the disease.
- Have ever been exposed to inhaled beryllium metal. (This type of metal is used to make aircrafts and weapons.)
- Have had contact with organic dust from birds or hay.

Exposure to beryllium metal and organic dust can cause inflamed lumps in your lungs that look like the granulomas from sarcoidosis. However, these lumps are signs of other conditions.

Physical Exam

Your doctor will check you for signs and symptoms of sarcoidosis. Signs and symptoms may include red bumps on your skin; swollen lymph nodes; an enlarged liver, spleen, or salivary glands; or redness in your eyes. Your doctor also will check for other causes of your symptoms.

Your doctor may listen to your lungs and heart. Abnormal breathing or heartbeat sounds could be a sign that sarcoidosis is affecting your lungs or heart.

Diagnostic Tests

You may have tests to confirm a diagnosis and to find out how sarcoidosis is affecting you. Tests include a chest X-ray, lung function tests, biopsy, and other tests to assess organ damage.

Chest X-Ray

A chest X-ray is a painless test that creates pictures of the structures inside your chest, such as your heart and lungs. The test may show granulomas or enlarged lymph nodes in your chest. About 95 percent of people who have sarcoidosis have abnormal chest X-rays.

Lung Function Tests

Lung function tests measure how much air you can breathe in and out, how fast you can breathe air out, and how well your lungs deliver oxygen to your blood. These tests can show whether sarcoidosis is affecting your lungs.

Biopsy

Your doctor may do a biopsy to confirm a diagnosis or rule out other causes of your symptoms. A biopsy involves taking a small sample of tissue from one of your affected organs.

Usually, doctors try to biopsy the organs that are easiest to access. Examples include the skin, tear glands, or the lymph nodes that are just under the skin.

If this isn't possible, your doctor may use a positron emission tomography (PET) scan to pinpoint areas for biopsy. For this test, a small amount of radioactive substance is injected into a vein, usually in your arm.

The substance, which releases energy, travels through the blood and collects in organs or tissues. Special cameras detect the energy and convert it into three-dimensional (3D) pictures.

If lung function tests or a chest X-ray shows signs of sarcoidosis in your lungs, your doctor may do a bronchoscopy to get a small sample of lung tissue.

During this procedure, a thin, flexible tube is passed through your nose (or sometimes your mouth), down your throat, and into the airways to reach your lung tissue.

Other Tests to Assess Organ Damage

You also may have other tests to assess organ damage and find out whether you need treatment. For example, your doctor may recommend blood tests and/or an EKG (electrocardiogram).

If you're diagnosed with sarcoidosis, you should see an ophthalmologist (eye specialist), even if you don't have eye symptoms. In sarcoidosis, eye damage can occur without symptoms.

How Is Sarcoidosis Treated?

Not everyone who has sarcoidosis needs treatment. Sometimes the disease goes away on its own. Whether you need treatment and what type of treatment you need depend on your signs and symptoms, which organs are affected, and whether those organs are working well.

If the disease affects certain organ—such as your eyes, heart, or brain—you'll need treatment even if you don't have any symptoms.

In either case, whether you have symptoms or not, you should see your doctor for ongoing care. He or she will want to check to make sure that the disease isn't damaging your organs. For example, you may need routine lung function tests to make sure that your lungs are working well.

If the disease isn't worsening, your doctor may watch you closely to see whether the disease goes away on its own. If the disease does start to get worse, your doctor can prescribe treatment.

The goals of treatment include:

- relieving symptoms

- improving organ function

- controlling inflammation and reducing the size of granulomas (inflamed lumps)

- preventing pulmonary fibrosis (lung scarring) if your lungs are affected

Your doctor may prescribe topical treatments and/or medicines to treat the disease.

Medicines

Prednisone

Prednisone, a type of steroid, is the main treatment for sarcoidosis. This medicine reduces inflammation. In most people, prednisone relieves symptoms within a couple of months.

Although most people need to take prednisone for 12 months or longer, your doctor may lower the dose within a few months after you start the medicine.

Long-term use of prednisone, especially at high doses, can cause serious side effects. Work with your doctor to decide whether the benefits of this medicine outweigh the risks. If your doctor prescribes this treatment, he or she will find the lowest dose that controls your disease.

When you stop taking prednisone, you should cut back slowly (as your doctor advises). This will help prevent flareups of sarcoidosis.

Cutting back slowly also allows your body to adjust to not having the medicine.

If a relapse or flareup occurs after you stop taking prednisone, you may need a second round of treatment. If you remain stable for more than 1 year after stopping this treatment, the risk of relapse is low.

Other Medicines

Other medicines, besides prednisone, also are used to treat sarcoidosis. Examples include:

- Hydroxychloroquine or chloroquine (known as antimalarial medicines). These medicines work best for treating sarcoidosis that affects the skin or brain. Your doctor also may prescribe an antimalarial if you have a high level of calcium in your blood due to sarcoidosis.

- Medicines that suppress the immune system, such as methotrexate, azathioprine, or leflunomide. These medicines work best for treating sarcoidosis that affects your lungs, eyes, skin, or joints.

Your doctor may prescribe these medicines if your sarcoidosis worsens while you're taking prednisone or if you can't handle prednisone's side effects.

If you have Lofgren syndrome with pain or fever, your doctor may prescribe nonsteroidal anti-inflammatory drugs (NSAIDs), such as ibuprofen.

If you're wheezing and coughing, you may need inhaled medicine to help open your airways. You take inhaled medicine using an inhaler. This device allows the medicine to go straight to your lungs.

Anti-tumor necrosis factor drugs, originally developed to treat arthritis, are being studied to treat sarcoidosis.

Living with Sarcoidosis

Sarcoidosis has no cure, but you can take steps to manage the disease. Get ongoing care and follow a healthy lifestyle. Talk with your doctor if you're pregnant or planning a pregnancy.

Ongoing Care

Ongoing care is important, even if you don't take medicine for your sarcoidosis. New symptoms can occur at any time. Also, the disease can slowly worsen without your noticing.

How often you need to see your doctor will depend on the severity of your symptoms, which organs are affected, which treatments you're using, and whether you have any side effects from treatment. Even if you don't have symptoms, you should see your doctor for ongoing care.

Your doctor may recommend routine tests, such as lung function tests and eye exams. He or she will want to check to make sure that the disease isn't damaging your organs.

Discuss with your doctor how often you need to have followup visits. You may have some followup visits with your primary care doctor and others with one or more specialists.

Make sure to take all of your medicines as your doctor prescribes.

Lifestyle Changes

Making lifestyle changes can help you manage your health. For example, follow a healthy diet and be as physically active as you can. A healthy diet includes a variety of fruits, vegetables, and whole grains.

It also includes lean meats, poultry, fish, beans, and fat-free or low-fat milk or milk products. A healthy diet is low in saturated fat, *trans* fat, cholesterol, sodium (salt), and added sugar.

If you smoke, quit. Talk with your doctor about programs and products that can help you quit. Also, try to avoid other lung irritants, such as dust, chemicals, and secondhand smoke.

If you have trouble quitting smoking on your own, consider joining a support group. Many hospitals, workplaces, and community groups offer classes to help people quit smoking.

Emotional Issues

Living with sarcoidosis may cause fear, anxiety, depression, and stress. Talk about how you feel with your healthcare team. Talking to a professional counselor also can help. If you're very depressed, your doctor may recommend medicines or other treatments that can improve your quality of life.

Joining a patient support group may help you adjust to living with sarcoidosis. You can see how other people who have the same symptoms have coped with them. Talk with your doctor about local support groups or check with an area medical center.

Support from family and friends also can help relieve stress and anxiety. Let your loved ones know how you feel and what they can do to help you.

Pregnancy

Many women who have sarcoidosis give birth to healthy babies. Women who have severe sarcoidosis, especially if they're older, may have trouble becoming pregnant. Sometimes sarcoidosis may get worse after the baby is delivered.

If you have sarcoidosis and are pregnant or planning a pregnancy, talk with your doctor about the risks involved. Also, if you become pregnant, it's important to get good prenatal care and regular sarcoidosis checkups during and after pregnancy.

Some sarcoidosis medicines are considered safe to use during pregnancy; others are not recommended.

Part Four

Other Conditions That Affect Respiration

Chapter 28

Cystic Fibrosis

What Is Cystic Fibrosis?

Cystic fibrosis, or CF, is an inherited disease of the secretory glands. Secretory glands include glands that make mucus and sweat.

"Inherited" means the disease is passed from parents to children through genes. People who have CF inherit two faulty genes for the disease—one from each parent. The parents likely don't have the disease themselves.

CF mainly affects the lungs, pancreas, liver, intestines, sinuses, and sex organs.

Other Names for Cystic Fibrosis?

- Cystic fibrosis of the pancreas

- Fibrocystic disease of the pancreas

- Mucoviscidosis

- Mucoviscidosis of the pancreas

- Pancreas fibrocystic disease

- Pancreatic cystic fibrosis

This chapter includes text excerpted from "Cystic Fibrosis," National Heart, Lung, and Blood Institute (NHLBI), December 26, 2013.

What Causes Cystic Fibrosis?

A defect in the *CFTR* gene causes CF. This gene makes a protein that controls the movement of salt and water in and out of your body's cells. In people who have CF, the gene makes a protein that doesn't work well. This causes thick, sticky mucus and very salty sweat.

Research suggests that the *CFTR* protein also affects the body in other ways. This may help explain other symptoms and complications of CF.

More than a thousand known defects can affect the *CFTR* gene. The type of defect you or your child has may affect the severity of CF. Other genes also may play a role in the severity of the disease.

How Is Cystic Fibrosis Inherited?

Every person inherits two *CFTR* genes—one from each parent. Children who inherit a faulty *CFTR* gene from each parent will have CF.

Children who inherit one faulty *CFTR* gene and one normal *CFTR* gene are "CF carriers." CF carriers usually have no symptoms of CF and live normal lives. However, they can pass the faulty CFTR gene to their children.

The image below shows how two parents who are both CF carriers can pass the faulty *CFTR* gene to their children.

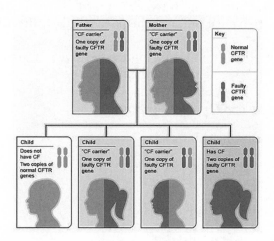

Figure 28.1. *Example of an Inheritance Pattern for Cystic Fibrosis*

The image shows how CFTR genes are inherited. A person inherits two copies of the CFTR gene—one from each parent. If each parent has a normal CFTR gene and a faulty CFTR gene, each child has a 25 percent chance of inheriting two normal genes; a 50 percent chance of inheriting one normal gene and one faulty gene; and a 25 percent chance of inheriting two faulty genes.

Who Is at Risk for Cystic Fibrosis?

CF affects both males and females and people from all racial and ethnic groups. However, the disease is most common among Caucasians of Northern European descent.

CF also is common among Latinos and American Indians, especially the Pueblo and Zuni. The disease is less common among African Americans and Asian Americans.

More than 10 million Americans are carriers of a faulty CF gene. Many of them don't know that they're CF carriers.

What Are the Signs and Symptoms of Cystic Fibrosis?

The signs and symptoms of CF vary from person to person and over time. Sometimes you'll have few symptoms. Other times, your symptoms may become more severe.

One of the first signs of CF that parents may notice is that their baby's skin tastes salty when kissed, or the baby doesn't pass stool when first born.

Most of the other signs and symptoms of CF happen later. They're related to how CF affects the respiratory, digestive, or reproductive systems of the body.

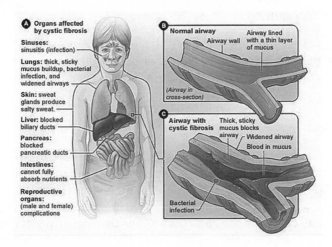

Figure 28.2. *Cystic Fibrosis*

Figure A shows the organs that cystic fibrosis can affect. Figure B shows a cross-section of a normal airway. Figure C shows an airway with cystic fibrosis. The widened airway is blocked by thick, sticky mucus that contains blood and bacteria.

People who have CF have thick, sticky mucus that builds up in their airways. This buildup of mucus makes it easier for bacteria to grow and cause infections. Infections can block the airways and cause frequent coughing that brings up thick sputum (spit) or mucus that's sometimes bloody.

People who have CF tend to have lung infections caused by unusual germs that don't respond to standard antibiotics. For example, lung infections caused by bacteria called mucoid *Pseudomonas* are much more common in people who have CF than in those who don't. An infection caused by these bacteria may be a sign of CF.

People who have CF have frequent bouts of sinusitis, an infection of the sinuses. The sinuses are hollow air spaces around the eyes, nose, and forehead. Frequent bouts of bronchitis and pneumonia also can occur. These infections can cause long-term lung damage.

As CF gets worse, you may have more serious problems, such as pneumothorax or bronchiectasis.

Some people who have CF also develop nasal polyps (growths in the nose) that may require surgery.

How Is Cystic Fibrosis Diagnosed?

Doctors diagnose CF based on the results from various tests.

Newborn Screening

All States screen newborns for CF using a genetic test or a blood test. The genetic test shows whether a newborn has faulty *CFTR* genes. The blood test shows whether a newborn's pancreas is working properly.

Sweat Test

If a genetic test or blood test suggests CF, a doctor will confirm the diagnosis using a sweat test. This test is the most useful test for diagnosing CF. A sweat test measures the amount of salt in sweat.

For this test, the doctor triggers sweating on a small patch of skin on an arm or leg. He or she rubs the skin with a sweat-producing chemical and then uses an electrode to provide a mild electrical current. This may cause a tingling or warm feeling.

Sweat is collected on a pad or paper and then analyzed. The sweat test usually is done twice. High salt levels confirm a diagnosis of CF.

Other Tests

If you or your child has CF, your doctor may recommend other tests, such as:

- Genetic tests to find out what type of *CFTR* defect is causing your CF.

- A chest X-ray. This test creates pictures of the structures in your chest, such as your heart, lungs, and blood vessels. A chest X-ray can show whether your lungs are inflamed or scarred, or whether they trap air.

- A sinus X-ray. This test may show signs of sinusitis, a complication of CF.

- Lung function tests. These tests measure how much air you can breathe in and out, how fast you can breathe air out, and how well your lungs deliver oxygen to your blood.

- A sputum culture. For this test, your doctor will take a sample of your sputum (spit) to see whether bacteria are growing in it. If you have bacteria called mucoid *Pseudomonas,* you may have more advanced CF that needs aggressive treatment.

Prenatal Screening

If you're pregnant, prenatal genetic tests can show whether your fetus has CF. These tests include amniocentesis and chorionic villus sampling (CVS).

In amniocentesis, your doctor inserts a hollow needle through your abdominal wall into your uterus. He or she removes a small amount of fluid from the sac around the baby. The fluid is tested to see whether both of the baby's *CFTR* genes are normal.

In CVS, your doctor threads a thin tube through the vagina and cervix to the placenta. The doctor removes a tissue sample from the placenta using gentle suction. The sample is tested to see whether the baby has CF.

Cystic Fibrosis Carrier Testing

People who have one normal *CFTR* gene and one faulty *CFTR* gene are CF carriers. CF carriers usually have no symptoms of CF and live normal lives. However, carriers can pass faulty *CFTR* genes on to their children.

If you have a family history of CF or a partner who has CF (or a family history of it) and you're planning a pregnancy, you may want to find out whether you're a CF carrier.

A genetics counselor can test a blood or saliva sample to find out whether you have a faulty CF gene. This type of testing can detect faulty CF genes in 9 out of 10 cases.

How Is Cystic Fibrosis Treated?

CF has no cure. However, treatments have greatly improved in recent years. The goals of CF treatment include:

- preventing and controlling lung infections

- loosening and removing thick, sticky mucus from the lungs

- preventing or treating blockages in the intestines

- providing enough nutrition

- preventing dehydration (a lack of fluid in the body)

Depending on the severity of CF, you or your child may be treated in a hospital.

Treatment for Lung Problems

The main treatments for lung problems in people who have CF are chest physical therapy (CPT), exercise, and medicines. Your doctor also may recommend a pulmonary rehabilitation (PR) program.

Chest Physical Therapy

CPT also is called chest clapping or percussion. It involves pounding your chest and back over and over with your hands or a device to loosen the mucus from your lungs so that you can cough it up.

You might sit down or lie on your stomach with your head down while you do CPT. Gravity and force help drain the mucus from your lungs.

Some people find CPT hard or uncomfortable to do. Several devices have been developed that may help with CPT, such as:

- An electric chest clapper, known as a mechanical percussor.

- An inflatable therapy vest that uses high-frequency airwaves to force the mucus that's deep in your lungs toward your upper airways so you can cough it up.

- A small, handheld device that you exhale through. The device causes vibrations that dislodge the mucus.

- A mask that creates vibrations that help break the mucus loose from your airway walls.

Breathing techniques also may help dislodge mucus so you can cough it up. These techniques include forcing out a couple of short breaths or deeper breaths and then doing relaxed breathing. This may help loosen the mucus in your lungs and open your airways.

Exercise

Aerobic exercise that makes you breathe harder can help loosen the mucus in your airways so you can cough it up. Exercise also helps improve your overall physical condition.

However, CF causes your sweat to become very salty. As a result, your body loses large amounts of salt when you sweat. Thus, your doctor may recommend a high-salt diet or salt supplements to maintain the balance of minerals in your blood.

If you exercise regularly, you may be able to cut back on your CPT. However, you should check with your doctor first.

Medicines

If you have CF, your doctor may prescribe antibiotics, anti-inflammatory medicines, bronchodilators, or medicines to help clear the mucus. These medicines help treat or prevent lung infections, reduce swelling and open up the airways, and thin mucus. If you have mutations in a gene called *G551D*, which occurs in about 5 percent of people who have CF, your doctor may prescribe the oral medicine ivacaftor (approved for people with CF who are 6 years of age and older).

Antibiotics are the main treatment to prevent or treat lung infections. Your doctor may prescribe oral, inhaled, or intravenous (IV) antibiotics.

Oral antibiotics often are used to treat mild lung infections. Inhaled antibiotics may be used to prevent or control infections caused by the bacteria mucoid *Pseudomonas*. For severe or hard-to-treat infections, you may be given antibiotics through an IV tube (a tube inserted into a vein). This type of treatment may require you to stay in a hospital.

Anti-inflammatory medicines can help reduce swelling in your airways due to ongoing infections. These medicines may be inhaled or oral.

Bronchodilators help open the airways by relaxing the muscles around them. These medicines are inhaled. They're often taken just before CPT to help clear mucus out of your airways. You also may take bronchodilators before inhaling other medicines into your lungs.

Your doctor may prescribe medicines to reduce the stickiness of your mucus and loosen it up. These medicines can help clear out mucus, improve lung function, and prevent worsening lung symptoms.

Treatments for Advanced Lung Disease

If you have advanced lung disease, you may need oxygen therapy. Oxygen usually is given through nasal prongs or a mask.

If other treatments haven't worked, a lung transplant may be an option if you have severe lung disease. A lung transplant is surgery to remove a person's diseased lung and replace it with a healthy lung from a deceased donor.

Pulmonary Rehabilitation

Your doctor may recommend PR as part of your treatment plan. PR is a broad program that helps improve the well-being of people who have chronic (ongoing) breathing problems.

PR doesn't replace medical therapy. Instead, it's used with medical therapy and may include:

- exercise training
- nutritional counseling
- education on your lung disease or condition and how to manage it
- energy-conserving techniques
- breathing strategies
- psychological counseling and/or group support

PR has many benefits. It can improve your ability to function and your quality of life. The program also may help relieve your breathing problems. Even if you have advanced lung disease, you can still benefit from PR.

Chapter 29

Hypersensitivity Pneumonitis

What Is Hypersensitivity Pneumonitis?

Hypersensitivity pneumonitis is a rare immune system disorder that affects the lungs. It occurs in some people after they breathe in certain substances they encounter in the environment. These substances trigger their immune systems, causing short- or long-term inflammation, especially in a part of the lungs called the interstitium. This inflammation makes it harder for the lungs to function properly and may even permanently damage the lungs. If diagnosed, some types of hypersensitivity pneumonitis are treatable by avoiding exposure to the environmental substances or with medicines such as corticosteroids that reduce inflammation. If the condition goes untreated or is not well controlled over time, the chronic inflammation can cause irreversible scarring of the lungs that may severely impair their ability to function.

Causes

Hypersensitivity pneumonitis is caused by repeated exposure to environmental substances that cause inflammation in the lungs when inhaled. These substances include certain:

- bacteria and mycobacteria

This chapter includes text excerpted from "Hypersensitivity Pneumonitis," National Heart, Lung, and Blood Institute (NHLBI), May 27, 2016.

- fungi or molds
- proteins
- chemicals

Where Can These Substances Be Found in the Environment?

Common environmental sources of substances that can cause hypersensitivity pneumonitis are:

- animal furs
- air conditioner, humidifier, and ventilation systems
- bird droppings and feathers
- contaminated foods such as cheese, grapes, barley, sugarcane
- contaminated industry products or materials such as sausage casings and corks
- contaminated metal working fluid
- hardwood dusts
- hay or grain animal feed
- hot tubs

Because this condition is caused by different substances found in many environmental sources, doctors once thought they were treating different lung diseases. Research has helped us understand hypersensitivity pneumonitis is triggered by different causative substances.

Why Does Hypersensitivity Pneumonitis Only Occur in Some People?

If you have hypersensitivity pneumonitis, your body's immune system reacts strongly to certain substances. Differences in our immune systems may explain why some people have strong reactions after breathing in certain substances, while others who breathe those same substances do not.

Tell Me More

Normally, the immune system in the lungs monitors inhaled substances. The immune system is activated when it recognizes a portion of the substance called the antigen as foreign. The activated immune system produces molecules that cause normal levels of inflammation, such as increased levels of immune cells and factors including antibodies that recognize and help clear the foreign substance. Normally after clearing the substance, the immune system shuts off and the inflammation stops. Usually, these processes are well controlled.

The immune systems of people with hypersensitivity pneumonitis are unable to shut down these normal inflammation processes, especially in the lung interstitium. The interstitium is a space where the lung's air sacs, called alveoli, come in contact with blood vessels and a small amount of connective tissue. When there is high level of inflammation in the lungs, immune cells begin to collect in this space. These uncontrolled levels of inflammation in the lungs cause the signs, symptoms, and complications of this condition.

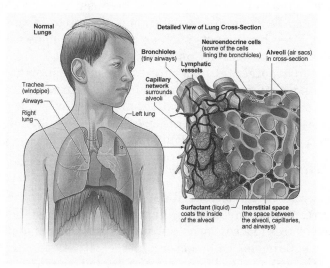

Figure 29.1. *Lymphatic Vessel*

In the lung interstitium, alveoli air sacs come into contact with the blood vessels and connective tissues of the lung. If you have hypersensitivity pneumonitis, your body's immune system reacts strongly to certain inhaled substances, causing inflammation especially in the interstitium or interstitial space.

Risk Factors

Certain factors affect your risk of developing hypersensitivity pneumonitis. These factors include age, environment or occupation, family history and genetics, lifestyle habits, other medical conditions, and sex or gender.

Age

Although hypersensitivity pneumonitis can occur at any age, people tend to be diagnosed with this condition between 50 and 55 years of age. Hypersensitivity pneumonitis is a common type of chronic interstitial lung disease in children.

Environment or Occupation

Repeated exposure to certain substances that cause the condition, possibly while working in occupations where environmental sources are common, can increase your risk of developing hypersensitivity pneumonitis. Certain occupations—such as farmers or people who breed animals or birds, cheese washers, woodworkers, and wine makers—have a greater chance of exposure to causative substances. However, you may be exposed to environmental sources in your home or elsewhere. Even having pets such as birds in the home can increase your risk of hypersensitivity pneumonitis.

Alone, environmental exposure to causative substances is not enough to cause hypersensitivity pneumonitis. An estimated 85 to 95 percent of people exposed to causative substances either never develop hypersensitivity pneumonitis or they experience a mild immune reaction with no obvious signs or symptoms or disease.

Family History and Genetics

Genetics is thought to predispose some people to have strong immune responses and develop hypersensitivity pneumonitis after repeat exposures to a causative substance. In some populations, family history of pulmonary fibrosis or hypersensitivity pneumonitis may increase the risk of developing hypersensitivity pneumonitis. When hypersensitivity pneumonitis occurs in relatives it is called familial hypersensitivity pneumonitis.

Researchers are beginning to map genetic variations in immune system proteins that may increase the risk for developing hypersensitivity pneumonitis. These differences may explain why immune cells respond differently between people who do or do not develop hypersensitivity pneumonitis after the same exposure to a causative substance.

Lifestyle Habits

Smoking is not thought to increase the risk of developing hypersensitivity pneumonitis. However, smoking can worsen chronic hypersensitivity pneumonitis and cause complications.

Other Medical Conditions

Some viral infections later in life may increase the risk of developing hypersensitivity pneumonitis.

Sex or Gender

Men and women can have hypersensitivity pneumonitis. Some small studies found this condition to be slightly more common in women.

Screening and Prevention

Currently, there are no screening methods to determine who will or will not develop hypersensitivity pneumonitis. you avoid common environmental sources of substances known to cause this condition. If you are at risk for hypersensitivity pneumonitis, your doctor may recommend you avoid common environmental sources of substances known to cause this condition.

Signs, Symptoms, and Complications

Signs and symptoms vary between acute, subacute, and chronic types of hypersensitivity pneumonitis. If your condition is not diagnosed or well controlled by treatment, it can lead to irreversible lung damage and other potentially fatal complications.

Signs and Symptoms

The following are common signs and symptoms of acute, subacute, and chronic hypersensitivity pneumonitis.

Type of Hypersensitivity Pneumonitis	Signs and Symptoms								
	Flu-like Illness (fever, chills, muscle or joint pain, headache)	Rales	Cough	Chronic Bronchitis	Shortness of Breath	Anorexia or Weight Loss	Fatigue	Lung Fibrosis	Clubbing of Fingers or Toes
Acute	✓		✓	✓					
Subacute		✓	✓	✓	✓	✓			
Chronic			✓	✓	✓	✓	✓	✓	✓

Figure 29.2. *Signs and Symptoms of Hypersensitivity*

Signs and symptoms of acute, subacute, and chronic hypersensitivity pneumonitis may include flu-like illness including fever, chills, muscle or joint pain, or headaches; rales; cough; chronic bronchitis; shortness of breath; anorexia or weight loss; fatigue; fibrosis of the lungs; and clubbing of fingers or toes.

While some signs and symptoms occur in several types of hypersensitivity pneumonitis, they may vary in severity. The exact signs and symptoms you experience also may vary.

Tell Me More

Acute hypersensitivity pneumonitis is the most common form of this condition. It is thought to occur as a result of a short period of exposure to a large amount of causative substance. Symptoms usually occur within 9 hours of being exposed again to a substance that triggers your immune system. If an additional exposure does not occur, symptoms usually resolve after a few days. Subacute and chronic forms of hypersensitivity pneumonitis occur after multiple or continuous exposures to small amounts of causative substance. Approximately 5 percent of patients develop chronic disease.

Complications

Hypersensitivity pneumonitis may cause the following potentially fatal complications if the condition is not diagnosed or well controlled by treatment.

- **Irreversible lung damage and permanently reduced lung function** because of severe fibrosis and impaired ability to oxygenate the blood during normal breathing.

- **Pulmonary hypertension** due to damage of blood vessels in the lungs.

- **Heart failure** because inflammation makes it harder for the heart to pump blood to and through the lungs.

Diagnosis

To diagnose hypersensitivity pneumonitis, your doctor will collect your medical history to understand your symptoms and see if you have an exposure history to possible causative substances. Your doctor will perform a physical exam and may order diagnostic tests and procedures. Based on this information, your doctor may able to determine whether you have acute, subacute, or chronic hypersensitivity pneumonitis.

Diagnostic Tests and Procedures

To diagnose hypersensitivity pneumonitis, your doctor may order:

- **Blood tests** to detect high levels of white blood cells and other immune cells and factors in your blood that indicate your immune system is activated and causing inflammation somewhere in your body.

- **Bronchoalveolar lavage (BAL)** to collect fluid from your lungs that can be tested for high levels of white blood cells and other immune cells. High levels of these cells mean your body is making an immune response in your lungs, but low levels do not rule out hypersensitivity pneumonitis.

- **Computed tomography (CT)** to image the lungs and look for inflammation or damage such as fibrosis. CT scans, particularly high-resolution ones, can help distinguish between types of hypersensitivity pneumonitis.

- **Inhalation challenge tests** to see if a controlled exposure to a suspected causative substance triggers your immune system and the onset of common signs and symptoms such as an increase in temperature, increase in white blood cell levels, rales that are heard during a physical exam, or reduced lung function. A positive test can confirm an inhaled substance triggers your immune system.

- **Lung biopsies** to see if your lung tissue shows signs of inflammation, fibrosis, or other changes known to occur in hypersensitivity pneumonitis.

- **Lung function tests** to see if you show signs of restriction such as reduced breathing capacity or abnormal blood oxygen levels and check if you have obstructed airways. These tests help assess the severity of your lung disease and when repeated they can help monitor whether your condition is stable or worsening over time. Lung function tests may be normal between acute flares.

- **Precipitin tests** to see if you have antibodies in your blood that recognize and bind to a causative substance. While a positive test means that you have been exposed to a substance, it cannot confirm you have hypersensitivity pneumonitis. This is because some people without this condition also have antibodies in their blood to these substances. If you have antibodies to a substance, your doctor may have you perform an inhalation challenge test to see if a new exposure to the same substance can activate your immune system and cause a new acute flare.

- **Chest X-rays** to image the lungs and look for inflammation or damage such as fibrosis in your lungs.

Is It Hard to Diagnose This Condition?

It can take months or even years for your doctor to diagnose hypersensitivity pneumonitis in you or your child. Learn why hypersensitivity pneumonitis can be hard to diagnose.

- **There are no clear exposure histories to potential causative substances before having symptoms.** This occurs in up to 50 percent of patients who are later diagnosed with hypersensitivity pneumonitis. Despite hypersensitivity pneumonitis being a common childhood interstitial lung disease, children are often diagnosed late after the condition has progressed to chronic disease. This is because children tend to be exposed to small amounts of causative substance over long periods of time, which does not trigger obvious acute symptoms and makes it very difficult to determine their exposure history.

- **Other conditions may cause similar signs and symptoms.** Before diagnosing hypersensitivity pneumonitis, your doctor must rule out: unintentional effects of medicines such as bleomycin, methotrexate, or nitrofurantoin; lung infections such as pneumonia or the flu (influenza); smoking-related lung disease; connective tissue disease; bleeding in the lungs; idiopathic pulmonary fibrosis; sarcoidosis; and lung cancer.

- **Diagnostic features seen in chest X-rays, CT scans, and lung biopsies may differ between children and adults.** Even when a person's exposure history is known or hypersensitivity pneumonitis is suspected, doctors look for diagnostic features in chest X-rays, CT scans, and lung biopsies that are indicators of the disease in adults. More research is needed to help map diagnostic features for children with this condition.

Treatment

Treatments for hypersensitivity pneumonitis usually include avoidance strategies and medicines. Occasionally, lung transplants are used to treat severe chronic disease in some patients.

Avoidance Strategies

If your doctor is able to identify the environmental substance that causes your hypersensitivity pneumonitis, he or she will recommend that you adopt the following avoidance strategies.

- **Remove** the causative substance if possible

- **Replace** workplace or other products with available alternatives that do not contain the substance responsible for your condition

- **Alter** work processes so you don't continue to breathe in the causative substance

- **Stay away** from known sources of your causative substance

Medicines

If avoidance strategies do not work for your condition, your doctor may prescribe corticosteroids or other immunosuppressive medicines to treat your condition. The choice, dose, and duration of these medicines will depend on your condition and medical history. Acute and subacute types of hypersensitivity pneumonitis usually respond well to these treatments.

Depending on your condition, your doctor also may prescribe some of the following supportive therapies.

- **Oxygen therapy** as needed for low levels of oxygen in the blood.

- **Bronchodilators** to relax the muscles in the airways and open your airways to make breathing easier.

- **Opioids** to control shortness of breath or chronic cough that is resistant to other treatments. Regular (e.g., several times a day, for several weeks or more) or longer use of opioids can lead to physical dependence and possibly addiction.

Lung Transplants

If your condition is not adequately controlled by avoidance strategies or medicines and you develop serious complications, you may be a candidate for a lung transplant. During this procedure, healthy donor lung will be transplanted into you to replace the damaged lung. Two important things to know:

- **This procedure is not a cure**. This is because your immune system will be the same after the procedure. This means that if you are exposed again to the substances that triggers your immune system, new inflammation may damage the transplanted donor lung tissue.

- **This procedure is not for everyone**. Even if you are a candidate for this procedure, it may be difficult to find a matching organ donor. Lung transplants are serious medical procedures with their own risks. Talk to your doctor about what procedures are right for you.

Tell Me More

Treatment is more successful when hypersensitivity pneumonitis is diagnosed in the early stages of the disease, before permanent irreversible lung damage has occurred. As new data emerges, doctors are becoming more aware of the unique treatment needs for children with hypersensitivity pneumonitis.

Chapter 30

Lung Cancer

The lungs are a pair of cone-shaped breathing organs inside the chest. The lungs bring oxygen into the body when breathing in and send carbon dioxide out of the body when breathing out. Each lung has sections called lobes. Two tubes called bronchi lead from the trachea (windpipe) to the lungs.

The two main types of lung cancer are non-small cell lung cancer and small cell lung cancer. The types are based on the way the cells look under a microscope. Non-small cell lung cancer is much more common than small cell lung cancer.

Tobacco smoking is the most common cause of lung cancer. Lung cancer is the leading cause of death from cancer in the United States and the number of deaths from lung cancer in women is increasing.

For most patients with lung cancer, current treatments do not cure the cancer.

Treatment

Non-Small Cell Lung Cancer Treatment

Non-Small Cell Lung Cancer Is a Disease in Which Malignant (Cancer) Cells Form in the Tissues of the Lung

The lungs are a pair of cone-shaped breathing organs in the chest. The lungs bring oxygen into the body as you breathe in. They release

This chapter includes text excerpted from "Lung Cancer—Patient Version," National Cancer Institute (NCI), October 30, 2015.

carbon dioxide, a waste product of the body's cells, as you breathe out. Each lung has sections called lobes. The left lung has two lobes. The right lung is slightly larger and has three lobes. Two tubes called bronchi lead from the trachea (windpipe) to the right and left lungs. The bronchi are sometimes also involved in lung cancer. Tiny air sacs called alveoli and small tubes called bronchioles make up the inside of the lungs.

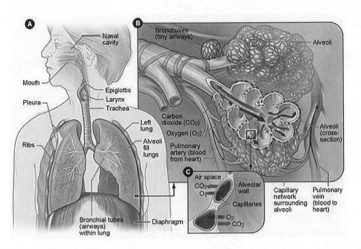

Figure 30.1. *Anatomy of the Respiratory System*

Figure A shows the location of the respiratory structures in the body. Figure B is an enlarged view of the airways, alveoli (air sacs), and capillaries (tiny blood vessels). Figure C is a closeup view of gas exchange between the capillaries and alveoli. CO_2 is carbon dioxide, and O_2 is oxygen.

(Source: "How the Lungs Work," National Heart, Lung, and Blood Institute (NHLBI), July 17, 2012.)

A thin membrane called the pleura covers the outside of each lung and lines the inside wall of the chest cavity. This creates a sac called the pleural cavity. The pleural cavity normally contains a small amount of fluid that helps the lungs move smoothly in the chest when you breathe.

There are two main types of lung cancer: non-small cell lung cancer and small cell lung cancer.

There Are Several Types of Non-Small Cell Lung Cancer

Each type of non-small cell lung cancer has different kinds of cancer cells. The cancer cells of each type grow and spread in different ways.

The types of non-small cell lung cancer are named for the kinds of cells found in the cancer and how the cells look under a microscope:

- Squamous cell carcinoma: Cancer that begins in squamous cells, which are thin, flat cells that look like fish scales. This is also called epidermoid carcinoma.

- Large cell carcinoma: Cancer that may begin in several types of large cells.

- Adenocarcinoma: Cancer that begins in the cells that line the alveoli and make substances such as mucus.

- Other less common types of non-small cell lung cancer are: pleomorphic, carcinoid tumor, salivary gland carcinoma, and unclassified carcinoma.

Smoking Is the Major Risk Factor for Non-Small Cell Lung Cancer

Anything that increases your chance of getting a disease is called a risk factor. Having a risk factor does not mean that you will get cancer; not having risk factors doesn't mean that you will not get cancer. Talk to your doctor if you think you may be at risk for lung cancer.

Risk factors for lung cancer include the following:

- Smoking cigarettes, pipes, or cigars, now or in the past. This is the most important risk factor for lung cancer. The earlier in life a person starts smoking, the more often a person smokes, and the more years a person smokes, the greater the risk of lung cancer.

- Being exposed to secondhand smoke.

- Being exposed to radiation from any of the following:
  - radiation therapy to the breast or chest
  - radon in the home or workplace
  - imaging tests such as CT scans
  - atomic bomb radiation

- Being exposed to asbestos, chromium, nickel, beryllium, arsenic, soot, or tar in the workplace.

- Living where there is air pollution.

- Having a family history of lung cancer.

- Being infected with the human immunodeficiency virus (HIV).

- Taking beta carotene supplements and being a heavy smoker.

Older age is the main risk factor for most cancers. The chance of getting cancer increases as you get older.

When smoking is combined with other risk factors, the risk of lung cancer is increased.

Signs of Non-Small Cell Lung Cancer Include a Cough That Doesn't Go Away and Shortness of Breath

Sometimes lung cancer does not cause any signs or symptoms. It may be found during a chest X-ray done for another condition. Signs and symptoms may be caused by lung cancer or by other conditions. Check with your doctor if you have any of the following:

- chest discomfort or pain
- a cough that doesn't go away or gets worse over time
- trouble breathing
- wheezing
- blood in sputum (mucus coughed up from the lungs)
- hoarseness
- loss of appetite
- weight loss for no known reason
- feeling very tired
- trouble swallowing
- swelling in the face and/or veins in the neck

Tests That Examine the Lungs Are Used to Detect (Find), Diagnose, and Stage Non-Small Cell Lung Cancer

Tests and procedures to detect, diagnose, and stage non-small cell lung cancer are often done at the same time. Some of the following tests and procedures may be used:

- Physical exam and history
- Laboratory tests
- Chest X-ray
- CT scan (CAT scan)
- Sputum cytology

- Fine-needle aspiration (FNA) biopsy of the lung

- Bronchoscopy

- Thoracoscopy

- Thoracentesis

- Light and electron microscopy

- Immunohistochemistry

Certain Factors Affect Prognosis (Chance of Recovery) and Treatment Options

- The prognosis (chance of recovery) and treatment options depend on the following:

- The stage of the cancer (the size of the tumor and whether it is in the lung only or has spread to other places in the body).

- The type of lung cancer.

- Whether the cancer has mutations (changes) in certain genes, such as the epidermal growth factor receptor (*EGFR*) gene or the anaplastic lymphoma kinase (*ALK*) gene.

- Whether there are signs and symptoms such as coughing or trouble breathing.

- The patient's general health.

For Most Patients with Non-Small Cell Lung Cancer, Current Treatments Do Not Cure the Cancer

If lung cancer is found, taking part in one of the many clinical trials being done to improve treatment should be considered. Clinical trials are taking place in most parts of the country for patients with all stages of non-small cell lung cancer.

Small Cell Lung Cancer Treatment

There Are Two Main Types of Small Cell Lung Cancer

These two types include many different types of cells. The cancer cells of each type grow and spread in different ways. The types of small cell lung cancer are named for the kinds of cells found in the cancer and how the cells look when viewed under a microscope:

1. Small cell carcinoma (oat cell cancer)

2. Combined small cell carcinoma

Tests and Procedures That Examine the Lungs Are Used to Detect (Find), Diagnose, and Stage Small Cell Lung Cancer

Physical exam and history

- Laboratory tests
- Chest X-ray
- CT scan (CAT scan) of the brain, chest, and abdomen
- Sputum cytology
- Biopsy
- Bronchoscopy
- Thoracoscopy
- Thoracentesis
- Mediastinoscopy
- Light and electron microscopy
- Immunohistochemistry

Certain Factors Affect Prognosis (Chance of Recovery) and Treatment Options

The prognosis (chance of recovery) and treatment options depend on the following:

- The stage of the cancer (whether it is in the chest cavity only or has spread to other places in the body).
- The patient's age, gender, and general health.

For certain patients, prognosis also depends on whether the patient is treated with both chemotherapy and radiation.

For Most Patients with Small Cell Lung Cancer, Current Treatments Do Not Cure the Cancer

If lung cancer is found, patients should think about taking part in one of the many clinical trials being done to improve treatment.

Clinical trials are taking place in most parts of the country for patients with all stages of small cell lung cancer.

Lung Cancer Prevention

Avoiding Risk Factors and Increasing Protective Factors May Help Prevent Lung Cancer

Avoiding cancer risk factors may help prevent certain cancers. Risk factors include smoking, being overweight, and not getting enough exercise. Increasing protective factors such as quitting smoking, eating a healthy diet, and exercising may also help prevent some cancers. Talk to your doctor or other healthcare professional about how you might lower your risk of cancer.

The Following Are Risk Factors for Lung Cancer

Cigarette, Cigar, and Pipe Smoking

Tobacco smoking is the most important risk factor for lung cancer. Cigarette, cigar, and pipe smoking all increase the risk of lung cancer. Tobacco smoking causes about 9 out of 10 cases of lung cancer in men and about 8 out of 10 cases of lung cancer in women.

Studies have shown that smoking low tar or low nicotine cigarettes does not lower the risk of lung cancer.

Studies also show that the risk of lung cancer from smoking cigarettes increases with the number of cigarettes smoked per day and the number of years smoked. People who smoke have about 20 times the risk of lung cancer compared to those who do not smoke.

Secondhand Smoke

Being exposed to secondhand tobacco smoke is also a risk factor for lung cancer. Secondhand smoke is the smoke that comes from a burning cigarette or other tobacco product, or that is exhaled by smokers. People who inhale secondhand smoke are exposed to the same cancer-causing agents as smokers, although in smaller amounts. Inhaling secondhand smoke is called involuntary or passive smoking.

Family History

Having a family history of lung cancer is a risk factor for lung cancer. People with a relative who has had lung cancer may be twice as likely to have lung cancer as people who do not have a relative who has had lung cancer. Because cigarette smoking tends to run in families and family members are exposed to secondhand smoke, it is hard to know whether the increased risk of lung cancer is from the family history of lung cancer or from being exposed to cigarette smoke.

HIV Infection

Being infected with the human immunodeficiency virus (HIV), the cause of acquired immunodeficiency syndrome (AIDS), is linked with a higher risk of lung cancer. People infected with HIV may have more than twice the risk of lung cancer than those who are not infected. Since smoking rates are higher in those infected with HIV than in those not infected, it is not clear whether the increased risk of lung cancer is from HIV infection or from being exposed to cigarette smoke.

Environmental Risk Factors

- **Radiation exposure:** Being exposed to radiation is a risk factor for lung cancer. Atomic bomb radiation, radiation therapy, imaging tests, and radon are sources of radiation exposure.

- **Workplace exposure:** Studies show that being exposed to the following substances increases the risk of lung cancer:
  - Asbestos
  - Arsenic
  - Chromium
  - Nickel
  - Beryllium
  - Cadmium
  - Tar and soot

  These substances can cause lung cancer in people who are exposed to them in the workplace and have never smoked. As the level of exposure to these substances increases, the risk of lung cancer also increases. The risk of lung cancer is even higher in people who are exposed and also smoke.

- **Air pollution:** Studies show that living in areas with higher levels of air pollution increases the risk of lung cancer.

Beta Carotene Supplements in Heavy Smokers

Taking beta carotene supplements (pills) increases the risk of lung cancer, especially in smokers who smoke one or more packs a day. The risk is higher in smokers who have at least one alcoholic drink every day.

The Following Are Protective Factors for Lung Cancer

Not Smoking

The best way to prevent lung cancer is to not smoke.

Quitting Smoking

Smokers can decrease their risk of lung cancer by quitting. In smokers who have been treated for lung cancer, quitting smoking lowers the risk of new lung cancers. Counseling, the use of nicotine replacement products, and antidepressant therapy have helped smokers quit for good.

In a person who has quit smoking, the chance of preventing lung cancer depends on how many years and how much the person smoked and the length of time since quitting. After a person has quit smoking for 10 years, the risk of lung cancer decreases 30 percent to 50 percent.

Lower Exposure to Workplace Risk Factors

Laws that protect workers from being exposed to cancer-causing substances, such as asbestos, arsenic, nickel, and chromium, may help lower their risk of developing lung cancer. Laws that prevent smoking in the workplace help lower the risk of lung cancer caused by secondhand smoke.

Lower Exposure to Radon

Lowering radon levels may lower the risk of lung cancer, especially among cigarette smokers. High levels of radon in homes may be reduced by taking steps to prevent radon leakage, such as sealing basements.

Chapter 31

Lymphangioleiomyomatosis (LAM)

What Is LAM?

LAM, or lymphangioleiomyomatosis, is a rare lung disease that mostly affects women of childbearing age.

In LAM, abnormal, muscle-like cells begin to grow out of control in certain organs or tissues, especially the lungs, lymph nodes, and kidneys.

Over time, these LAM cells can destroy the normal lung tissue. As a result, air can't move freely in and out of the lungs. In some cases, this means the lungs can't supply the body's other organs with enough oxygen.

What Causes LAM?

The cause of LAM and why it mainly affects women isn't known. Recent studies show that sporadic LAM has some of the same traits as another rare disease called tuberous sclerosis complex (TSC). This has begun to provide some valuable clues about what causes LAM.

This chapter includes text excerpted from "LAM," National Heart, Lung, and Blood Institute (NHLBI), December 26, 2013.

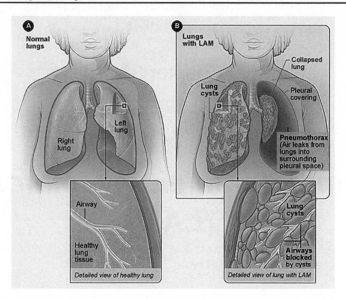

Figure 31.1. *Normal Lungs and Lungs with LAM*

Figure A shows the location of the lungs and airways in the body. The inset image shows a cross-section of a healthy lung. Figure B shows a view of the lungs with LAM and a collapsed lung (pneumothorax). The inset image shows a cross-section of a lung with LAM.

The common features of sporadic LAM and TSC are:

- Kidney growths. People who have TSC get growths in their kidneys. These growths are the same as the angiomyolipomas that many women who have LAM get in their kidneys.

- Lung cysts. Some women who have TSC get cysts in their lungs. These cysts are the same as the ones that women who have sporadic LAM get in their lungs. When a woman who has TSC gets cysts in her lungs, the lung disease is called TSC-associated LAM or TSC–LAM.

TSC is a genetic disease. A defect in one of two genes causes the disease. These genes are called *TSC1* and *TSC2*. They normally make proteins that control cell growth and movement in the body. In people who have TSC, the genes are faulty. The proteins that the genes make can't control cell growth and movement.

Women who have LAM also have abnormal *TSC1* and *TSC2* genes. Researchers have found that these genes play a role in causing LAM. This finding is leading to new treatments for LAM.

Because LAM affects women, the hormone estrogen also may play a role in causing the disease.

Who Is at Risk for LAM?

LAM is a rare disease that mostly affects women of childbearing age. Many women who develop LAM are between the ages of 20 and 40 when they begin to have symptoms. LAM can occur in older women as well, although this is less common.

Some women might have LAM and not know it. Many of LAM's signs and symptoms are the same as those of other diseases, such as asthma, emphysema, and bronchitis.

LAM affects about 3 out of every 10 women who have tuberous sclerosis complex (TSC). Some of these women may have mild cases of LAM that don't cause symptoms. Not everyone who has TSC and LAM has lung symptoms.

In rare cases, LAM has been reported in men.

What Are the Signs and Symptoms of LAM?

The uncontrolled growth of LAM cells and their effect on nearby body tissues causes the signs and symptoms of LAM. The most common signs and symptoms are:

- Shortness of breath, especially during activity. At first, shortness of breath may occur only during high-energy activities. Over time, you may have trouble breathing during simple activities, such as dressing and showering.

- Chest pain or aches. This pain might be worse when you breathe in.

- Frequent cough. This may occur with bloody phlegm (a sticky fluid).

- Wheezing (a whistling sound when you breathe).

Other signs and symptoms of LAM include:

- Pneumothorax, or collapsed lung. In LAM, a pneumothorax can occur if lung cysts rupture through the lining of a lung. Air that collects in the space between the lung and chest wall must be removed to reinflate the lung.

- Pleural effusions. This condition can occur if bodily fluids collect in the space between the lung and the chest wall. Often the fluid contains a milky substance called chyle (kile). The excess fluid in the chest may cause shortness of breath because the lung has less room to expand.

- Blood in the urine. This sign may occur in women who have kidney tumors called angiomyolipomas.

- Enlarged lymph nodes. These usually occur in the abdomen or the chest. Very rarely, enlarged lymph nodes may occur in locations where they can be felt, such as the neck or under the arms.

- Abdominal swelling, sometimes with pain.

- Swelling in the legs, ankles, or feet.

Other diseases also can cause many of these signs and symptoms. If you're having any of these problems, see your doctor. He or she can help find the cause of your symptoms.

How Is LAM Diagnosed?

Methods for diagnosing LAM have improved. It's now possible for doctors to diagnose the disease at an early stage.

LAM is diagnosed based on your signs and symptoms and the results from tests and procedures. If you have LAM, you may need to see a pulmonologist. This is a doctor who specializes in lung diseases and conditions.

Signs and Symptoms

Your doctor will ask about your signs and symptoms related to LAM. He or she may ask how long you've had symptoms, and whether they've become worse over time.

Many of LAM's signs and symptoms are the same as those of other diseases, such as asthma, emphysema, and bronchitis. Your doctor will want to rule out those conditions before making a final diagnosis.

Diagnostic Tests and Procedures

Your doctor may recommend tests to show how well your lungs are working and what your lung tissue looks like.

These tests can show whether your lungs are delivering enough oxygen to your blood. You also may have tests to check for complications of LAM.

Tests for Lung Function

Lung function tests. For lung function tests, you breathe through a mouthpiece into a machine called a spirometer. The spirometer measures the amount of air you breathe in and out.

Other lung function tests can show about how much air your lungs can hold and how well your lungs deliver oxygen to your blood.

Blood tests. Your doctor may take a blood sample from a vein in your arm to look at your blood cells and blood chemistry.

Pulse oximetry. For this test, a small sensor is attached to your finger or ear. The sensor uses light to estimate how much oxygen is in your blood.

Tests to Check for Complications or Detect LAM Cells

Chest X-ray. A chest X-ray creates a picture of the structures in your chest, such as your heart and lungs. The test can show a collapsed lung or fluid in your chest. In the early stages of LAM, your chest X-rays may look normal. As the disease gets worse, the X-rays may show cysts in your lungs.

High-resolution CT (HRCT) scan. The most useful imaging test for diagnosing LAM is an HRCT scan. This test creates a computer-generated picture of your lungs. The picture shows more detail than the pictures from a chest X-ray.

An HRCT scan can show cysts, shadows of cell clusters, excess fluid, a collapsed lung, and enlarged lymph nodes. The test also can show how much normal lung tissue has been replaced by the LAM cysts.

HRCT scans of your abdomen and pelvis can show whether you have growths in your kidneys, other abdominal organs, or lymph nodes.

Procedures to Look for LAM Cells

The results from the above tests—along with information about your signs, symptoms, and medical history—might be enough for your doctor to diagnose LAM.

However, if your doctor needs more information, the most useful method involves looking at samples of your lung tissue for LAM cells.

You may want to see a doctor who specializes in LAM for this test. Several procedures can be used to get a sample of lung tissue.

Video-assisted thoracoscopy. In this procedure, also called VAT, your doctor inserts a small, lighted tube into little cuts made in your chest wall. This lets him or her look inside your chest and snip out a few small pieces of lung tissue.

VAT is done in a hospital. The procedure isn't major surgery, but it does require general anesthesia (that is, you're given medicine to make you sleep during the procedure).

Open lung biopsy. In this procedure, your doctor removes a few small pieces of lung tissue through a cut made in your chest wall between your ribs. An open lung biopsy is done in a hospital. You'll be given medicine to make you sleep during the procedure.

Open lung biopsies are rarely done anymore because the recovery time is much longer than the recovery time from VAT.

Transbronchial biopsy. In this procedure, your doctor inserts a long, narrow, flexible, lighted tube down your windpipe and into your lungs. He or she then snips out bits of lung tissue using a tiny device.

This procedure usually is done in a hospital. Your mouth and throat are numbed to prevent pain.

The amount of tissue that your doctor removes is very small, so this test doesn't always provide enough information.

Other biopsies. Your doctor also can diagnose LAM using the results from other tissue biopsies, such as biopsies of lymph nodes or lymphatic tumors called lymphangiomyomas.

Other Tests

If you're diagnosed with sporadic LAM, your doctor may advise you to have a computed tomography (CT) scan or magnetic resonance imaging (MRI) scan of your head. These tests can help screen for underlying tuberous sclerosis complex (TSC).

CT and MRI scans will reveal TSC in only a small number of people who are initially diagnosed with sporadic LAM.

Researchers are exploring other tests that may help diagnose LAM. These tests include blood tests for the LAM cells or a blood vessel growth factor called VEGF-D.

How Is LAM Treated?

Currently, no treatment is available to stop the growth of the cysts and cell clusters that occur in LAM. Most treatments for LAM are aimed at easing symptoms and preventing complications.

The main treatments are:

- medicines to improve air flow in the lungs and reduce wheezing
- oxygen therapy
- procedures to remove fluid from the chest or abdomen and stop it from building up again
- procedures to shrink angiomyolipomas (AMLs)
- lung transplant
- hormone therapy

Medicines

Medicines That Help You Breathe Better

If you're having trouble breathing, your doctor may prescribe bronchodilators. These medicines relax the muscles around the airways. This helps the airways open up, making it easier for you to breathe.

Lung function tests can sometimes show whether these medicines are likely to help you.

Medicines That Prevent Bone Loss

Women who have LAM are at risk for a bone-weakening condition called osteoporosis. This is in part because many LAM therapies block the estrogen action needed to keep bones strong.

To prevent osteoporosis, your doctor may measure your bone density. If you have lost bone density, your doctor may prescribe medicines to prevent bone loss. He or she also may prescribe calcium and vitamin D supplements.

Rapamycin (Sirolimus)

Sirolimus was originally developed to prevent the immune system from rejecting kidney transplants. However, studies have shown that the medicine helps regulate the abnormal growth and movement of LAM cells.

Research suggests that sirolimus may shrink tumors in the kidneys of women who have LAM.

A study funded in part by the National Institutes of Health (NIH) showed that sirolimus also helps stabilize lung function, reduce symptoms, and improve quality of life for people who have LAM.

Sirolimus does have side effects, some of which can be serious. If you have LAM, talk with your doctor about the benefits and risks of this medicine, and whether it's an option for you.

Oxygen Therapy

If the level of oxygen in your blood is low, your doctor may suggest oxygen therapy. Oxygen usually is given through nasal prongs or a mask. At first, you may need oxygen only while exercising. It also may help to use it while sleeping. Over time, you may need full-time oxygen therapy.

A standard exercise stress test or a 6-minute walk test can show whether you need oxygen while exercising. A 6-minute walk test measures the distance you can walk in 6 minutes. An exercise stress test measures how well your lungs and heart work while you walk on a treadmill or pedal a stationary bike.

You also may need a blood test to show your blood oxygen level and how much oxygen you need.

Procedures to Remove Air or Fluid from the Chest or Abdomen

Several procedures can remove excess air or fluid from your chest and abdomen. These procedures also help prevent air or fluid from building up again.

Removing fluid from your chest or abdomen may help relieve discomfort and shortness of breath. The procedure to remove fluid from the chest is called thoracentesis. The procedure to remove fluid from the abdomen is called paracentesis.

Your doctor often can remove the fluid with a needle and syringe. If large amounts of fluid build up in your chest, your doctor may have to insert a tube into your chest to remove the fluid.

Removing air from your chest may relieve shortness of breath and chest pain caused by a collapsed lung. Your doctor usually can remove the air with a tube. The tube is inserted into your chest between your side ribs. Often, the tube is attached to a suction device. If this procedure doesn't work, or if your lungs collapse often, you may need surgery.

If fluid and air often leak into your chest, your doctor may inject a chemical at the site of the leakage. The chemical fuses your lung and chest wall together. This removes the space for leakage.

Your doctor may do this procedure at your bedside in the hospital. You will be given medicine to prevent pain. The procedure also can be done in an operating room using video-assisted thoracoscopy. In this case, you will be given medicine to make you sleep during the procedure.

Procedures to Remove or Shrink Angiomyolipomas

AMLs often don't cause symptoms, but sometimes they can cause ongoing pain or bleeding. If this happens, you may need surgery to remove some of the tumors.

If bleeding isn't too severe, a radiologist often can block the blood vessels feeding the AMLs. This may cause them to shrink.

Lung Transplant

Lung transplants can improve lung function and quality of life in patients who have advanced LAM.

However, lung transplants have a high risk of complications, including infections and rejection of the transplanted lung by the body.

Studies suggest that more than three-quarters of women with LAM who receive a lung transplant survive for at least 3 years.

In a few cases, doctors have found LAM cells in the newly transplanted lungs and other parts of the body. However, the LAM cells don't seem to stop the transplanted lung from working.

Hormone Therapy

Estrogen is thought to play a role in causing LAM. Thus, your doctor may want to treat you with hormone therapy that limits the effects of estrogen on your body. Hormone therapy is given in pill form or as injections.

Some doctors also suggest surgery to remove the ovaries. This causes menopause and greatly reduces estrogen levels in the body.

Unfortunately, at this time, no clear evidence shows that this type of treatment works for women who have LAM.

Chapter 32

Nasal Polyps

What Is a Nasal Polyp?

Nasal polyps are small, polypoidal, noncancerous growths that can occur anywhere in the mucous membranes lining the nose or the paranasal sinuses. They may occur singly or in clusters, and they usually form where the sinuses open into the nasal cavity. While small polyps may not cause problems as they are freely movable, larger ones can block the sinuses or the nasal airway.

Nasal polyps can develop at any age, but they are most common in adults over age 40. Men are more prone to this disease, while it is uncommon in children under ten years. When young children are diagnosed with nasal polyps, in fact, doctors should conduct further tests to rule out cystic fibrosis, a genetic disorder characterized by a buildup of mucus in the lungs. Nasal polyps occur in nearly two-thirds of cystic fibrosis patients.

Causes

It is not entirely clear why some people develop nasal polyps and others do not. Although there is no definite cause of nasal polyposis, some factors may contribute to an increased risk of developing nasal polyps. One of the most common triggers is nasal congestion arising from chronic inflammation of the sinuses, which may be caused by

"Nasal Polyps," © 2016 Omnigraphics. Reviewed September 2016.

allergies or recurring sinus infections. A certain degree of genetic predisposition has been observed in patients with nasal polyps, and it may explain why the mucosa in some people reacts differently to inflammation. Polyps are also commonly seen in patients with late onset of asthma and aspirinsensitivity, allergic rhinitis, and sinusitis.

Types of Nasal Polyps

Nasal polyps can be classified as a) Antrochoanal and b) Ethmoidal.

Antrochoanal nasal polyp is single, unilateral, and originates from maxillary sinus; it is mostly found in children. Ethmoidal polyps are bilateral and usually found in adults.

Symptoms and Diagnosis

Polyposis may be asymptomatic in some people, particularly if the polyps are small. Larger polyps are usually associated with catarrh (excessive secretion of mucus), breathing difficulties, inflammation of the paranasal cavities, and loss of smell and taste. Other symptoms of nasal polyps may include postnasal drip (drainage of mucous down the back of the throat) and a dull, achy feeling in the face because of fluid buildup.

Diagnosis of nasal polyps is generally made using a procedure called nasal endoscopy. Although a routine examination with a rhinoscope (a lighted device fitted with a lens that can be inserted into the nose) can find polyps located in the nasal cavity, an endoscope (a long, flexible tool fitted with a miniature camera on its end) is required to find polyps that are deep-seated in the sinuses. The doctor may also request a Computerized Tomography (CT) scan to diagnose polyps and additional tests such as biopsy to rule out nasal and sinus cancer, and non-malignant conditions such as nasal papilloma.

Treatment Options

Although various forms of medicine can alleviate symptoms associated with nasal polyps, they may provide only temporary relief. The first line of treatment is usually nasal drops or sprays containing steroids. Steroid treatment is often beneficial if the polyps are small, and the patient is likely to experience marked improvement in breathing as the polyps shrink and free up the airways. Tapered oral steroid medications can prevent sinus inflammation associated with allergies and effectively reduce the size of inflammatory polyps, but these drugs are used sparingly because they may increase the risk of such health concerns as diabetes, high blood pressure, and osteoporosis. Steroids, both topical and oral, are also frequently used after surgery to prevent the recurrence of polyps.

- Doctors may also prescribe antibiotics to treat chronic sinusitis that may be associated with nasal polyps.

- Endoscopic nasal surgery is the most commonly used treatment option for polyposis when the polyps are too large to respond to corticosteroids. This minimally invasive surgical procedure, known as a polypectomy, is performed with a nasal endoscope and can be done on an outpatient basis. The procedure, which is done in approximately 45 minutes to an hour, is carried out under general anaesthesia using a suction device or a microdebrider (a minuscule, motorized shaver) to remove the polyps. If there is no bleeding, the patient is discharged after a few hours of observation. Antibiotics are usually prescribed to prevent infection at the site of surgery.

- Although surgery can provide symptomatic relief for a few years, the nasal polyps grow back in at least 15 percent of patients. In such cases, postoperative use of steroidal sprays and saline washes is usually prescribed to extend the period before the polyps recur.

References

1. Case-Lo, Christine. "Nasal Polyps," Healthline, October 5, 2015.

2. "Nasal Polyps—Treatment," NHS Choices, February 12, 2015.

Chapter 33

Neuromuscular and Kidney Diseases That Impact Lung Function

Chapter Contents

Section 33.1

Amyotrophic Lateral Sclerosis

This section includes text excerpted from "Amyotrophic Lateral
Sclerosis (ALS) Fact Sheet," National Institute of Neurological
Disorders and Stroke (NINDS), March 14, 2016.

What Is Amyotrophic Lateral Sclerosis?

Amyotrophic lateral sclerosis (ALS), sometimes called Lou Gehrig
disease, is a rapidly progressive, invariably fatal neurological disease
that attacks the nerve cells (*neurons*) responsible for controlling voluntary muscles (muscle action we are able to control, such as those in
the arms, legs, and face). The disease belongs to a group of disorders
known as *motor neuron diseases*, which are characterized by the gradual degeneration and death of motor neurons.

Motor neurons are nerve cells located in the brain, brain stem, and
spinal cord that serve as controlling units and vital communication
links between the nervous system and the voluntary muscles of the
body. Messages from motor neurons in the brain (called *upper motor
neurons*) are transmitted to motor neurons in the spinal cord (called
lower motor neurons) and from them to particular muscles. In ALS,
both the upper motor neurons and the lower motor neurons degenerate
or die, and stop sending messages to muscles. Unable to function, the
muscles gradually weaken, waste away (*atrophy*), and have very fine
twitches (called *fasciculations*). Eventually, the ability of the brain to
start and control voluntary movement is lost.

ALS causes weakness with a wide range of disabilities. Eventually,
all muscles under voluntary control are affected, and individuals lose
their strength and the ability to move their arms, legs, and body. When
muscles in the diaphragm and chest wall fail, people lose the ability
to breathe without ventilatory support. Most people with ALS die
from respiratory failure, usually within 3 to 5 years from the onset of
symptoms. However, about 10 percent of those with ALS survive for
10 or more years.

Although the disease usually does not impair a person's mind or
intelligence, several recent studies suggest that some persons with

ALS may have depression or alterations in cognitive functions involving decision-making and memory.

ALS does not affect a person's ability to see, smell, taste, hear, or recognize touch. Patients usually maintain control of eye muscles and bladder and bowel functions, although in the late stages of the disease most individuals will need help getting to and from the bathroom.

What Are the Symptoms?

The onset of ALS may be so subtle that the symptoms are overlooked. The earliest symptoms may include fasciculations, cramps, tight and stiff muscles (*spasticity*), muscle weakness affecting an arm or a leg, slurred and nasal speech, or difficulty chewing or swallowing. These general complaints then develop into more obvious weakness or atrophy that may cause a physician to suspect ALS.

The parts of the body showing early symptoms of ALS depend on which muscles in the body are affected. Many individuals first see the effects of the disease in a hand or arm as they experience difficulty with simple tasks requiring manual dexterity such as buttoning a shirt, writing, or turning a key in a lock. In other cases, symptoms initially affect one of the legs, and people experience awkwardness when walking or running or they notice that they are tripping or stumbling more often. When symptoms begin in the arms or legs, it is referred to as "limb onset" ALS. Other individuals first notice speech problems, termed "bulbar onset" ALS.

Regardless of the part of the body first affected by the disease, muscle weakness and atrophy spread to other parts of the body as the disease progresses. Individuals may develop problems with moving, swallowing (*dysphagia*), and speaking or forming words (*dysarthria*). Symptoms of upper motor neuron involvement include spasticity and exaggerated reflexes (*hyperreflexia*) including an overactive gag reflex. An abnormal reflex commonly called Babinski sign (the large toe extends upward as the sole of the foot is stimulated in a certain way) also indicates upper motor neuron damage. Symptoms of lower motor neuron degeneration include muscle weakness and atrophy, muscle cramps, and fasciculations.

To be diagnosed with ALS, people must have signs and symptoms of both upper and lower motor neuron damage that cannot be attributed to other causes.

Although the sequence of emerging symptoms and the rate of disease progression vary from person to person, eventually individuals will not be able to stand or walk, get in or out of bed on their own, or use their hands and arms. Difficulty swallowing and chewing impair the person's ability to eat normally and increase the risk of choking. Maintaining weight will then become a problem. Because cognitive abilities are relatively intact, people are aware of their progressive loss of function and may become anxious and depressed. A small percentage of individuals may experience problems with memory or decision-making, and there is growing evidence that some may even develop a form of dementia over time. Healthcare professionals need to explain the course of the disease and describe available treatment options so that people can make informed decisions in advance. In later stages of the disease, individuals have difficulty breathing as the muscles of the respiratory system weaken. They eventually lose the ability to breathe on their own and must depend on ventilatory support for survival. Affected individuals also face an increased risk of pneumonia during later stages of ALS.

What Causes ALS?

The cause of ALS is not known, and scientists do not yet know why ALS strikes some people and not others. An important step toward answering this question was made in 1993 when scientists supported by the National Institute of Neurological Disorders and Stroke (NINDS) discovered that mutations in the gene that produces the SOD1 enzyme were associated with some cases of familial ALS. Although it is still not clear how mutations in the *SOD1* gene lead to motor neuron degeneration, there is increasing evidence that mutant SOD1 protein can become toxic.

Since then, over a dozen additional genetic mutations have been identified, many through NINDS-supported research, and each of these gene discoveries has provided new insights into possible mechanisms of ALS.

For example, the discovery of certain genetic mutations involved in ALS suggests that changes in the processing of RNA molecules (involved with functions including gene regulation and activity) may lead to ALS-related motor neuron degeneration. Other gene mutations implicate defects in protein recycling. And still others point to possible defects in the structure and shape of motor neurons, as well as increased susceptibility to environmental toxins. Overall, it is becoming increasingly clear that a number of cellular defects can lead to motor neuron degeneration in ALS.

Another research advance was made in 2011 when scientists found that a defect in the *C9orf72* gene is not only present in a significant subset of ALS patients but also in some patients who suffer from a type of frontotemporal dementia (FTD). This observation provides evidence for genetic ties between these two neurodegenerative disorders. In fact, some researchers are proposing that ALS and some forms of FTD are related disorders with genetic, clinical, and pathological overlap.

In searching for the cause of ALS, researchers are also studying the role of environmental factors such as exposure to toxic or infectious agents, as well as physical trauma or behavioral and occupational factors. For example, studies of populations of military personnel who were deployed to the Gulf region during the 1991 war show that those veterans were more likely to develop ALS compared to military personnel who were not in the region.

Future research may show that many factors, including a genetic predisposition, are involved in the development of ALS.

How Is ALS Treated?

No cure has yet been found for ALS. However, the U.S. Food and Drug Administration (FDA) approved the first drug treatment for the disease—riluzole (Rilutek)—in 1995. Riluzole is believed to reduce damage to motor neurons by decreasing the release of glutamate. Clinical trials with ALS patients showed that riluzole prolongs survival by several months, mainly in those with difficulty swallowing. The drug also extends the time before an individual needs ventilation support. Riluzole does not reverse the damage already done to motor neurons, and persons taking the drug must be monitored for liver damage and other possible side effects. However, this first disease-specific therapy offers hope that the progression of ALS may one day be slowed by new medications or combinations of drugs.

Other treatments for ALS are designed to relieve symptoms and improve the quality of life for individuals with the disorder. This supportive care is best provided by multidisciplinary teams of healthcare professionals such as physicians; pharmacists; physical, occupational, and speech therapists; nutritionists; and social workers and home care and hospice nurses. Working with patients and caregivers, these teams can design an individualized plan of medical and physical therapy and provide special equipment aimed at keeping patients as mobile and comfortable as possible.

Physicians can prescribe medications to help reduce fatigue, ease muscle cramps, control spasticity, and reduce excess saliva and phlegm. Drugs also are available to help patients with pain, depression, sleep disturbances, and constipation. Pharmacists can give advice on the proper use of medications and monitor a patient's prescriptions to avoid risks of drug interactions.

Physical therapy and special equipment can enhance an individual's independence and safety throughout the course of ALS. Gentle, low-impact aerobic exercise such as walking, swimming, and stationary bicycling can strengthen unaffected muscles, improve cardiovascular health, and help patients fight fatigue and depression. Range of motion and stretching exercises can help prevent painful spasticity and shortening (contracture) of muscles. Physical therapists can recommend exercises that provide these benefits without overworking muscles. Occupational therapists can suggest devices such as ramps, braces, walkers, and wheelchairs that help individuals conserve energy and remain mobile.

People with ALS who have difficulty speaking may benefit from working with a speech therapist. These health professionals can teach individuals adaptive strategies such as techniques to help them speak louder and more clearly. As ALS progresses, speech therapists can help people develop ways for responding to yes-or-no questions with their eyes or by other nonverbal means and can recommend aids such as speech synthesizers and computer-based communication systems. These methods and devices help people communicate when they can no longer speak or produce vocal sounds.

Nutritional support is an important part of the care of people with ALS. Individuals and caregivers can learn from speech therapists and nutritionists how to plan and prepare numerous small meals throughout the day that provide enough calories, fiber, and fluid and how to avoid foods that are difficult to swallow. People may begin using suction devices to remove excess fluids or saliva and prevent choking. When individuals can no longer get enough nourishment from eating, doctors may advise inserting a feeding tube into the stomach. The use of a feeding tube also reduces the risk of choking and pneumonia that can result from inhaling liquids into the lungs. The tube is not painful and does not prevent individuals from eating food orally if they wish.

Managing Respiratory Problems

When the muscles that assist in breathing weaken, use of nocturnal ventilatory assistance (*intermittent positive pressure ventilation* [IPPV] or *bilevel positive airway pressure* [BIPAP]) may be used to aid breathing during sleep. Such devices artificially inflate the person's lungs from various external sources that are applied directly to the face or body. Individuals with ALS will have breathing tests on a regular basis to determine when to start non-invasive ventilation (NIV). When muscles are no longer able to maintain normal oxygen and carbon dioxide levels, these devices may be used full-time. The NeuRx Diaphragm Pacing System, which uses implanted electrodes and a battery pack to cause the diaphragm (breathing muscle) to contract, has been approved by the FDA to help certain individuals who have ALS and breathing problems an average benefit of up to 16 months before onset of severe respiratory failure.

Individuals may eventually consider forms of mechanical ventilation (respirators) in which a machine inflates and deflates the lungs. To be effective, this may require a tube that passes from the nose or mouth to the windpipe (trachea) and for long-term use, an operation such as a tracheostomy, in which a plastic breathing tube is inserted directly in the patient's windpipe through an opening in the neck. Patients and their families should consider several factors when deciding whether and when to use one of these options. Ventilation devices differ in their effect on the person's quality of life and in cost. Although ventilation support can ease problems with breathing and prolong survival, it does not affect the progression of ALS. People need to be fully informed about these considerations and the long-term effects of life without movement before they make decisions about ventilation support.

Social workers and home care and hospice nurses help patients, families, and caregivers with the medical, emotional, and financial challenges of coping with ALS, particularly during the final stages of the disease. Respiratory therapists can help caregivers with tasks such as operating and maintaining respirators, and home care nurses are available not only to provide medical care but also to teach caregivers about giving tube feedings and moving patients to avoid painful skin problems and contractures. Home hospice nurses work in consultation with physicians to ensure proper medication and pain control.

Section 33.2

Goodpasture Syndrome

This section includes text excerpted from "Goodpasture
Syndrome," Genetic and Rare Diseases Information
Center (GARD), September 22, 2015.

What Is Goodpasture Syndrome?

Goodpasture syndrome is an autoimmune disease of unknown
cause that affects the lungs and kidneys and is characterized by pulmonary alveolar hemorrhage (bleeding in the lungs), and a kidney
disease known as glomerulonephritis. Some use the term "Goodpasture syndrome" for the findings of glomerulonephritis and pulmonary
hemorrhage and the term "Goodpasture disease" for those patients
with glomerulonephritis, pulmonary hemorrhage, and anti-GBM antibodies. Currently, the preferred term for both conditions is "anti-GBM
antibody disease."

Circulating antibodies are directed against the collagen of the part
of the kidney known as the glomerular basement membrane (GBM),
thereby resulting in acute or rapidly progressive glomerulonephritis.
Antibodies also attack the collagen of the air sacs of the lung (alveolus)
resulting in bleeding of the lung (pulmonary hemorrhage). Anti-GBM
antibody disease is most often idiopathic, although it can occasionally
follow pulmonary infections or be associated with pulmonary injury.
Diagnosis is confirmed with the presence of anti-GBM antibody in
blood or in the kidney. The treatment of choice is plasmapheresis in
conjunction with prednisone and cyclophosphamide.

Symptoms

The signs and symptoms related to the lung disease may include:

- Hemoptysis (bleeding from the nose): In about two thirds of
  cases, precedes the kidney disease by 8–12 months. Present in
  82–90 percent of the adults

- Cough (40–60 percent of the cases)

374

- Breathing difficulty (dyspnea) in about 57–72 percent of the cases

- Pallor (the most common clinical sign)

- Crackles and rhonchi (low-pitched, rattling sound)

- Heart murmur (20–25 percent of the cases)

- Hepatomegaly (enlarged liver)

- Edema

Prompt diagnosis of pulmonary hemorrhage is vital because it is the principal cause of early death in patients with anti-GBM disease.

The signs and symptoms related to the kidney disease may include:

- Blood in urine (hematuria)

- Protein in urine (proteinuria)

- Abnormal kidney function

- Hypertension (high blood pressure) can be present but is not very common (reported in 4–17 percent of adult patients and extremely rare in children)

Signs and Symptoms

- Anemia
- Autoimmunity
- Chest pain
- Glomerulopathy
- Hemoptysis
- Proteinuria
- Pulmonary embolism
- Pulmonary infiltrates
- Respiratory insufficiency
- Vasculitis
- Hematuria
- Abnormality of temperature regulation
- Arthralgia
- Arthritis
- Myalgia
- Renal insufficiency
- Retinal detachment
- Subcutaneous hemorrhage
- Autosomal recessive inheritance
- Dyspnea
- Lomerulonephritis

Cause

There is still much to learn about the cause of Goodpasture syndrome. It is thought that a combination of genetic and environmental factors, such as cigarette smoke, inhaled hydrocarbons, and viruses play a role in the development of this autoimmune condition.

In autoimmune disorders, the body makes antibodies that attacks its own tissues. In the case of Goodpasture syndrome, antibodies form against a certain type of protein called collagen. Collagen is present in many tissues in the body. In Goodpasture syndrome, collagen in the alveoli (tiny air sacs in the lungs) and in the glomeruli (the filtering units of the kidney) is attacked. This leads to bleeding in the air sacs and inflammation in the glomeruli of the kidney. Symptoms of the antibody attack may include shortness of breath, cough, and bloody sputum, blood and protein in the urine, and kidney failure.

Genetic predisposition to Goodpasture syndrome involves the human leukocyte antigen (HLA) system. The HLA system is involved in helping our immune system know the difference between "self" and "non-self." Human leukocyte antigens determine a person's tissue type. Each person has 3 pairs of major HLA antigens. We inherit one set from each of our parents (and pass one of our two sets on to each of our children).

Diagnosis

A diagnosis of anti-GBM disease is made when a patient presents with lung hemorrhage, urinary findings such as proteinuria and hematuria, which are indicative of acute glomerulonephritis, and circulating anti–glomerular basement membrane (anti-GBM) antibodies.

A kidney biopsy is the best method for detecting anti-GBM antibodies in tissues. Some recommend doing a kidney biopsy in all cases while others suggest only doing the biopsy when the diagnosis is still in doubt. Light microscopy usually shows a feature known as crescentic glomerulonephritis, whereas immunofluorescence microscopy demonstrates a finding that is characteristic of this disease, of "linear deposition of IgG along the glomerular capillaries." Patients in whom the diagnosis of lung hemorrhage is still unclear should have bronchoscopy.

In children, the most consistent feature is 'crescentic glomerulonephritis' with either circulating anti-GBM antibodies or linear staining of IgG on the immunofluorescence. Clinical features include severe kidney malfunction in all patients and lung hemorrhage in half of them.

It is essential to promptly diagnose pulmonary hemorrhage because this is the principal cause of early death when untreated.

Conditions that affect the lung and kidney (pulmonary-renal syndromes) are important to consider and need to be ruled out when the diagnosis is not confirmed. These include granulomatosis with polyangiitis (Wegener granulomatosis), Churg-Strauss syndrome, systemic lupus erythematosus, microscopic polyangiitis, rheumathoid arthritis, IgA-mediated disorders (e.g., IgA nephropathy or Henoch-Schönlein purpura) and of immune complex–mediated renal disease (e.g., essential mixed cryoglobulinemia), community-acquired pneumonia and undifferentiated connective-tissue disease.

In children also consider Behcet Syndrome, hemosiderosis (bleeding into the lung and iron accumulation) and legionella infection.

Treatment

The treatment of choice is plasmapheresis in conjunction with prednisone and cyclophosphamide. The three main goals for the treatment are:

1. Rapidly remove circulating antibody, primarily by plasmapheresis.

2. Stop further production of antibodies using immunosuppression with medications, namely, corticosteroids (e.g., prednisone) and cyclophosphamide. In children, plasmapheresis is done together with corticosteroids and cyclophosphamide. The duration of the immunosuppressive treatment varies but is typically 6 months for corticosteroids and 3 months for cyclophosphamide.

3. Remove offending agents that may have initiated the antibody production.

After hospital discharge, patients require long-term regular visits for monitoring kidney function and for immunosuppressive therapy. If kidney function does not return, dialysis is continued indefinitely and the patient should be referred for kidney transplantation.

If the person smokes, it is recommended he or she stop. Also, if the patient is exposed to hydrocarbon in his or her occupation, he or she should consider changing jobs, as exposure to hydrocarbon has been shown to increase a person's chances of disease recurrence.

Section 33.3

Muscular Dystrophy

This section includes text excerpted from "Muscular Dystrophy:
Hope through Research," National Institute of Neurological
Disorders and Stroke (NINDS), March 4, 2016.

What Is Muscular Dystrophy?

Muscular dystrophy (MD) refers to a group of more than 30 genetic
diseases that cause progressive weakness and degeneration of skeletal muscles used during voluntary movement. The word dystrophy is
derived from the Greek *dys*, which means "difficult" or "faulty," and
troph, or "nourish." These disorders vary in age of onset, severity, and
pattern of affected muscles. All forms of MD grow worse as muscles
progressively degenerate and weaken. Many individuals eventually
lose the ability to walk.

Some types of MD also affect the heart, gastrointestinal system,
endocrine glands, spine, eyes, brain, and other organs. Respiratory
and cardiac diseases may occur, and some people may develop a swallowing disorder. MD is not contagious and cannot be brought on by
injury or activity.

What Causes MD?

All of the muscular dystrophies are inherited and involve a mutation in one of the thousands of genes that program proteins critical to
muscle integrity. The body's cells don't work properly when a protein
is altered or produced in insufficient quantity (or sometimes missing
completely). Many cases of MD occur from spontaneous mutations
that are not found in the genes of either parent, and this defect can
be passed to the next generation.

Genes are like blueprints: they contain coded messages that determine a person's characteristics or traits. They are arranged along 23
rod-like pairs of chromosomes, with one half of each pair being inherited from each parent. Each half of a chromosome pair is similar to the

other, except for one pair, which determines the sex of the individual. Muscular dystrophies can be inherited in three ways:

- *Autosomal dominant* inheritance occurs when a child receives a normal gene from one parent and a defective gene from the other parent. Autosomal means the genetic mutation can occur on any of the 22 non-sex chromosomes in each of the body's cells. Dominant means only one parent needs to pass along the abnormal gene in order to produce the disorder. In families where one parent carries a defective gene, each child has a 50 percent chance of inheriting the gene and therefore the disorder. Males and females are equally at risk and the severity of the disorder can differ from person to person.

- *Autosomal recessive* inheritance means that both parents must carry and pass on the faulty gene. The parents each have one defective gene but are not affected by the disorder. Children in these families have a 25 percent chance of inheriting both copies of the defective gene and a 50 percent chance of inheriting one gene and therefore becoming a carrier, able to pass along the defect to their children. Children of either sex can be affected by this pattern of inheritance.

- *X-linked* (or sex-linked) *recessive* inheritance occurs when a mother carries the affected gene on one of her two X chromosomes and passes it to her son (males always inherit an X chromosome from their mother and a Y chromosome from their father, while daughters inherit an X chromosome from each parent). Sons of carrier mothers have a 50 percent chance of inheriting the disorder. Daughters also have a 50 percent chance of inheriting the defective gene but usually are not affected, since the healthy X chromosome they receive from their father can offset the faulty one received from their mother. Affected fathers cannot pass an X-linked disorder to their sons but their daughters will be carriers of that disorder. Carrier females occasionally can exhibit milder symptoms of MD.

How Many People Have MD?

MD occurs worldwide, affecting all races. Its incidence varies, as some forms are more common than others. Its most common form in children, Duchenne muscular dystrophy, affects approximately 1 in every 3,500 to 6,000 male births each year in the United States. Some types of MD are more prevalent in certain countries and regions of the world. Many muscular dystrophies are familial, meaning there is some family history of the disease. Duchenne cases often have no prior family history. This is likely due to the large size of the dystrophin gene that is implicated in the disorder, making it a target for spontaneous mutations.

How Does MD Affect Muscles?

Muscles are made up of thousands of muscle fibers. Each fiber is actually a number of individual cells that have joined together during development and are encased by an outer membrane. Muscle fibers that make up individual muscles are bound together by connective tissue.

Muscles are activated when an impulse, or signal, is sent from the brain through the spinal cord and peripheral nerves (nerves that connect the central nervous system to sensory organs and muscles) to the neuromuscular junction (the space between the nerve fiber and the muscle it activates). There, a release of the chemical acetylcholine triggers a series of events that cause the muscle to contract.

The muscle fiber membrane contains a group of proteins—called the *dystrophin-glycoprotein* complex—which prevents damage as muscle fibers contract and relax. When this protective membrane is damaged, muscle fibers begin to leak the protein *creatine kinase* (needed for the chemical reactions that produce energy for muscle contractions) and take on excess calcium, which causes further harm. Affected muscle fibers eventually die from this damage, leading to progressive muscle degeneration.

Although MD can affect several body tissues and organs, it most prominently affects the integrity of muscle fibers. The disease causes muscle degeneration, progressive weakness, fiber death, fiber branching and splitting, phagocytosis (in which muscle fiber material is broken down and destroyed by scavenger cells), and, in some cases, chronic or permanent shortening of tendons and muscles. Also, overall muscle strength and tendon reflexes are usually lessened or lost due to replacement of muscle by connective tissue and fat.

Are There Other MD-Like Conditions?

There are many other heritable diseases that affect the muscles, the nerves, or the neuromuscular junction. Such diseases as inflammatory *myopathy*, progressive muscle weakness, and cardiomyopathy (heart muscle weakness that interferes with pumping ability) may produce symptoms that are very similar to those found in some forms of MD), but they are caused by different genetic defects. The differential diagnosis for people with similar symptoms includes congenital myopathy, spinal muscular atrophy, and congenital myasthenic syndromes. The sharing of symptoms among multiple neuromuscular diseases, and the prevalence of sporadic cases in families not previously affected by MD, often makes it difficult for people with MD to obtain a quick diagnosis. Gene testing can provide a definitive diagnosis for many types of MD, but not all genes have been discovered that are responsible for some types of MD. Some individuals may have signs of MD, but carry none of the currently recognized genetic mutations. Studies of other related muscle diseases may, however, contribute to what we know about MD.

How Are the Muscular Dystrophies Diagnosed?

Both the individual's medical history and a complete family history should be thoroughly reviewed to determine if the muscle disease is secondary to a disease affecting other tissues or organs or is an inherited condition. It is also important to rule out any muscle weakness resulting from prior surgery, exposure to toxins, or current medications that may affect the person's functional status or rule out many acquired muscle diseases. Thorough clinical and neurological exams can rule out disorders of the central and/or peripheral nervous systems, identify any patterns of muscle weakness and atrophy, test reflex responses and coordination, and look for contractions.

Various laboratory tests may be used to confirm the diagnosis of MD.

Blood and urine tests can detect defective genes and help identify specific neuromuscular disorders.

Exercise tests can detect elevated rates of certain chemicals following exercise and are used to determine the nature of the MD or other muscle disorder.

Genetic testing looks for genes known to either cause or be associated with inherited muscle disease.

Genetic counseling can help parents who have a family history of MD determine if they are carrying one of the mutated genes that cause the disorder.

Diagnostic imaging can help determine the specific nature of a disease or condition. One such type of imaging, called magnetic resonance imaging (MRI), is used to examine muscle quality, any atrophy or abnormalities in size, and fatty replacement of muscle tissue, as well as to monitor disease progression.

Muscle biopsies are used for diagnostic purposes, and in research settings, to monitor the course of disease and treatment effectiveness.

Immunofluorescence testing can detect specific proteins such as dystrophin within muscle fibers. Following biopsy, fluorescent markers are used to stain the sample that has the protein of interest.

Electron microscopy can identify changes in subcellular components of muscle fibers. Electron microscopy can also identify changes that characterize cell death, mutations in muscle cell mitochondria, and an increase in connective tissue seen in muscle diseases such as MD. Changes in muscle fibers that are evident in a rare form of distal MD can be seen using an electron microscope.

Neurophysiology studies can identify physical and/or chemical changes in the nervous system.

How Are the Muscular Dystrophies Treated?

There is no specific treatment that can stop or reverse the progression of any form of MD. All forms of MD are genetic and cannot be prevented at this time, aside from the use of prenatal screening interventions. However, available treatments are aimed at keeping the person independent for as long as possible and prevent complications that result from weakness, reduced mobility, and cardiac and respiratory difficulties. Treatment may involve a combination of approaches, including physical therapy, drug therapy, and surgery. The available treatments are sometimes quite effective and can have a significant impact on life expectancy and quality of life.

Section 33.4

Myasthenia Gravis

This section includes text excerpted from "Myasthenia Gravis
Fact Sheet," National Institute of Neurological Disorders and
Stroke (NINDS), May 10, 2016.

What Is Myasthenia Gravis?

Myasthenia gravis is a chronic autoimmune neuromuscular disease
characterized by varying degrees of weakness of the skeletal (voluntary) muscles of the body. The name myasthenia gravis, which is Latin
and Greek in origin, literally means "grave muscle weakness." With
current therapies, however, most cases of myasthenia gravis are not as
"grave" as the name implies. In fact, most individuals with myasthenia
gravis have a normal life expectancy.

The hallmark of myasthenia gravis is muscle weakness that
increases during periods of activity and improves after periods of rest.
Certain muscles such as those that control eye and eyelid movement,
facial expression, chewing, talking, and swallowing are often, but not
always, involved in the disorder. The muscles that control breathing
and neck and limb movements may also be affected.

What Causes Myasthenia Gravis?

Myasthenia gravis is caused by a defect in the transmission of
nerve impulses to muscles. It occurs when normal communication
between the nerve and muscle is interrupted at the neuromuscular
junction—the place where nerve cells connect with the muscles they
control. Normally when impulses travel down the nerve, the nerve
endings release a neurotransmitter substance called acetylcholine.
Acetylcholine travels from the neuromuscular junction and binds to
acetylcholine receptors which are activated and generate a muscle
contraction.

In myasthenia gravis, antibodies block, alter, or destroy the receptors for acetylcholine at the neuromuscular junction, which prevents
the muscle contraction from occurring. These antibodies are produced

by the body's own immune system. Myasthenia gravis is an autoimmune disease because the immune system—which normally protects the body from foreign organisms—mistakenly attacks itself.

What Is the Role of the Thymus Gland in Myasthenia Gravis?

The thymus gland, which lies in the chest area beneath the breastbone, plays an important role in the development of the immune system in early life. Its cells form a part of the body's normal immune system. The gland is somewhat large in infants, grows gradually until puberty, and then gets smaller and is replaced by fat with age. In adults with myasthenia gravis, the thymus gland remains large and is abnormal. It contains certain clusters of immune cells indicative of lymphoid hyperplasia—a condition usually found only in the spleen and lymph nodes during an active immune response. Some individuals with myasthenia gravis develop thymomas (tumors of the thymus gland). Thymomas are generally benign, but they can become malignant.

The relationship between the thymus gland and myasthenia gravis is not yet fully understood. Scientists believe the thymus gland may give incorrect instructions to developing immune cells, ultimately resulting in autoimmunity and the production of the acetylcholine receptor antibodies, thereby setting the stage for the attack on neuromuscular transmission.

What Are the Symptoms of Myasthenia Gravis?

Although myasthenia gravis may affect any voluntary muscle, muscles that control eye and eyelid movement, facial expression, and swallowing are most frequently affected. The onset of the disorder may be sudden and symptoms often are not immediately recognized as myasthenia gravis.

In most cases, the first noticeable symptom is weakness of the eye muscles. In others, difficulty in swallowing and slurred speech may be the first signs. The degree of muscle weakness involved in myasthenia gravis varies greatly among individuals, ranging from a localized form limited to eye muscles (ocular myasthenia), to a severe or generalized form in which many muscles—sometimes including those that control breathing—are affected. Symptoms, which vary in type and severity, may include a drooping of one or both eyelids (ptosis), blurred or double vision (diplopia) due to weakness of the muscles that control eye movements, unstable or waddling gait, a change in facial expression, difficulty in swallowing, shortness of breath, impaired speech (dysarthria), and weakness in the arms, hands, fingers, legs, and neck.

Who Gets Myasthenia Gravis?

Myasthenia gravis occurs in all ethnic groups and both genders. It most commonly affects young adult women (under 40) and older men (over 60), but it can occur at any age.

In neonatal myasthenia, the fetus may acquire immune proteins (antibodies) from a mother affected with myasthenia gravis. Generally, cases of neonatal myasthenia gravis are temporary and the child's symptoms usually disappear within 2–3 months after birth. Other children develop myasthenia gravis indistinguishable from adults. Myasthenia gravis in juveniles is uncommon.

Myasthenia gravis is not directly inherited nor is it contagious. Occasionally, the disease may occur in more than one member of the same family.

Rarely, children may show signs of congenital myasthenia or congenital myasthenic syndrome. These are not autoimmune disorders, but are caused by defective genes that produce abnormal proteins instead of those which normally would produce acetylcholine, acetylcholinesterase (the enzyme that breaks down acetylcholine), or the acetylcholine receptor and other proteins present along the muscle membrane.

How Is Myasthenia Gravis Diagnosed?

Because weakness is a common symptom of many other disorders, the diagnosis of myasthenia gravis is often missed or delayed (sometimes up to two years) in people who experience mild weakness or in those individuals whose weakness is restricted to only a few muscles.

The first steps of diagnosing myasthenia gravis include a review of the individual's medical history, and physical and neurological examinations. The physician looks for impairment of eye movements or muscle weakness without any changes in the individual's ability to feel things. If the doctor suspects myasthenia gravis, several tests are available to confirm the diagnosis.

A special blood test can detect the presence of immune molecules or acetylcholine receptor antibodies. Most patients with myasthenia gravis have abnormally elevated levels of these antibodies. Recently, a second antibody—called the anti-MuSK antibody—has been found in about 30 to 40 percent of individuals with myasthenia gravis who do not have acetylcholine receptor antibodies. This antibody can also be tested for in the blood. However, neither of these antibodies is present in some individuals with myasthenia gravis, most often in those with ocular myasthenia gravis.

The edrophonium test uses intravenous administration of edrophonium chloride to very briefly relieve weakness in people with myasthenia gravis. The drug blocks the degradation (breakdown) of acetylcholine and temporarily increases the levels of acetylcholine at the neuromuscular junction. Other methods to confirm the diagnosis include a version of nerve conduction study which tests for specific muscle "fatigue" by repetitive nerve stimulation. This test records weakening muscle responses when the nerves are repetitively stimulated by small pulses of electricity. Repetitive stimulation of a nerve during a nerve conduction study may demonstrate gradual decreases of the muscle action potential due to impaired nerve-to-muscle transmission.

Single fiber electromyography (EMG) can also detect impaired nerve-to-muscle transmission. EMG measures the electrical potential of muscle cells when single muscle fibers are stimulated by electrical impulses. Muscle fibers in myasthenia gravis, as well as other neuromuscular disorders, do not respond as well to repeated electrical stimulation compared to muscles from normal individuals.

Diagnostic imaging of the chest, using computed tomography (CT) or magnetic resonance imaging (MRI), may be used to identify the presence of a thymoma.

Pulmonary function testing, which measures breathing strength, helps to predict whether respiration may fail and lead to a myasthenic crisis.

How Is Myasthenia Gravis Treated?

There are several therapies available to help reduce and improve muscle weakness. Medications used to treat the disorder include anticholinesterase agents such as neostigmine and pyridostigmine, which help improve neuromuscular transmission and increase muscle strength. Immunosuppressive drugs such as prednisone, azathioprine, cyclosporin, mycophenolate mofetil, and tacrolimus may also be used. These medications improve muscle strength by suppressing the production of abnormal antibodies. Their use must be carefully monitored by a physician because they may cause major side effects.

Thymectomy, the surgical removal of the thymus gland (which often is abnormal in individuals with myasthenia gravis), reduces symptoms in some individuals without thymoma and may cure some people, possibly by re-balancing the immune system. Thymectomy is recommended for individuals with thymoma. Other therapies used to treat myasthenia gravis include plasmapheresis, a procedure in which serum containing the abnormal antibodies is removed from the blood while cells are replaced, and high-dose intravenous immune globulin, which temporarily modifies the immune system by infusing antibodies from donated blood. These therapies may be used to help individuals during especially difficult periods of weakness. A neurologist will determine which treatment option is best for each individual depending on the severity of the weakness, which muscles are affected, and the individual's age and other associated medical problems.

What Are Myasthenic Crises?

A myasthenic crisis occurs when the muscles that control breathing weaken to the point that ventilation is inadequate, creating a medical emergency and requiring a respirator for assisted ventilation. In individuals whose respiratory muscles are weak, crises—which generally call for immediate medical attention—may be triggered by infection, fever, or an adverse reaction to medication.

Chapter 34

Obesity Hypoventilation Syndrome (Pickwickian Syndrome)

What Is Obesity Hypoventilation Syndrome?

Obesity hypoventilation syndrome (OHS) is a breathing disorder that affects some obese people. In OHS, poor breathing results in too much carbon dioxide (hypoventilation) and too little oxygen in the blood (hypoxemia).

OHS sometimes is called Pickwickian syndrome.

What Causes Obesity Hypoventilation Syndrome?

Obesity hypoventilation syndrome (OHS) is a breathing disorder that affects some obese people. Why these people develop OHS isn't fully known. Researchers think that several factors may work together to cause OHS. These factors include:

- A respiratory system that has to work harder than normal and perhaps differently because of excess body weight. (The

This chapter includes text excerpted from "Obesity Hypoventilation Syndrome," National Heart, Lung, and Blood Institute (NHLBI), January 27, 2012. Reviewed September 2016.

respiratory system is a group of organs and tissues, including the lungs, that helps you breathe.)

- A slow response by the body to fix the problem of too much carbon dioxide and too little oxygen in the blood.

- The presence of sleep apnea, usually obstructive sleep apnea.

Who Is at Risk for Obesity Hypoventilation Syndrome?

People who are obese are at risk for obesity hypoventilation syndrome (OHS). "Obesity" refers to having too much body fat. People who are obese have body weight that's greater than what is considered healthy for a certain height.

The most useful measure of obesity is body mass index (BMI). BMI is calculated from your height and weight. In adults, a BMI of 30 or more is considered obese.

If you are obese, you're at greater risk for OHS if your BMI is 40 or higher. You're also at greater risk if most of your excess weight is around your waist, rather than at your hips. This is referred to as "abdominal obesity."

OHS tends to occur more often in men than women. At the time of diagnosis, most people are 40 to 60 years old.

What Are the Signs and Symptoms of Obesity Hypoventilation Syndrome?

Many of the signs and symptoms of obesity hypoventilation syndrome (OHS) are the same as those of obstructive sleep apnea. This is because many people who have OHS also have obstructive sleep apnea.

One of the most common signs of obstructive sleep apnea is loud and chronic (ongoing) snoring. Pauses may occur in the snoring. Choking or gasping may follow the pauses.

Other symptoms include:

- daytime sleepiness

- morning headaches

- memory, learning, or concentration problems

- feeling irritable or depressed, or having mood swings or personality changes

You also may have rapid, shallow breathing. During a physical exam, your doctor might hear abnormal heart sounds while listening to your heart with a stethoscope. He or she also might notice that the opening to your throat is small and your neck is larger than normal.

Complications of Obesity Hypoventilation Syndrome

When left untreated, OHS can cause serious problems, such as:

- Leg edema, which is swelling in the legs caused by fluid in the body's tissues.

- Pulmonary hypertension, which is increased pressure in the pulmonary arteries. These arteries carry blood from your heart to your lungs to pick up oxygen.

- Cor pulmonale, which is failure of the right side of the heart.

- Secondary erythrocytosis, which is a condition in which the body makes too many red blood cells.

How Is Obesity Hypoventilation Syndrome Diagnosed?

Obesity hypoventilation syndrome (OHS) is diagnosed based on your medical history, signs and symptoms, and test results.

How Is Obesity Hypoventilation Syndrome Treated?

Treatments for obesity hypoventilation syndrome (OHS) include breathing support, weight loss, and medicines.
The goals of treating OHS may include:

- supporting and aiding your breathing
- achieving major weight loss
- treating underlying and related conditions

Medicines

Your doctor may prescribe medicines to treat OHS (although this treatment is less common than others).

Your doctor also may advise you to avoid certain substances and medicines that can worsen OHS. Examples include alcohol, sedatives, and narcotics. They can interfere with how well your body is able to maintain normal carbon dioxide and oxygen levels.

If you're having surgery, make sure you tell your surgeon and healthcare team that you have OHS. Some medicines routinely used for surgery can worsen your condition.

How Can Obesity Hypoventilation Syndrome Be Prevented?

You can prevent obesity hypoventilation syndrome (OHS) by maintaining a healthy weight. However, not everyone who is obese develops OHS. Researchers don't fully know why only some people who are obese develop the condition.

To adopt other healthy lifestyle habits, follow these tips:

- Focus on portion size. Watch the portion sizes in fast food and other restaurants. The portions served often are enough for two or three people. Children's portion sizes should be smaller than those for adults. Cutting back on portion sizes will help you manage your calorie intake.

- Be physically active. Make personal and family time as active as possible. Find activities that everyone will enjoy. For example, go for a brisk walk, bike or rollerblade, or train together for a walk or run.

- Reduce screen time. Limit the use of TVs, computers, DVDs, and videogames; they cut back on the time for physical activity. Health experts recommend 2 hours or less a day of screen time that's not work- or homework-related.

- Keep track of your weight and body mass index (BMI). BMI is calculated from your height and weight. In adults, a BMI of 30 or more is considered obese.

Even if you have OHS, you might be able to prevent the condition from worsening. For example, avoid alcohol, sedatives, and narcotics. These substances can interfere with how well your body is able to maintain normal carbon dioxide and oxygen levels.

Chapter 35

Pulmonary Edema

Pulmonary edema, also known as lung congestion, is a medical condition in which excess fluid accumulates in the lungs. The lungs are made up of alveoli, small sacs that expand and contract with each breath. The function of alveoli is to take in oxygen and release carbon dioxide during breathing. In healthy people, this exchange of oxygen and carbon dioxide occurs naturally and without problems. For people with pulmonary edema, the alveoli accumulate fluid that prevents the exchange of oxygen and carbon dioxide. This fluid prevents oxygen from being released into the bloodstream, causing a feeling of shortness of breath.

Pulmonary edema is usually classified as cardiogenic (related to a heart problem, also known as congestive heart failure) or non-cardiogenic (caused by a health problem not related to the heart). Cardiogenic pulmonary edema is the more common form of pulmonary edema and affects an estimated two percent of Americans.

Causes

Cardiogenic pulmonary edema develops when the heart is unable to move enough blood from the lungs into the bloodstream. This causes uneven pressure inside the chambers of the heart, which in turn causes fluid to be pushed back into the lungs. This fluid fills the alveoli and prevents the lungs from functioning properly.

Cardiogenic pulmonary edema can be caused by:

- heart attack
- heart disease
- abnormal heart valve function
- abnormal arterial function
- uncontrolled hypertension (high blood pressure)

Non-cardiogenic pulmonary edema develops when the blood vessels in the lungs become damaged, causing fluid to leak from the blood vessels into the alveoli. This fluid leakage can be caused by a variety of factors, including:

- abnormal thyroid function
- kidney failure
- lung damage or pulmonary embolism
- adult respiratory distress syndrome (ARDS)
- bacterial or viral infection (pneumonia, hanta virus, dengue virus)
- major bodily injury or trauma (head injury, seizure, brain hemorrhage)
- use/abuse of certain drugs (aspirin, chemotherapy, cocaine, heroin)
- inhaled toxins (ammonia, chlorine gas, smoke inhalation)
- inhaled water (when swimming or nearly drowning)
- exposure to altitude above 8,000 feet without proper acclimation

Symptoms

Pulmonary edema symptoms may begin suddenly or develop gradually over time. Symptoms include:

- shortness of breath (the most common symptom)
- difficulty breathing when lying flat that improves upon sitting up or standing
- gasping for breath, wheezing, gurgling, feeling of drowning
- inability to speak due to shortness of breath

- difficulty breathing with exertion or exercise
- coughing up blood, bloody froth
- chest pain, irregular or rapid heartbeat
- fatigue
- swelling of abdomen or legs
- unnatural skin tone, grey or blue appearance
- excessive sweating
- anxiety, restlessness
- decreased alertness, impaired thought, poor decision making
- headache
- vomiting

Complications

If left untreated, pulmonary edema can result in severe complications. Hypertension due to pulmonary edema can increase pressure on the pulmonary artery, causing the heart to weaken and fail. This in turn can lead to swelling of the legs and abdomen, liver congestion and swelling, and accumulation of fluid in the membranes surrounding the lungs. These complications can be fatal if uncontrolled.

Diagnosis

A doctor or other health care provider can diagnose pulmonary edema using a variety of assessments and tests. A physical exam is performed to check for abnormal heart sounds, rapid or irregular heart rate, abnormal lung sounds, rapid or irregular breathing, abnormal appearance of veins in the neck, swelling of legs or abdomen, and abnormal skin color. Diagnostic blood tests, X-rays, echocardiogram, electrocardiogram, cardiac catheterization, or coronary angiogram may also be performed.

Treatment

Treatment of pulmonary edema varies depending on the nature and severity of symptoms. Common treatments include the use of supplemental oxygen, breathing assistance via mechanical ventilator, diuretic medications to reduce pressure caused by the accumulation of fluid in the lungs, narcotic medications to reduce shortness of breath and anxiety, medications to dilate blood vessels to relieve pressure on the heart, and/or medications to regulate blood pressure.

Prevention

Pulmonary edema is preventable through the maintenance of a healthy lifestyle and controlling certain health conditions. Hypertension and diabetes are two common causes of pulmonary edema and should be regulated through proper screening and health care. People at risk for pulmonary edema should follow the treatment plan prescribed by their doctor, including taking all prescription medications as directed. Following a diet that is low in salt and fat, quitting smoking, maintaining a healthy weight, getting regular exercise, and avoiding triggers such as allergens are important factors in limiting the development of pulmonary edema. Another common recommendation is to reduce or manage stress in order to limit the risk of heart problems.

References

1. "Diseases and Conditions: Pulmonary Edema," Mayo Clinic, July 24, 2014.

2. "Pulmonary Edema," Medline Plus, February 24, 2016.

3. "Pulmonary Edema," WebMD, April 15, 2016.

Chapter 36

Pulmonary Embolism

What Is Pulmonary Embolism?

Pulmonary embolism, or PE, is a sudden blockage in a lung artery. The blockage usually is caused by a blood clot that travels to the lung from a vein in the leg.

A clot that forms in one part of the body and travels in the bloodstream to another part of the body is called an embolus.

PE is a serious condition that can:

- Damage part of your lung because of a lack of blood flow to your lung tissue. This damage may lead to pulmonary hypertension (increased pressure in the pulmonary arteries).

- Cause low oxygen levels in your blood.

- Damage other organs in your body because of a lack of oxygen.

If a blood clot is large, or if there are many clots, PE can cause death.

Other Names for Pulmonary Embolism

Venous thromboembolism (VTE). This term is used for both pulmonary embolism and deep vein thrombosis (DVT).

This chapter includes text excerpted from "Pulmonary Embolism," National Center for Biotechnology Information (NCBI), U.S. National Library of Medicine (NLM), June 11, 2014.

What Causes Pulmonary Embolism?

Major Causes

PE usually begins as a blood clot in a deep vein of the leg. This condition is called deep vein thrombosis. The clot can break free, travel through the bloodstream to the lungs, and block an artery.

Blood clots can form in the deep veins of the legs if blood flow is restricted and slows down. This can happen if you don't move around for long periods, such as:

- after some types of surgery

- during a long trip in a car or airplane

- if you must stay in bed for an extended time

Blood clots are more likely to develop in veins damaged from surgery or injured in other ways.

Other Causes

Rarely, an air bubble, part of a tumor, or other tissue travels to the lungs and causes PE. Also, if a large bone in the body (such as the thigh bone) breaks, fat from the bone marrow can travel through the blood. If the fat reaches the lungs, it can cause PE.

Who Is at Risk for Pulmonary Embolism?

PE occurs equally in men and women. The risk increases with age. For every 10 years after age 60, the risk of having PE doubles.

Certain inherited conditions, such as factor V Leiden, increase the risk of blood clotting and PE.

Major Risk Factors

Your risk for PE is high if you have DVT or a history of DVT. In DVT, blood clots form in the deep veins of the body—most often in the legs. These clots can break free, travel through the bloodstream to the lungs, and block an artery.

Your risk for PE also is high if you've had the condition before.

Other Risk Factors

Other factors also can increase the risk for PE, such as:

- being bedridden or unable to move around much

- having surgery or breaking a bone (the risk goes up in the weeks following the surgery or injury)

- having certain diseases or conditions, such as a stroke, paralysis (an inability to move), chronic heart disease, or high blood pressure

- smoking

People who have recently been treated for cancer or who have a central venous catheter are more likely to develop DVT, which increases their risk for PE. A central venous catheter is a tube placed in a vein to allow easy access to the bloodstream for medical treatment.

Other risk factors for DVT include sitting for long periods (such as during long car or airplane rides), pregnancy and the 6-week period after pregnancy, and being overweight or obese. Women who take hormone therapy pills or birth control pills also are at increased risk for DVT.

The risk of developing blood clots increases as your number of risk factors increases.

What Are the Signs and Symptoms of Pulmonary Embolism?

Major Signs and Symptoms

Signs and symptoms of PE include unexplained shortness of breath, problems breathing, chest pain, coughing, or coughing up blood. An arrhythmia (irregular heartbeat) also may suggest that you have PE.

Sometimes the only signs and symptoms are related to DVT. These include swelling of the leg or along a vein in the leg, pain or tenderness in the leg, a feeling of increased warmth in the area of the leg that's swollen or tender, and red or discolored skin on the affected leg.

See your doctor right away if you have any signs or symptoms of PE or DVT. It's also possible to have PE and not have any signs or symptoms.

Other Signs and Symptoms

Some people who have PE have feelings of anxiety or dread, light-headedness or fainting, rapid breathing, sweating, or an increased heart rate.

How Is Pulmonary Embolism Diagnosed?

PE is diagnosed based on your medical history, a physical exam, and test results.

Doctors who treat patients in the emergency room often are the ones to diagnose PE with the help of a radiologist. A radiologist is a doctor who deals with X-rays and other similar tests.

Medical History and Physical Exam

To diagnose PE, the doctor will ask about your medical history. He or she will want to:

- Find out your DVT and PE risk factors

- See how likely it is that you could have PE

- Rule out other possible causes for your symptoms

Your doctor also will do a physical exam. During the exam, he or she will check your legs for signs of DVT. He or she also will check your blood pressure and your heart and lungs.

Diagnostic Tests

Many tests can help diagnose PE. Which tests you have will depend on how you feel when you get to the hospital, your risk factors, available testing options, and other conditions you could possibly have. You may have one or more of the following tests.

Ultrasound

Doctors can use ultrasound to look for blood clots in your legs. Ultrasound uses sound waves to check blood flow in your veins.

For this test, gel is put on the skin of your legs. A hand-held device called a transducer is moved back and forth over the affected areas. The transducer gives off ultrasound waves and detects their echoes as they bounce off the vein walls and blood cells.

A computer turns the echoes into a picture on a computer screen, allowing the doctor to see blood flow in your legs. If the doctor finds blood clots in the deep veins of your legs, he or she will recommend treatment.

DVT and PE both are treated with the same medicines.

Computed Tomography Scans

Doctors can use computed tomography scans, or CT scans, to look for blood clots in the lungs and legs.

For this test, dye is injected into a vein in your arm. The dye makes the blood vessels in your lungs and legs show up on X-ray images. You'll lie on a table, and an X-ray tube will rotate around you. The tube will take pictures from many angles.

This test allows doctors to detect most cases of PE. The test only takes a few minutes. Results are available shortly after the scan is done.

Lung Ventilation / Perfusion Scan

A lung ventilation/perfusion scan, or VQ scan, uses a radioactive substance to show how well oxygen and blood are flowing to all areas of your lungs. This test can help detect PE.

Pulmonary Angiography

Pulmonary angiography is another test used to diagnose PE. This test isn't available at all hospitals, and a trained specialist must do the test.

For this test, a flexible tube called a catheter is threaded through the groin (upper thigh) or arm to the blood vessels in the lungs. Dye is injected into the blood vessels through the catheter.

X-ray pictures are taken to show blood flowing through the blood vessels in the lungs. If a blood clot is found, your doctor may use the catheter to remove it or deliver medicine to dissolve it.

Blood Tests

Certain blood tests may help your doctor find out whether you're likely to have PE.

A D-dimer test measures a substance in the blood that's released when a blood clot breaks down. High levels of the substance may mean a clot is present. If your test is normal and you have few risk factors, PE isn't likely.

Other blood tests check for inherited disorders that cause blood clots. Blood tests also can measure the amount of oxygen and carbon dioxide in your blood. A clot in a blood vessel in your lungs may lower the level of oxygen in your blood.

Other Tests

To rule out other possible causes of your symptoms, your doctor may use one or more of the following tests.

- Echocardiography (echo). This test uses sound waves to create a moving picture of your heart. Doctors use echo to check heart function and detect blood clots inside the heart.

- EKG (electrocardiogram). An EKG is a simple, painless test that detects and records the heart's electrical activity.

- Chest X-ray. This test creates pictures of your lungs, heart, large arteries, ribs, and diaphragm (the muscle below your lungs).

- Chest MRI (magnetic resonance imaging). This test uses radio waves and magnetic fields to create pictures of organs and structures inside the body. MRI often can provide more information than an X-ray.

How Is Pulmonary Embolism Treated?

PE is treated with medicines, procedures, and other therapies. The main goals of treating PE are to stop the blood clot from getting bigger and keep new clots from forming.

Treatment may include medicines to thin the blood and slow its ability to clot. If your symptoms are life threatening, your doctor may give you medicine to quickly dissolve the clot. Rarely, your doctor may use surgery or another procedure to remove the clot.

Medicines

Anticoagulants, or blood thinners, decrease your blood's ability to clot. They're used to stop blood clots from getting larger and prevent clots from forming. Blood thinners don't break up blood clots that have already formed. (The body dissolves most clots with time.)

You can take blood thinners as either a pill, an injection, or through a needle or tube inserted into a vein (called intravenous, or IV, injection). Warfarin is given as a pill. (Coumadin® is a common brand name for warfarin.) Heparin is given as an injection or through an IV tube.

Your doctor may treat you with both heparin and warfarin at the same time. Heparin acts quickly. Warfarin takes 2 to 3 days before it starts to work. Once warfarin starts to work, heparin usually is stopped.

Pregnant women usually are treated with heparin only, because warfarin is dangerous for the pregnancy.

If you have DVT, treatment with blood thinners usually lasts for 3 to 6 months. If you've had blood clots before, you may need a longer period of treatment. If you're being treated for another illness, such as cancer, you may need to take blood thinners as long as PE risk factors are present.

The most common side effect of blood thinners is bleeding. This can happen if the medicine thins your blood too much. This side effect can be life threatening.

Sometimes the bleeding is internal, which is why people treated with blood thinners usually have routine blood tests. These tests, called PT and PTT tests, measure the blood's ability to clot. These tests also help your doctor make sure you're taking the right amount of medicine. Call your doctor right away if you're bruising or bleeding easily.

Thrombin inhibitors are a newer type of blood-thinning medicine. They're used to treat some types of blood clots in people who can't take heparin.

Emergency Treatment

When PE is life threatening, a doctor may use treatments that remove or break up the blood clot. These treatments are given in an emergency room or hospital.

Thrombolytics are medicines that can quickly dissolve a blood clot. They're used to treat large clots that cause severe symptoms. Because thrombolytics can cause sudden bleeding, they're used only in life-threatening situations.

Sometimes a doctor may use a catheter (a flexible tube) to reach the blood clot. The catheter is inserted into a vein in the groin (upper thigh) or arm and threaded to the clot in the lung. The doctor may use the catheter to remove the clot or deliver medicine to dissolve it.

Rarely, surgery may be needed to remove the blood clot.

Other Types of Treatment

If you can't take medicines to thin your blood, or if the medicines don't work, your doctor may suggest a vena cava filter. This device keeps blood clots from traveling to your lungs.

The filter is inserted inside a large vein called the inferior vena cava. (This vein carries blood from the body back to the heart.) The filter catches clots before they travel to the lungs. This type of treatment can prevent PE, but it won't stop other blood clots from forming.

Graduated compression stockings can reduce the chronic (ongoing) swelling that a blood clot in the leg may cause.

Graduated compression stockings are worn on the legs from the arch of the foot to just above or below the knee. These stockings are tight at the ankle and become looser as they go up the leg. This causes gentle compression (pressure) up the leg. The pressure keeps blood from pooling and clotting.

How Can Pulmonary Embolism Be Prevented?

PE begins with preventing DVT. Knowing whether you're at risk for DVT and taking steps to lower your risk are important.

- Exercise your lower leg muscles if you're sitting for a long time while traveling.

- Get out of bed and move around as soon as you're able after having surgery or being ill. The sooner you move around, the better your chance is of avoiding a blood clot.

- Take medicines to prevent clots after some types of surgery (as your doctor prescribes).

- Follow up with your doctor.

If you've already had DVT or PE, you can take more steps to prevent new blood clots from forming. Visit your doctor for regular checkups. Also, use compression stockings to prevent chronic (ongoing) swelling in your legs from DVT (as your doctor advises).

Contact your doctor right away if you have any signs or symptoms of DVT or PE.

Chapter 37

Pulmonary Hypertension

What Is Pulmonary Hypertension?

Pulmonary hypertension, or PH, is increased pressure in the pulmonary arteries. These arteries carry blood from your heart to your lungs to pick up oxygen.

PH causes symptoms such as shortness of breath during routine activity (for example, climbing two flights of stairs), tiredness, chest pain, and a racing heartbeat. As the condition worsens, its symptoms may limit all physical activity.

Types of Pulmonary Hypertension

The World Health Organization divides pulmonary hypertension (PH) into five groups. These groups are organized based on the cause of the condition.

In all groups, the average pressure in the pulmonary arteries is higher than 25 mmHg at rest or 30 mmHg during physical activity. The pressure in normal pulmonary arteries is 8–20 mmHg at rest.

(Note that group 1 is called pulmonary arterial hypertension (PAH) and groups 2 through 5 are called pulmonary hypertension. However, together all groups are called pulmonary hypertension.)

This chapter includes text excerpted from "Pulmonary Hypertension," National Heart, Lung, and Blood Institute (NHLBI), August 2, 2011. Reviewed September 2016.

Group 1 Pulmonary Arterial Hypertension

Group 1 PAH includes:

- PAH that has no known cause

- PAH that's inherited (passed from parents to children through genes)

- PAH that's caused by drugs or toxins, such as street drugs and certain diet medicines

- PAH that's caused by conditions such as:

  - Connective tissue diseases. (Connective tissue helps support all parts of your body, including your skin, eyes, and heart.)

  - HIV infection

  - Liver disease

  - Congenital heart disease. This is heart disease that's present at birth.

  - Sickle cell disease

  - Schistosomiasis. This is an infection caused by a parasite. Schistosomiasis is one of the most common causes of PAH in many parts of the world.

  - PAH that's caused by conditions that affect the veins and small blood vessels of the lungs.

Group 2 Pulmonary Hypertension

Group 2 includes PH with left heart disease. Conditions that affect the left side of the heart, such as mitral valve disease or long-term high blood pressure, can cause left heart disease and PH. Left heart disease is likely the most common cause of PH.

Group 3 Pulmonary Hypertension

Group 3 includes PH associated with lung diseases, such as COPD (chronic obstructive pulmonary disease) and interstitial lung diseases. Interstitial lung diseases cause scarring of the lung tissue.

Group 3 also includes PH associated with sleep-related breathing disorders, such as sleep apnea.

Group 4 Pulmonary Hypertension

Group 4 includes PH caused by blood clots in the lungs or blood clotting disorders.

Group 5 Pulmonary Hypertension

Group 5 includes PH caused by various other diseases or conditions. Examples include:

- Blood disorders, such as polycythemia vera and essential thrombocythemia.

- Systemic disorders, such as sarcoidosis and vasculitis. Systemic disorders involve many of the body's organs.

- Metabolic disorders, such as thyroid disease and glycogen storage disease. (In glycogen storage disease, the body's cells don't use a form of glucose (sugar) properly.)

- Other conditions, such as tumors that press on the pulmonary arteries and kidney disease.

Other Names for Pulmonary Hypertension

Group 1 pulmonary arterial hypertension (PAH) that occurs without a known cause often is called primary PAH or idiopathic PAH.

Group 1 PAH that occurs with a known cause often is called associated PAH. For example, PAH that occurs in a person who has scleroderma might be called "PAH occurring in association with scleroderma," or simply "scleroderma-associated PAH."

Groups 2–5 pulmonary hypertension (PH) sometimes are called secondary PH.

What Causes Pulmonary Hypertension?

Pulmonary hypertension (PH) begins with inflammation and changes in the cells that line your pulmonary arteries. Other factors also can affect the pulmonary arteries and cause PH. For example, the condition may develop if:

- The walls of the arteries tighten.

- The walls of the arteries are stiff at birth or become stiff from an overgrowth of cells.

- Blood clots form in the arteries.

407

These changes make it hard for your heart to push blood through your pulmonary arteries and into your lungs. Thus, the pressure in the arteries rises, causing PH.

Many factors can contribute to the process that leads to the different types of PH.

Group 1 pulmonary arterial hypertension (PAH) may have no known cause, or the condition may be inherited. ("Inherited" means the condition is passed from parents to children through genes.)

Some diseases and conditions also can cause group 1 PAH. Examples include HIV infection, congenital heart disease, and sickle cell disease. Also, the use of street drugs (such as cocaine) and certain diet medicines can lead to PAH.

Many diseases and conditions can cause groups 2 through 5 PH (often called secondary PH), including:

- mitral valve disease

- lung diseases, such as COPD (chronic obstructive pulmonary disease)

- sleep apnea

- sarcoidosis

Who Is at Risk for Pulmonary Hypertension?

The exact number of people who have pulmonary hypertension (PH) isn't known.

Group 1 pulmonary arterial hypertension (PAH) without a known cause is rare. It affects women more often than men. People who have group 1 PAH tend to be overweight.

PH that occurs with another disease or condition is more common.

PH usually develops between the ages of 20 and 60, but it can occur at any age. People who are at increased risk for PH include:

- Those who have a family history of the condition.

- Those who have certain diseases or conditions, such as heart and lung diseases, liver disease, HIV infection, or blood clots in the pulmonary arteries.

- Those who use street drugs (such as cocaine) or certain diet medicines.

- Those who live at high altitudes.

What Are the Signs and Symptoms of Pulmonary Hypertension

Signs and symptoms of pulmonary hypertension (PH) may include:

- shortness of breath during routine activity, such as climbing two flights of stairs
- tiredness
- chest pain
- a racing heartbeat
- pain on the upper right side of the abdomen
- decreased appetite

As PH worsens, you may find it hard to do any physical activities. At this point, other signs and symptoms may include:

- feeling light-headed, especially during physical activity
- fainting at times
- swelling in your legs and ankles
- a bluish color on your lips and skin

How Is Pulmonary Hypertension Diagnosed?

Your doctor will diagnose pulmonary hypertension (PH) based on your medical and family histories, a physical exam, and the results from tests and procedures.

PH can develop slowly. In fact, you may have it for years and not know it. This is because the condition has no early signs or symptoms.

When symptoms do occur, they're often like those of other heart and lung conditions, such as asthma. This makes PH hard to diagnose.

Medical and Family Histories

Your doctor may ask about your signs and symptoms and how and when they began. He or she also may ask whether you have other medical conditions that can cause PH.

Your doctor will want to know whether you have any family members who have or have had PH. People who have a family history of PH are at higher risk for the condition.

Physical Exam

During the physical exam, your doctor will listen to your heart and lungs with a stethoscope. He or she also will check your ankles and legs for swelling and your lips and skin for a bluish color. These are signs of PH.

Diagnostic Tests and Procedures

Your doctor may recommend tests and procedures to confirm a diagnosis of PH and to look for its underlying cause. Your doctor also will use test results to find out the severity of your PH.

Tests and Procedures to Confirm a Diagnosis

- Echocardiography
- Chest X-ray
- Electrocardiogram (EKG)
- Right heart catheterization

Tests to Look for the Underlying Cause of Pulmonary Hypertension

- Chest CT scan
- Chest MRI
- Lung function tests
- Polysomnogram (PSG)
- Lung ventilation/perfusion (VQ) scan
- Blood tests

Finding out the Severity of Pulmonary Hypertension

Exercise testing is used to find out the severity of PH. This testing consists of either a 6-minute walk test or a cardiopulmonary exercise test.

A 6-minute walk test measures the distance you can quickly walk in 6 minutes. A cardiopulmonary exercise test measures how well your lungs and heart work while you exercise on a treadmill or bicycle.

During exercise testing, your doctor will rate your activity level. Your level is linked to the severity of your PH. The rating system ranges from class 1 to class 4.

- Class 1 has no limits. You can do regular physical activities, such as walking or climbing stairs. These activities don't cause PH symptoms, such as tiredness, shortness of breath, or chest pain.

- Class 2 has slight or mild limits. You're comfortable while resting, but regular physical activity causes PH symptoms.

- Class 3 has marked or noticeable limits. You're comfortable while resting. However, walking even one or two blocks or climbing one flight of stairs can cause PH symptoms.

- Class 4 has severe limits. You're not able to do any physical activity without discomfort. You also may have PH symptoms while at rest.

Over time, you may need more exercise tests to find out how well your treatments are working. Each time testing is done, your doctor will compare your activity level with the previous one.

How Is Pulmonary Hypertension Treated?

Pulmonary hypertension (PH) has no cure. However, treatment may help relieve symptoms and slow the progress of the disease.

PH is treated with medicines, procedures, and other therapies. Treatment will depend on what type of PH you have and its severity.

Group 1 Pulmonary Arterial Hypertension

Group 1 pulmonary arterial hypertension (PAH) includes PH that's inherited, that has no known cause, or that's caused by certain drugs or conditions. Treatments for group 1 PAH include medicines and medical procedures.

Medicines

Your doctor may prescribe medicines to relax the blood vessels in your lungs and reduce excess cell growth in the blood vessels. As the blood vessels relax, more blood can flow through them.

Your doctor may prescribe medicines that are taken by mouth, inhaled, or injected.

Examples of medicines for group 1 PAH include:

- phosphodiesterase-5 inhibitors, such as sildenafil

- prostanoids, such as epoprostenol

- endothelin receptor antagonists, such as bosentan and ambrisentan

- calcium channel blockers, such as diltiazem

Your doctor may prescribe one or more of these medicines. To find out which of these medicines works best, you'll likely have an acute vasoreactivity test. This test shows how the pressure in your pulmonary arteries reacts to certain medicines. The test is done during right heart catheterization.

Medical and Surgical Procedures

If you have group 1 PAH, your doctor may recommend one or more of the following procedures.

Atrial septostomy. For this procedure, a thin, flexible tube called a catheter is put into a blood vessel in your leg and threaded to your heart. The tube is then put through the wall that separates your right and left atria (the upper chambers of your heart). This wall is called the septum. A tiny balloon on the tip of the tube is inflated. This creates an opening between the atria. This procedure relieves the pressure in the right atria and increases blood flow. Atrial septostomy is rarely done in the United States.

Lung transplant. A lung transplant is surgery to replace a person's diseased lung with a healthy lung from a deceased donor. This procedure may be used for people who have severe lung disease that's causing PAH.

Heart–lung transplant. A heart–lung transplant is surgery in which both the heart and lung are replaced with healthy organs from a deceased donor.

Group 2 Pulmonary Hypertension

Conditions that affect the left side of the heart, such as mitral valve disease, can cause group 2 PH. Treating the underlying condition will help treat PH. Treatments may include lifestyle changes, medicines, and surgery.

Group 3 Pulmonary Hypertension

Lung diseases, such as COPD (chronic obstructive pulmonary disease) and interstitial lung disease, can cause group 3 PH. Certain sleep disorders, such as sleep apnea, also can cause group 3 PH.

If you have this type of PH, you may need oxygen therapy. This treatment raises the level of oxygen in your blood. You'll likely get the oxygen through soft, plastic prongs that fit into your nose. Oxygen therapy can be done at home or in a hospital.

Your doctor also may recommend other treatments if you have an underlying lung disease.

Group 4 Pulmonary Hypertension

Blood clots in the lungs or blood clotting disorders can cause group 4 PH. If you have this type of PH, your doctor will likely prescribe blood-thinning medicines. These medicines prevent clots from forming or getting larger.

Sometimes doctors use surgery to remove scarring in the pulmonary arteries due to old blood clots.

Group 5 Pulmonary Hypertension

Various diseases and conditions, such as thyroid disease and sarcoidosis, can cause group 5 PH. An object, such as a tumor, pressing on the pulmonary arteries also can cause group 5 PH.

Group 5 PH is treated by treating its cause.

All Types of Pulmonary Hypertension

Several treatments may be used for all types of PH. These treatments include:

- Diuretics, also called water pills. These medicines help reduce fluid buildup in your body, including swelling in your ankles and feet.

- Blood-thinning medicines. These medicines help prevent blood clots from forming or getting larger.

- Digoxin. This medicine helps the heart beat stronger and pump more blood. Digoxin sometimes is used to control the heart rate if abnormal heart rhythms, such as atrial fibrillation or atrial flutter, occur.

- Oxygen therapy. This treatment raises the level of oxygen in your blood.

- Physical activity. Regular activity may help improve your ability to be active. Talk with your doctor about a physical activity plan that's safe for you.

Chapter 38

Traumatic Lung Disorders

Chapter Contents

Section 38.1

Acute Respiratory Distress Syndrome (ARDS)

This section includes text excerpted from "ARDS," National
Heart, Lung, and Blood Institute (NHLBI), January 12, 2012.
Reviewed September 2016.

What Is ARDS?

ARDS, or acute respiratory distress syndrome, is a lung condition
that leads to low oxygen levels in the blood. ARDS can be life threatening because your body's organs need oxygen-rich blood to work well.

People who develop ARDS often are very ill with another disease
or have major injuries. They might already be in the hospital when
they develop ARDS.

Other Names for ARDS

- Acute lung injury

- Adult respiratory distress syndrome

- Increased-permeability pulmonary edema

- Noncardiac pulmonary edema

In the past, ARDS was called stiff lung, shock lung, and wet lung.

What Causes ARDS?

Many conditions or factors can directly or indirectly injure the lungs
and lead to ARDS. Some common ones are:

- Sepsis. This is a condition in which bacteria infect the
  bloodstream.

- Pneumonia. This is an infection in the lungs.

- Severe bleeding caused by an injury to the body.

- An injury to the chest or head, like a severe blow.

- Breathing in harmful fumes or smoke.

- Inhaling vomited stomach contents from the mouth.

It's not clear why some very sick or seriously injured people develop ARDS and others don't.

Who Is at Risk for ARDS?

People at risk for ARDS have a condition or illness that can directly or indirectly injure their lungs.

Direct Lung Injury

Conditions that can directly injure the lungs include:

- Pneumonia. This is an infection in the lungs.

- Breathing in harmful fumes or smoke.

- Inhaling vomited stomach contents from the mouth.

- Using a ventilator. This is a machine that helps people breathe; rarely, it can injure the lungs.

- Nearly drowning.

Indirect Lung Injury

Conditions that can indirectly injure the lungs include:

- Sepsis. This is a condition in which bacteria infect the bloodstream.

- Severe bleeding caused by an injury to the body or having many blood transfusions.

- An injury to the chest or head, such as a severe blow.

- Pancreatitis. This is a condition in which the pancreas becomes irritated or infected. The pancreas is a gland that releases enzymes and hormones.

- Fat embolism. This is a condition in which fat blocks an artery. A physical injury, like a broken bone, can lead to a fat embolism.

- Drug reaction.

What Are the Signs and Symptoms of ARDS?

The first signs and symptoms of ARDS are feeling like you can't get enough air into your lungs, rapid breathing, and a low blood oxygen level.

Other signs and symptoms depend on the cause of ARDS. They may occur before ARDS develops. For example, if pneumonia is causing ARDS, you may have a cough and fever before you feel short of breath.

Sometimes people who have ARDS develop signs and symptoms such as low blood pressure, confusion, and extreme tiredness. This may mean that the body's organs, such as the kidneys and heart, aren't getting enough oxygen-rich blood.

People who develop ARDS often are in the hospital for other serious health problems. Rarely, people who aren't hospitalized have health problems that lead to ARDS, such as severe pneumonia.

If you have trouble breathing, call your doctor right away. If you have severe shortness of breath, call 9–1–1.

Complications from ARDS

If you have ARDS, you can develop other medical problems while in the hospital. The most common problems are:

- Infections. Being in the hospital and lying down for a long time can put you at risk for infections, such as pneumonia. Being on a ventilator also puts you at higher risk for infections.

- A pneumothorax (collapsed lung). This is a condition in which air or gas collects in the space around the lungs. This can cause one or both lungs to collapse. The air pressure from a ventilator can cause this condition.

- Lung scarring. ARDS causes the lungs to become stiff (scarred). It also makes it hard for the lungs to expand and fill with air. Being on a ventilator also can cause lung scarring.

- Blood clots. Lying down for long periods can cause blood clots to form in your body. A blood clot that forms in a vein deep in your body is called a deep vein thrombosis. This type of blood clot can break off, travel through the bloodstream to the lungs, and block blood flow. This condition is called pulmonary embolism.

How Is ARDS Diagnosed?

Your doctor will diagnose ARDS based on your medical history, a physical exam, and test results.

Medical History

Your doctor will ask whether you have or have recently had conditions that could lead to ARDS.

Your doctor also will ask whether you have heart problems, such as heart failure. Heart failure can cause fluid to build up in your lungs.

Physical Exam

ARDS may cause abnormal breathing sounds, such as crackling. Your doctor will listen to your lungs with a stethoscope to hear these sounds.

He or she also will listen to your heart and look for signs of extra fluid in other parts of your body. Extra fluid may mean you have heart or kidney problems.

Your doctor will look for a bluish color on your skin and lips. A bluish color means your blood has a low level of oxygen. This is a possible sign of ARDS.

Diagnostic Tests

You may have ARDS or another condition that causes similar symptoms. To find out, your doctor may recommend one or more of the following tests.

Initial Tests

The first tests done are:

- An arterial blood gas test. This blood test measures the oxygen level in your blood using a sample of blood taken from an artery. A low blood oxygen level might be a sign of ARDS.

- Chest X-ray. This test creates pictures of the structures in your chest, such as your heart, lungs, and blood vessels. A chest X-ray can show whether you have extra fluid in your lungs.

- Blood tests, such as a complete blood count, blood chemistries, and blood cultures. These tests help find the cause of ARDS, such as an infection.

- A sputum culture. This test is used to study the spit you've coughed up from your lungs. A sputum culture can help find the cause of an infection.

Other Tests

Other tests used to diagnose ARDS include:

- Chest computed tomography scan, or chest CT scan. This test uses a computer to create detailed pictures of your lungs. A chest CT scan may show lung problems, such as fluid in the lungs, signs of pneumonia, or a tumor.

- Heart tests that look for signs of heart failure. Heart failure is a condition in which the heart can't pump enough blood to meet the body's needs. This condition can cause fluid to build up in your lungs.

How Is ARDS Treated?

ARDS is treated in a hospital's intensive care unit. Current treatment approaches focus on improving blood oxygen levels and providing supportive care. Doctors also will try to pinpoint and treat the underlying cause of the condition.

Oxygen Therapy

One of the main goals of treating ARDS is to provide oxygen to your lungs and other organs (such as your brain and kidneys). Your organs need oxygen to work properly.

Oxygen usually is given through nasal prongs or a mask that fits over your mouth and nose. However, if your oxygen level doesn't rise or it's still hard for you to breathe, your doctor will give you oxygen through a breathing tube. He or she will insert the flexible tube through your mouth or nose and into your windpipe.

Before inserting the tube, your doctor will squirt or spray a liquid medicine into your throat (and possibly your nose) to make it numb. Your doctor also will give you medicine through an intravenous (IV) line in your bloodstream to make you sleepy and relaxed.

The breathing tube will be connected to a machine that supports breathing (a ventilator). The ventilator will fill your lungs with oxygen-rich air.

Your doctor will adjust the ventilator as needed to help your lungs get the right amount of oxygen. This also will help prevent injury to your lungs from the pressure of the ventilator.

You'll use the breathing tube and ventilator until you can breathe on your own. If you need a ventilator for more than a few days, your doctor may do a tracheotomy.

This procedure involves making a small cut in your neck to create an opening to the windpipe. The opening is called a tracheostomy. Your doctor will place the breathing tube directly into the windpipe. The tube is then connected to the ventilator.

Supportive Care

Supportive care refers to treatments that help relieve symptoms, prevent complications, or improve quality of life. Supportive approaches used to treat ARDS include:

- Medicines to help you relax, relieve discomfort, and treat pain.

- Ongoing monitoring of heart and lung function (including blood pressure and gas exchange).

- Nutritional support. People who have ARDS often suffer from malnutrition. Thus, extra nutrition may be given through a feeding tube.

- Treatment for infections. People who have ARDS are at higher risk for infections, such as pneumonia. Being on a ventilator also increases the risk of infections. Doctors use antibiotics to treat pneumonia and other infections.

- Prevention of blood clots. Lying down for long periods can cause blood clots to form in the deep veins of your body. These clots can travel to your lungs and block blood flow (a condition called pulmonary embolism). Blood-thinning medicines and other treatments, such as compression stocking (stockings that create gentle pressure up the leg), are used to prevent blood clots.

- Prevention of intestinal bleeding. People who receive long-term support from a ventilator are at increased risk of bleeding in the intestines. Medicines can reduce this risk.

- Fluids. You may be given fluids to improve blood flow through your body and to provide nutrition. Your doctor will make sure you get the right amount of fluids. Fluids usually are given through an IV line inserted into one of your blood vessels.

Section 38.2

Atelectasis

This section includes text excerpted from "Atelectasis," National Heart, Lung, and Blood Institute (NHLBI), January 13, 2012. Reviewed September 2016.

What Is Atelectasis?

Atelectasis is a condition in which one or more areas of your lungs collapse or don't inflate properly. If only a small area or a few small areas of the lungs are affected, you may have no signs or symptoms.

If a large area or several large areas of the lungs are affected, they may not be able to deliver enough oxygen to your blood. This can cause symptoms and complications.

Other Names for Atelectasis

• Closed lung

• Partial lung collapse

What Causes Atelectasis?

Atelectasis can occur if the lungs can't fully expand and fill with air. Atelectasis has many causes.

Conditions and Factors That Prevent Deep Breathing and Coughing

Conditions and factors that prevent deep breathing and coughing can cause atelectasis. For example, if you're taking shallow breaths or breathing with the help of a ventilator, your lungs don't fill with air in the normal way.

Normally, when you take a deep breath, the base (bottom) and the back of your lungs fill with air first. However, if you're taking shallow breaths or using a ventilator, air may not make it all the way to the air sacs at the bottom of your lungs. Thus, these air sacs won't inflate properly.

Atelectasis is very common after surgery. The medicine used during surgery to temporarily put you to sleep can decrease or stop your normal effort to breathe and urge to cough. Sometimes, especially after chest or abdominal surgery, pain may keep you from wanting to take deep breaths. As a result, part of your lung may collapse or not inflate right.

Pressure from outside the lungs also may make it hard to take deep breaths. A number of factors can cause pressure outside the lungs. Examples include a tumor, a tight body cast, a bone deformity, or pleural effusion (fluid buildup between the ribs and the lungs).

Lung conditions and other medical disorders that affect your ability to breathe deeply or cough and clear mucus from your lungs also may lead to atelectasis. One example is respiratory distress syndrome (RDS).

RDS is a breathing disorder that affects some newborns. It's more common in premature infants because their lungs aren't able to make enough surfactant. Surfactant is a liquid that coats the inside of the lungs and helps keep the air sacs open. Without enough surfactant, part of the lungs may collapse.

Other lung conditions and medical disorders that can cause atelectasis include pneumonia, lung cancer, and neuromuscular diseases. Rarely, asthma, COPD (chronic obstructive pulmonary disease), and cystic fibrosis are associated with atelectasis.

Migrating atelectasis in newborns is rare and may be caused by neuromuscular diseases. "Migrating" means that the part of the lung that collapses will change depending on the position of the baby.

An Airway Blockage

An airway blockage also can cause atelectasis. A blockage may be due to a foreign object (such as an inhaled peanut), a mucus plug, lung cancer, or a poorly placed breathing tube from a ventilator.

When a blockage occurs, the air that's already in the air sacs is absorbed into the bloodstream. New air can't get past the blockage to refill the air sacs, so the affected area of lung deflates.

Who Is at Risk for Atelectasis?

You might be at risk for atelectasis if you can't take deep breaths or cough, or if you have an airway blockage.

Conditions that can increase your risk for atelectasis include:

- Surgery in which you're given medicine to make you sleep. This medicine can decrease or stop your normal effort to breathe and urge to cough.

- Any condition or factor that causes pain when you breathe. Examples include surgery on your chest or abdomen, trauma, broken ribs, or pleurisy (inflammation of the membrane that surrounds your lungs and lines your chest cavity).

- Being on a ventilator (a machine that supports breathing).

- A blockage in your airway due to a foreign object, a mucus plug, lung cancer, or a poorly placed breathing tube.

- Lung conditions and other medical disorders that affect your ability to breathe deeply or cough. Examples include respiratory distress syndrome, pneumonia, lung cancer, and neuromuscular diseases. Rarely, asthma, COPD (chronic obstructive pulmonary disease), and cystic fibrosis are associated with atelectasis.

People who have one of the conditions above and who smoke or are obese are at greater risk for atelectasis than people who don't smoke or aren't obese.

Infants and toddlers (birth to 3 years old) who have risk factors for atelectasis seem to develop the condition more easily than adults.

What Are the Signs and Symptoms of Atelectasis?

Atelectasis likely won't cause signs or symptoms if it only affects a small area of lung.

If atelectasis affects a large area of lung, especially if it occurs suddenly, it may cause a low level of oxygen in your blood. As a result, you may feel short of breath. Your heart rate and breathing rate may increase, and your skin and lips may turn blue.

Other symptoms might be related to the underlying cause of the atelectasis (for example, chest pain due to surgery).

If your child has atelectasis, you may notice that he or she seems agitated, anxious, or scared.

How Is Atelectasis Diagnosed?

Your doctor will diagnose atelectasis based on your signs and symptoms and the results from tests and procedures. Atelectasis might be detected as a result of a chest X-ray done for an underlying lung condition.

Atelectasis usually is diagnosed by a radiologist, pulmonologist (lung specialist), emergency medicine physician, or a primary care doctor (such as a pediatrician, internal medicine specialist, or family practitioner).

Diagnostic Tests and Procedures

The most common test used to diagnose atelectasis is a chest X-ray. A chest X-ray is a painless test that creates pictures of the structures inside your chest, such as your heart, lungs, and blood vessels.

Your doctor also may recommend a chest computed tomography scan, or chest CT scan. This test creates precise pictures of the structures in your chest. A chest CT scan is a type of X-ray. However, the pictures from a chest CT scan show more details than pictures from a standard chest X-ray.

Atelectasis often resolves without treatment. If the condition is severe or lasts a long time and your doctor thinks it's caused by an airway blockage, he or she may use bronchoscopy. This procedure is used to look inside your airway.

During the procedure, your doctor passes a thin, flexible tube called a bronchoscope through your nose (or sometimes your mouth), down your throat, and into your airway. If you have a breathing tube, the bronchoscope can be passed through the tube to your airway.

A light and small camera on the bronchoscope allow your doctor to see inside your airway. Your doctor also can remove blockages during the procedure.

How Is Atelectasis Treated?

The main goals of treating atelectasis are to treat the cause of the condition and to reexpand the collapsed lung tissue. Treatment may vary based on the underlying cause of the atelectasis.

Atelectasis Caused by Surgery

If atelectasis is caused by surgery, your doctor may recommend that you take the following steps to fully expand your lungs:

- Perform deep breathing exercises. This is very important after surgery. While in the hospital, you may use a device called an incentive spirometer. This device measures how much air you're breathing in and how fast you're breathing in. Using this device encourages you to breathe in deeply and slowly.

- Change your position. Sit up or walk around as soon as possible after surgery with your doctor's permission.

- Make an effort to cough. Coughing helps clear mucus and other substances from your airways.

Your doctor also may suggest using positive end-expiratory pressure (PEEP) or continuous positive airway pressure (CPAP). Both devices use mild air pressure to help keep the airways and air sacs open.

Atelectasis Caused by Pressure from outside the Lungs

If pressure from outside the lungs causes atelectasis, your doctor will treat the cause of the pressure. For example, if the cause is a tumor or fluid buildup, your doctor will remove the tumor or fluid. This will allow your lung to fully expand.

Atelectasis Caused by a Blockage

If a blockage causes atelectasis, you'll receive treatment to remove the blockage or relieve it. If the blockage is from an inhaled object, such as a peanut, your doctor will remove it during bronchoscopy.

If a mucus plug is blocking your airways, your doctor may use suction to remove it. Other treatments also can help clear excess mucus from the lungs, such as:

- Chest clapping or percussion. This treatment involves pounding your chest and back over and over with your hands or a device to loosen the mucus from your lungs so you can cough it up.

- Postural drainage. For this treatment, your bed may be tilted so that your head is lower than your chest. This allows mucus to drain more easily.

- Medicines. Your doctor may prescribe medicines to help open your airways or to loosen mucus.

Atelectasis Caused by a Lung Condition or Other Medical Disorder

If a lung condition or other medical disorder causes atelectasis, your doctor will treat the underlying cause with medicines, procedures, or other therapies.

How Can Atelectasis Be Prevented?

Not smoking before surgery can lower your risk of atelectasis. If you smoke, ask your doctor how far in advance of your surgery you should quit smoking.

After surgery, your doctor may recommend that you take the following steps to fully expand your lungs:

- Perform deep breathing exercises. These exercises are very important after surgery. While in the hospital, you may use a device called an incentive spirometer. This device measures how much air you're breathing in and how fast you're breathing in. Using this device encourages you to breathe deeply and slowly.

- Change your position. Sit up or walk around as soon as possible after surgery (with your doctor's permission).

- Make an effort to cough. Coughing helps clear mucus and other substances from your airways.

If deep breathing is painful, your doctor may prescribe medicines to control the pain. This can make it easier for you to take deep breaths and fully expand your lungs.

Section 38.3

Primary Spontaneous Pneumothorax

This section includes text excerpted from "Primary Spontaneous Pneumothorax," Genetics Home Reference (GHR), National Institute of Health (NIH), November 2012. Reviewed September 2016.

Primary spontaneous pneumothorax is an abnormal accumulation of air in the space between the lungs and the chest cavity (called the pleural space) that can result in the partial or complete collapse of a lung. This type of pneumothorax is described as primary because it occurs in the absence of lung disease such as emphysema. Spontaneous means the pneumothorax was not caused by an injury such as a rib fracture. Primary spontaneous pneumothorax is likely due to the formation of small sacs of air (blebs) in lung tissue that rupture, causing air to leak into the pleural space. Air in the pleural space creates pressure on the lung and can lead to its collapse. A person with this condition may feel chest pain on the side of the collapsed lung and shortness of breath.

Blebs may be present on an individual's lung (or lungs) for a long time before they rupture. Many things can cause a bleb to rupture, such as changes in air pressure or a very sudden deep breath. Often, people who experience a primary spontaneous pneumothorax have no prior sign of illness; the blebs themselves typically do not cause any symptoms and are visible only on medical imaging. Affected individuals may have one bleb to more than thirty blebs. Once a bleb ruptures and causes a pneumothorax, there is an estimated 13 to 60 percent chance that the condition will recur.

Frequency

Primary spontaneous pneumothorax is more common in men than in women. This condition occurs in 7.4 to 18 per 100,000 men each year and 1.2 to 6 per 100,000 women each year.

Genetic Changes

Mutations in the *FLCN* gene can cause primary spontaneous pneumothorax, although these mutations appear to be a very rare cause of this condition. The *FLCN* gene provides instructions for making a protein called folliculin. In the lungs, folliculin is found in the connective tissue cells that allow the lungs to contract and expand when breathing. Folliculin is also produced in cells that line the small air sacs (alveoli). Researchers have not determined the protein's function, but they believe it may help control the growth and division of cells. Folliculin may play a role in repairing and re-forming lung tissue following damage. Researchers have not determined how *FLCN* gene mutations lead to the formation of blebs and increase the risk of primary spontaneous pneumothorax. One theory is that the altered folliculin protein may trigger inflammation within the lung tissue that could alter and damage the tissue, causing blebs.

Primary spontaneous pneumothorax most often occurs in people without an identified gene mutation. The cause of the condition in these individuals is often unknown. Tall young men are at increased risk of developing primary spontaneous pneumothorax; researchers suggest that rapid growth of the chest during growth spurts may increase the likelihood of forming blebs. Smoking can also contribute to the development of primary spontaneous pneumothorax.

Mutations in the *FLCN* gene can cause primary spontaneous pneumothorax, although these mutations appear to be a very rare cause of this condition. The *FLCN* gene provides instructions for making a protein called folliculin. In the lungs, folliculin is found in the connective tissue cells that allow the lungs to contract and expand when breathing. Folliculin is also produced in cells that line the small air sacs (alveoli). Researchers have not determined the protein's function, but they believe it may help control the growth and division of cells. Folliculin may play a role in repairing and re-forming lung tissue following damage. Researchers have not determined how *FLCN* gene mutations lead to the formation of blebs and increase the risk of primary spontaneous pneumothorax. One theory is that the altered folliculin protein may trigger inflammation within the lung tissue that could alter and damage the tissue, causing blebs.

Primary spontaneous pneumothorax most often occurs in people without an identified gene mutation. The cause of the condition in these individuals is often unknown. Tall young men are at increased risk of developing primary spontaneous pneumothorax; researchers suggest that rapid growth of the chest during growth spurts may increase the likelihood of forming blebs. Smoking can also contribute to the development of primary spontaneous pneumothorax.

Inheritance Pattern

When this condition is caused by mutations in the *FLCN* gene, it is inherited in an autosomal dominant pattern, which means one copy of the altered gene in each cell is sufficient to cause the disorder. In most cases, a person inherits the *FLCN* gene mutation from an affected parent. People who have an *FLCN* gene mutation associated with primary spontaneous pneumothorax all appear to develop blebs, but it is estimated that only 40 percent of those individuals go on to have a primary spontaneous pneumothorax.

Other Names for This Condition

- Pneumothorax
- PSP
- Spontaneous pneumothorax

Chapter 39

Respiratory Conditions in Travelers

Chapter Contents

Section 39.1

Respiratory Infections

This section includes text excerpted from "Respiratory Infections," Centers for Disease Control and Prevention (CDC), July 10, 2015.

Respiratory infection is a leading cause of seeking medical care in returning travelers. Respiratory infections occur in up to 20 percent of all travelers, which is almost as common as travelers diarrhea. Upper respiratory infection is more common than lower respiratory infection. In general, the types of respiratory infections that affect travelers are similar to those in nontravelers, and exotic causes are rare. Clinicians must inquire about history of travel when evaluating a patient for respiratory infections.

Infectious Agent

Viral pathogens are the most common cause of respiratory infection in travelers; causative agents include rhinovirus, respiratory syncytial virus, influenza virus, parainfluenza virus, human metapneumovirus, measles, mumps, adenovirus, and coronavirus. Clinicians also need to consider novel viral causes of respiratory infection in travelers, including Middle East Respiratory Syndrome (MERS) Coronavirus, avian influenza H5N1, and avian influenza H7N9. Respiratory infection due to viral pathogens may lead to bacterial sinusitis, bronchitis, or pneumonia. Bacterial pathogens are less common but can include *Streptococcus pneumoniae, Mycoplasma pneumoniae, Haemophilus influenzae,* and *Chlamydophila pneumoniae. Coxiella burnetii* and *Legionella pneumophila* can also cause outbreaks and sporadic cases of respiratory illness.

Risk for Travelers

Reported outbreaks are usually associated with common exposure in hotels and cruise ships or among tour groups. A few pathogens have been associated with outbreaks in travelers, including influenza virus, *L. pneumophila,* and *Histoplasma capsulatum.* The peak influenza season in the temperate Northern Hemisphere is December through February. In the temperate Southern Hemisphere, the peak influenza season is June through August. Travelers to tropical zones are at risk all year. Exposure to an infected person from another hemisphere, such as on a cruise ship or package tour, can lead to an outbreak of influenza at any time or place.

Air-pressure changes during ascent and descent of aircraft can facilitate the development of sinusitis and otitis media. Direct airborne transmission aboard commercial aircraft is unusual because of frequent air recirculation and filtration, although influenza, tuberculosis, measles, and other diseases have resulted from transmission in modern aircraft. Transmission may occur between passengers who are seated near one another, usually through direct contact or droplets. Intermingling of large numbers of people in locations such as airports, cruise ships, and hotels can also facilitate transmission of respiratory pathogens.

The air quality at many travel destinations may not be optimal, and exposure to sulfur dioxide, nitrogen dioxide, carbon monoxide, ozone, and particulate matter is associated with a number of health risks, including respiratory tract inflammation, exacerbations of asthma and chronic obstructive pulmonary disease, impaired lung function, bronchitis, and pneumonia. Certain travelers have a higher risk for respiratory tract infection, including children, the elderly, and people with comorbid pulmonary conditions, such as asthma and chronic obstructive pulmonary disease (COPD).

The risk for tuberculosis among most travelers is low.

Diagnosis

Identifying a specific etiologic agent, especially in the absence of pneumonia or serious disease, is not always clinically necessary. If indicated, the following methods of diagnosis can be used:

- Molecular methods are available to detect a number of respiratory viruses, including influenza virus, parainfluenza virus, adenovirus, human metapneumovirus, and respiratory syncytial virus, and for certain nonviral pathogens.

- Rapid tests are also available to detect some pathogens such as respiratory syncytial virus, influenza virus, *L. pneumophila*, and group A *Streptococcus*.

- Microbiologic culturing of sputum and blood, although insensitive, can help identify a causative respiratory pathogen.

- Special consideration should be given to diagnosing patients with suspected MERS, H5N1, or H7N9.

Clinical Presentation

Most respiratory tract infections, especially those of the upper respiratory tract, are mild and not incapacitating. Upper respiratory tract infections often cause rhinorrhea or pharyngitis. Lower respiratory tract infections, particularly pneumonia, can be more severe. Lower respiratory tract infections are more likely to cause fever, dyspnea, or chest pain than upper respiratory tract infections. Cough is often present in either upper or lower tract infections. People with influenza commonly have acute onset of fever, myalgia, headache, and cough. At present, MERS should be considered in travelers who develop fever and pneumonia within 14 days after traveling from countries in or near the Arabian Peninsula or who have close contact with such travelers. Practitioners should be aware that regions associated with MERS may expand or change. H5N1 and H7N9 should be considered in patients with new-onset severe acute respiratory illness requiring hospitalization when no alternative etiology has been identified and if the patient has recently (within 10 days) been to a country with recently confirmed human or animal cases of H5N1 or H7N9 or has had close contact with an ill person who has traveled to these areas in the last 10 days. Pulmonary embolism should be considered in the differential diagnosis of travelers who present with dyspnea, cough, or pleurisy and fever, especially those who have recently been on long car or plane rides.

Treatment

Affected travelers are usually managed similarly to nontravelers, although travelers with progressive or severe illness should be evaluated for illnesses specific to their travel destinations and exposure history. Most respiratory infections are due to viruses, are mild, and do not require specific treatment or antibiotics. Self-treatment with antibiotics during travel can be considered for higher-risk travelers with symptoms of lower respiratory tract infection. A respiratory-spectrum fluoroquinolone such as levofloxacin or a macrolide such as azithromycin may be prescribed to the traveler for this purpose before travel.

The rate of influenza among travelers is not known. The difficulty in self-diagnosing influenza makes it problematic to decide whether to prescribe travelers a neuraminidase inhibitor for self-treatment.

This practice should probably be limited to travelers with a specific underlying condition that may predispose them to severe influenza.

Specific situations that may require medical intervention include the following:

- Pharyngitis without rhinorrhea, cough, or other symptoms that may indicate infection with group A *Streptococcus*.

- Sudden onset of cough, chest pain, and fever that may indicate pneumonia (or pulmonary embolism), resulting in a situation where the traveler may be sick enough to seek medical care right away.

- Travelers with underlying medical conditions, such as asthma, pulmonary disease, or heart disease, who may need to seek medical care earlier than otherwise healthy travelers.

Prevention

Vaccines are available to prevent a number of respiratory diseases, including influenza, *S. pneumoniae* infection, *H. influenzae* type B infection (in young children), pertussis, diphtheria, varicella, and measles. Unless contraindicated, travelers should be vaccinated against influenza and be up-to-date on other routine immunizations. Preventing respiratory illness while traveling may not be possible, but common-sense preventive measures include the following:

- Minimizing close contact with people who are coughing and sneezing.

- Frequent handwashing, either with soap and water or alcohol-based hand sanitizers (containing ≥60% alcohol) when soap and water are not available.

- Using a vasoconstricting nasal spray immediately before air travel, if the traveler has a preexisting eustachian tube dysfunction, may help lessen the likelihood of otitis or barotrauma.

Section 39.2

Altitude Sickness

This section includes text excerpted from "Altitude Illness," Centers for Disease Control and Prevention (CDC), July 10, 2015.

The high-altitude environment exposes travelers to cold, low humidity, increased ultraviolet radiation, and decreased air pressure, all of which can cause problems. The biggest concern, however, is hypoxia. At 10,000 ft, for example, the inspired PO^2 is only 69 percent of sea-level value. The magnitude of hypoxic stress depends on altitude, rate of ascent, and duration of exposure. Sleeping at high altitude produces the most hypoxemia; day trips to high altitude with return to low altitude are much less stressful on the body. Typical high-altitude destinations include Cusco, La Paz, Lhasa, Everest Base Camp, and Kilimanjaro.

The human body adjusts very well to moderate hypoxia, but requires time to do so. The process of acute acclimatization to high altitude takes 3–5 days; therefore, acclimatizing for a few days at 8,000–9,000 ft before proceeding to a higher altitude is ideal. Acclimatization prevents altitude illness, improves sleep, and increases comfort and well-being, although exercise performance will always be reduced compared with low altitude. Increase in ventilation is the most important factor in acute acclimatization; therefore, respiratory depressants must be avoided. Increased red-cell production does not play a role in acute acclimatization.

Tips for Acclimatization

Ascend gradually, if possible. Avoid going directly from low altitude to more than 9,000 ft sleeping altitude in 1 day. Once above 9,000 ft, move sleeping altitude no higher than 1,600 ft per day, and plan an extra day for acclimatization every 3,300 ft.

- Consider using acetazolamide to speed acclimatization, if abrupt ascent is unavoidable.

- Avoid alcohol for the first 48 hours.

- Participate in only mild exercise for the first 48 hours.

- Having a high-altitude exposure at more than 9,000 ft for 2 nights or more, within 30 days before the trip, is useful.

Risk for Travelers

Inadequate acclimatization may lead to altitude illness in any traveler going to 8,000 ft or higher, and sometimes even at lower altitude. Susceptibility and resistance to altitude illness are genetic traits, and no simple screening tests are available to predict risk. Risk is not affected by training or physical fitness. Children are equally susceptible as adults; people aged >50 years have slightly lower risk. How a traveler has responded to high altitude previously is the most reliable guide for future trips, but is not infallible. However, given certain baseline susceptibility, risk is largely influenced by rate of ascent and exertion. Determining an itinerary that will avoid any occurrence of altitude illness is difficult because of variations in individual susceptibility, as well as in starting points and terrain. The goal for the traveler may not be to avoid all symptoms of altitude illness but to have no more than mild illness.

Table 39.1. Risk Categories for Acute Mountain Sickness

Risk Category	Description	Prophylaxis Recommendations
Low	People with no prior history of altitude illness and ascending to less than 9,000 ft (2,750 m) People taking more than 2 days to arrive at 8,200–9,800 ft (2,500–3,000 m), with subsequent increases in sleeping elevation less than 1,600 ft (500 m) per day, and an extra day for acclimatization every 3,300 ft (1,000 m)	Acetazolamide prophylaxis generally not indicated.
Moderate	People with prior history of AMS and ascending to 8,200–9,100 ft (2,500–2,800 m) or higher in 1 day No history of AMS and ascending to more than 9,100 ft (2,800 m) in 1 day All people ascending more than 1,600 ft (500 m) per day (increase in sleeping elevation) at altitudes above 9,900 ft (3,000 m), but with an extra day for acclimatization every 3,300 ft (1,000 m)	Acetazolamide prophylaxis would be beneficial and should be considered.

Table 39.1. Continued

Risk Category	Description	Prophylaxis Recommendations
High	History of AMS and ascending to more than 9,100 ft (2,800 m) in 1 day All people with a prior history of HACE or HAPE All people ascending to more than 11,400 ft (3,500 m) in 1 day All people ascending more than 1,600 ft (500 m) per day (increase in sleeping elevation) above 9,800 ft (3,000 m), without extra days for acclimatization Very rapid ascents (such as less than 7-day ascents of Mount Kilimanjaro)	Acetazolamide prophylaxis strongly recommended.

Clinical Presentation

Altitude illness is divided into 3 syndromes: acute mountain sickness (AMS), high-altitude cerebral edema (HACE), and high-altitude pulmonary edema (HAPE).

Acute Mountain Sickness

AMS is the most common form of altitude illness, affecting, for example, 25 percent of all visitors sleeping above 8,000 ft (2,500 m) in Colorado. Symptoms are those of an alcohol hangover: headache is the cardinal symptom, sometimes accompanied by fatigue, loss of appetite, nausea, and occasionally vomiting. Headache onset is usually 2–12 hours after arrival at a higher altitude and often during or after the first night. Preverbal children may develop loss of appetite, irritability, and pallor. AMS generally resolves with 24–72 hours of acclimatization.

High-Altitude Cerebral Edema

HACE is a severe progression of AMS and is rare; it is most often associated with HAPE. In addition to AMS symptoms, lethargy becomes profound, with drowsiness, confusion, and ataxia on tandem gait test. A person with HACE requires immediate descent; death from HACE can ensue within 24 hours of developing ataxia, if the person fails to descend.

High-Altitude Pulmonary Edema

HAPE can occur by itself or in conjunction with AMS and HACE; incidence is 1 per 10,000 skiers in Colorado and up to 1 per 100 climbers at more than 14,000 ft. Initial symptoms are increased breathlessness with exertion, and eventually increased breathlessness at rest, associated with weakness and cough. Oxygen or descent is life-saving. HAPE can be more rapidly fatal than HACE.

Preexisting Medical Problems

Travelers with medical conditions, such as heart failure, myocardial ischemia (angina), sickle cell disease, or any form of pulmonary insufficiency, should be advised to consult a physician familiar with high-altitude medical issues before undertaking high-altitude travel. The risk for new ischemic heart disease in previously healthy travelers does not appear to be increased at high altitudes. People with diabetes can travel safely to high altitudes, but they must be accustomed to exercise and carefully monitor their blood glucose. Diabetic ketoacidosis may be triggered by altitude illness and may be more difficult to treat in those on acetazolamide. Not all glucose meters read accurately at high altitudes.

Most people do not have visual problems at high altitudes. However, at very high altitudes some people who have had radial keratotomy may develop acute farsightedness and be unable to care for themselves. LASIK and other newer procedures may produce only minor visual disturbances at high altitudes.

There are no studies or case reports of harm to a fetus if the mother travels briefly to high altitudes during pregnancy. However, it may be prudent to recommend that pregnant women do not stay at sleeping altitudes higher than 12,000 ft, if possible. The dangers of having a pregnancy complication in remote, mountainous terrain should also be discussed.

Diagnosis and Treatment

Acute Mountain Sickness / High-Altitude Cerebral Edema

The differential diagnosis of AMS/HACE includes dehydration, exhaustion, hypoglycemia, hypothermia, or hyponatremia. Focal neurologic symptoms, or seizures, are rare in HACE and should lead to suspicion of an intracranial lesion or seizure disorder. Patients with AMS can descend ≥300 m, and symptoms will rapidly abate. Alternatively, supplemental oxygen at 2 L per minute will relieve headache quickly and resolve AMS over hours, but it is rarely available. People with AMS can also safely remain at their current altitude and treat symptoms with nonopiate analgesics and antiemetics, such as ondansetron. They may also take acetazolamide, which speeds acclimatization and effectively treats AMS, but is better for prophylaxis than treatment. Dexamethasone is more effective than acetazolamide at rapidly relieving the symptoms of moderate to severe AMS. If symptoms are getting worse while the traveler is resting at the same altitude, he or she must descend.

HACE is an extension of AMS characterized by neurologic findings, particularly ataxia, confusion, or altered mental status. HACE may also occur in the presence of HAPE. People developing HACE in populated areas with access to medical care can be treated at altitude with supplemental oxygen and dexamethasone. In remote areas, descent should be initiated in any person suspected of having HACE. If descent is not feasible because of logistical issues, supplemental oxygen or a portable hyperbaric chamber can be lifesaving.

High-Altitude Pulmonary Edema

Although the progression of decreased exercise tolerance, increased breathlessness, and breathlessness at rest is almost always recognizable as HAPE, the differential diagnosis includes pneumonia, bronchospasm, myocardial infarction, or pulmonary embolism. Descent in this situation is urgent and mandatory, and should be accomplished with as little exertion as is feasible for the patient. If descent is not immediately possible, supplemental oxygen or a portable hyperbaric chamber is critical. Patients with mild HAPE who have access to oxygen (at a hospital or high-altitude medical clinic, for example) may not need to descend to lower elevation and can be treated with oxygen at the current elevation. In the field setting, where resources are limited and there is a lower margin for error, nifedipine can be used as an adjunct to descent, oxygen, or portable hyperbaric therapy. A phosphodiesterase inhibitor may be used if nifedipine is not available, but concurrent use of multiple pulmonary vasodilators is not recommended.

Medications

In addition to the discussion below, recommendations for the usage and dosing of medications to prevent and treat altitude illness are outlined in Table 38.2.

Acetazolamide

Acetazolamide prevents AMS when taken before ascent and can speed recovery if taken after symptoms have developed. The drug works by acidifying the blood, which causes an increase in respiration and arterial oxygenation and thus aids acclimatization. An effective dose that minimizes the common side effects of increased urination and paresthesias of the fingers and toes is 125 mg every 12 hours, beginning the day before ascent and continuing the first 2 days at altitude, or longer if ascent continues. Allergic reactions to acetazolamide are uncommon. As a nonantimicrobial sulfonamide, it does not cross-react with antimicrobial sulfonamides. However, it is best avoided by people with history of anaphylaxis to any sulfa. People with history of severe penicillin allergy have occasionally had allergic reactions to acetazolamide. The pediatric dose is 5 mg/kg/day in divided doses, up to 125 mg twice a day.

Dexamethasone

Dexamethasone is effective for preventing and treating AMS and HACE, and perhaps HAPE as well. Unlike acetazolamide, if the drug is discontinued at altitude before acclimatization, rebound can occur. Acetazolamide is preferable to prevent AMS while ascending, with dexamethasone reserved for treatment, as an adjunct to descent. The adult dose is 4 mg every 6 hours. An increasing trend is to use dexamethasone for "summit day" on high peaks such as Kilimanjaro and Aconcagua, in order to prevent abrupt altitude illness.

Nifedipine

Nifedipine prevents HAPE and ameliorates it as well. For prevention, it is generally reserved for people who are particularly susceptible to the condition. The adult dose for prevention or treatment is 30 mg of extended release every 12 hours, or 20 mg every 8 hours.

Other Medications

Phosphodiesterase-5 inhibitors can also selectively lower pulmonary artery pressure, with less effect on systemic blood pressure. Tadalafil, 10 mg twice a day, during ascent can prevent HAPE and is being studied for treatment. When taken before ascent, gingko biloba, 100–120 mg twice a day, was shown to reduce AMS in adults in some trials, but it was not effective in others, probably due to variation in ingredients. Ibuprofen 600 mg every 8 hours was recently found to help prevent AMS, although it was not as effective as acetazolamide. However, it is over-the-counter, inexpensive, and well-tolerated.

Table 39.2. Recommended Medication Doses to Prevent and Treat Altitude Illness

Medication	Indication	Route	Dose
Acetazolamide	AMS, HACE prevention	Oral	125 mg twice a day; 250 mg twice a day if >100 kg. Pediatrics: 2.5 mg/kg every 12 h
	AMS treatment	Oral	250 mg twice a day Pediatrics: 2.5 mg/kg every 12 h
Dexamethasone	AMS, HACE prevention	Oral	2 mg every 6 h or 4 mg every 12 h Pediatrics: should not be used for prophylaxis
	AMS, HACE treatment	Oral, IV, IM	AMS: 4 mg every 6 h HACE: 8 mg once, then 4 mg every 6 h Pediatrics: 0.15 mg/kg/dose every 6 h up to 4 mg
Nifedipine	HAPE prevention	Oral	30 mg SR version every 12 h, or 20 mg SR version every 8 h
	HAPE treatment	Oral	30 mg SR version every 12 h, or 20 mg SR version every 8 h
Tadalafil	HAPE prevention	Oral	10 mg twice a day
Sildenafil	HAPE prevention	Oral	50 mg every 8 h
Salmeterol	HAPE prevention	Inhaled	125 µg twice a day

Prevention of Severe Altitude Illness or Death

The main point of instructing travelers about altitude illness is not to eliminate the possibility, but to prevent death or evacuation due to altitude illness. Since the onset of symptoms and the clinical course are sufficiently slow and predictable, there is no reason for anyone to die from altitude illness, unless trapped by weather or geography in a situation in which descent is impossible. Three rules can prevent death or serious consequences from altitude illness:

- Know the early symptoms of altitude illness, and be willing to acknowledge when they are present.

- Never ascend to sleep at a higher altitude when experiencing symptoms of altitude illness, no matter how minor they seem.

- Descend if the symptoms become worse while resting at the same altitude.

For trekking groups and expeditions going into remote high-altitude areas, where descent to a lower altitude could be problematic, a pressurization bag (such as the Gamow bag) can be beneficial. A foot pump produces an increased pressure of 2 lb/in, mimicking a descent of 5,000–6,000 ft depending on the starting altitude. The total packed weight of bag and pump is about 14 lb (6.5 kg).

Section 39.3

Scuba Diving

This section includes text excerpted from "Scuba Diving," Centers for Disease Control and Prevention (CDC), July 10, 2015.

Published estimates report anywhere from one-half to 4 million people who participate in recreational diving in the United States, and many travel to tropical areas of the world to dive. Traveling divers can face a variety of medical challenges, but because dive injuries are generally rare, few clinicians are trained in their diagnosis and treatment. Therefore, the recreational diver must be able to recognize the signs of injury and find qualified dive medicine help when needed.

Preparing for Dive Travel

Planning for dive-related travel should take into account any recent changes in health, including injuries or surgery, and medication use. Respiratory disorders (such as asthma), disorders that affect higher function and consciousness (such as diabetes or seizures), psychological problems (such as anxiety), cardiovascular disease, and pregnancy raise special concerns about diving fitness.

Special mention must be made regarding cardiovascular fitness. Diving should be considered a potentially strenuous activity that can make substantial demands on the cardiovascular system. People with known risk factors for coronary disease who wish to either begin a dive program or continue diving should undergo a physical examination with assessment of their cardiovascular fitness. This may include an electrocardiogram and exercise treadmill test.

Diving Disorders

Barotrauma

Ear and Sinus

Ear barotrauma is the most common injury in divers. On descent, failure to equalize pressure changes in the middle ear space creates a pressure gradient across the eardrum. This pressure change must be controlled through proper equalization techniques to avoid bleeding or fluid accumulation in the middle ear and avoid stretching or rupture of the eardrum and the membranes covering the windows of the inner ear. Symptoms of barotrauma include the following:

- pain
- tinnitus (ringing in the ears)
- vertigo (dizziness or sensation of spinning)
- sensation of fullness
- effusion (fluid accumulation in the ear)
- decreased hearing

Paranasal sinuses, because of their relatively narrow connecting passageways, are especially susceptible to barotrauma, generally on descent. With small changes in pressure (depth), symptoms are usually mild and subacute but can be exacerbated by continued diving. Larger pressure changes, especially with forceful attempts at equilibration (such as the Valsalva maneuver), can be more injurious. Additional risk factors for ear and sinus barotrauma include the following:

- earplugs
- medications

- ear or sinus surgery

- nasal deformity

- disease

A diver who may have sustained ear or sinus barotrauma should discontinue diving and seek medical attention.

Pulmonary

A scuba diver must reduce the risk of lung overpressure problems by breathing normally and ascending slowly when breathing compressed gas. Overinflation of the lungs can result if a scuba diver ascends toward the surface without exhaling, which may happen, for example, when a novice diver panics. During ascent, compressed gas trapped in the lung increases in volume until the expansion exceeds the elastic limit of lung tissue, causing damage and allowing gas bubbles to escape into 1 or more of 3 possible locations:

- Gas entering the pleural space can cause lung collapse or pneumothorax.

- Gas entering the space around the heart, trachea, and esophagus (the mediastinum) causes mediastinal emphysema and frequently tracks under the skin (subcutaneous emphysema) or into the tissue around the larynx, sometimes precipitating a change in voice characteristics.

- Gas rupturing the alveolar walls can enter the pulmonary capillaries and pass via the pulmonary veins to the left side of the heart, where it is distributed according to relative blood flow, resulting in arterial gas embolism (AGE).

While mediastinal or subcutaneous emphysema may resolve spontaneously, pneumothorax generally requires specific treatment to remove the air and reinflate the lung. AGE is a medical emergency, requiring intervention, which includes recompression treatment with hyperbaric oxygen.

Lung overinflation injuries from scuba diving can range from dramatic and life threatening to mild symptoms of chest pain and dyspnea. Although pulmonary barotrauma is relatively uncommon in divers, prompt medical evaluation is necessary, and evidence for this condition should always be considered in the presence of respiratory or neurologic symptoms following a dive.

Decompression Illness

Decompression illness (DCI) is an all-inclusive term that describes the dysbaric injuries (AGE) and decompression sickness (DCS). Because the 2 diseases are considered to result from separate causes, they are described here separately. However, from a clinical and practical standpoint, distinguishing between them in the field may be impossible and unnecessary, since the initial treatment is the same for both. DCI can occur even in divers who have carefully followed the standard decompression tables and the principles of safe diving. Serious permanent injury may result from either AGE or DCS.

Arterial Gas Embolism

Gas entering the arterial blood through ruptured pulmonary vessels can distribute bubbles into the body tissues, including the heart and brain, where they can disrupt circulation or damage vessel walls. AGE may cause minimal neurologic symptoms, dramatic symptoms that require immediate attention, or death. Common signs and symptoms include the following:

- numbness
- weakness
- tingling
- dizziness
- blurred vision
- chest pain
- personality change
- paralysis or seizures
- loss of consciousness

In general, any scuba diver who surfaces unconscious or loses consciousness within 10 minutes after surfacing should be suspected to have AGE. Intervention with basic life support is indicated, including the administration of the highest fraction of oxygen, followed by rapid evacuation to a hyperbaric oxygen treatment facility.

Decompression Sickness

Breathing air under pressure causes excess inert gas (usually nitrogen) to dissolve in body tissues. The amount of gas dissolved is proportional to and increases with depth and time. As the diver ascends back to the surface, the excess dissolved gas must be cleared through respiration via the bloodstream. Depending on the amount dissolved and the rate of ascent, some gas can supersaturate tissues, where it separates from solution to form bubbles, interfering with blood flow and tissue oxygenation and causing the following signs and symptoms of DCS:

- joint aches or pain
- numbness or tingling
- mottling or marbling of skin
- coughing spasms or shortness of breath
- itching
- unusual fatigue
- dizziness
- weakness
- personality changes
- loss of bowel or bladder function
- staggering, loss of coordination, or tremors
- paralysis
- collapse or unconsciousness

Flying after Diving

The risk of developing decompression sickness is increased when divers are exposed to increased altitude too soon after a dive. The cabin pressure of commercial aircraft may be the equivalent of 6,000–8,000 ft. Thus, divers should avoid flying or an altitude exposure >2,000 ft (610 m) for

- ≥12 hours after surfacing from a single no-decompression dive
- ≥18 hours after repetitive dives or multiple days of diving
- substantially longer than 18 hours after dives where decompression stops were required

These recommended preflight surface intervals do not eliminate risk of DCS, and longer surface intervals will further reduce this risk.

447

Preventing Diving Disorders

Recreational divers should dive conservatively and well within the no-decompression limits of their dive tables or computers. Risk factors for DCI are primarily dive depth, dive time, and rate of ascent. Additional factors such as repetitive dives, strenuous exercise, dives to depths >60 ft, altitude exposure soon after a dive, and certain physiological variables also increase risk. Divers should be cautioned to stay hydrated and rested and dive within the limits of their training. Diving is a skill that requires training and certification and should be done with a companion.

Treatment of Diving Disorders

Definitive treatment of DCI begins with early recognition of symptoms, followed by recompression with hyperbaric oxygen. A high concentration (100%) of supplemental oxygen is recommended. Surface-level oxygen given for first aid may relieve the signs and symptoms of DCI and should be administered as soon as possible. Divers are often dehydrated, either because of incidental causes, immersion, or DCI itself, which can cause capillary leakage. Administration of isotonic glucose-free intravenous fluid is recommended in most cases. Oral rehydration fluids may also be helpful, provided they can be safely administered (for example, if the diver is conscious). The definitive treatment of DCI is recompression and oxygen administration in a hyperbaric chamber.

Divers Alert Network (DAN) maintains 24-hour emergency consultation and evacuation assistance at 919-684-9111 (collect calls are accepted). DAN will help with managing the injured diver, help decide if recompression is needed, provide the location of the closest recompression facility, and help arrange patient transport. DAN can also be contacted for routine, nonemergency consultation by telephone at 919-684-2948, extension 222.

Travelers who plan to scuba dive may want to ascertain whether there are recompression facilities at their destination before embarking on their trip.

Hazardous Marine Life

The oceans and waterways are filled with creatures and, although some are capable of wounding and poisoning, most marine animals are generally harmless unless threatened. Most injuries are the result of chance encounters or defensive maneuvers. Resulting wounds have many common characteristics: bacterial contamination, foreign bodies, and occasionally venom.

Part Five

Pediatric Respiratory Disorders

Chapter 40

Asthma in Children

About Asthma[1]

Asthma is a common lung condition in kids and teens. It causes breathing problems, with symptoms like coughing, wheezing, and shortness of breath. Anyone can have asthma, even babies, and the tendency to develop it often runs in families.

Asthma affects the bronchial tubes, or airways. When someone breathes normally, air goes in through the nose or mouth and then into the trachea (windpipe), through the bronchial tubes, into the lungs, and finally back out again.

But people with asthma have inflamed airways that produce lots of thick mucus. The airways also are overly sensitive (or hyperreactive) to certain things, like exercise, dust, or cigarette smoke. This hyperreactivity makes the smooth muscle that surrounds the airways tighten up. The combination of airway inflammation and muscle tightening narrows the airways and makes it hard for air to move through.

More than 25 million people have asthma in the United States. In fact, it's the No. 1 reason kids chronically miss school. And flare-ups are the most common cause of pediatric emergency room visits due to a chronic illness.

This chapter includes text excerpted from documents published by two sources. Text under headings marked 1 are excerpted from "Asthma Basics," © 1995–2016. The Nemours Foundation/KidsHealth®. Reprinted with permission; text under heading marked 2 is excerpted from "Exercise-Induced Asthma," © 1995–2016. The Nemours Foundation/KidsHealth®. Reprinted with permission.

Some kids have only mild, occasional symptoms or only show symptoms after exercising. Others have severe asthma that, if not treated, can greatly limit how active they are and cause changes in lung function.

But thanks to new medicines and treatment strategies, kids with asthma don't need to sit on the sidelines and their parents don't need to worry constantly. With knowledge and the right asthma management plan, families can learn to better control symptoms and asthma flare-ups, letting kids do just about anything they want.

About Asthma Flare-Ups[1]

Many kids with asthma can breathe normally for weeks or months between **asthma flare-ups** (also called asthma attacks, flares, episodes, or exacerbations) that cause the airways to narrow and become blocked, making it hard for air to move through them.

Flare-ups often seem to happen without warning, but they usually develop over time during a complicated process of increasing airway blockage.

All children with asthma have airways that are inflamed, which means that they swell and produce lots of thick mucus. And their airways are overly sensitive, or **hyperreactive**, to certain asthma triggers.

When exposed to these triggers, the muscles surrounding the airways tend to tighten, which makes the already clogged airways even narrower. Things that trigger flare-ups differ from person to person. Some common triggers are exercise, allergies, viral infections, and smoke.

So an asthma flare-up is caused by three important changes in the airways:

1. **swelling** of the lining of the airways

2. **excess mucus** that causes congestion and mucus "plugs" that get caught in the narrowed airways

3. **bronchoconstriction**, the tightening of the muscles around the airways

Together, the swelling, excess mucus, and bronchoconstriction narrow the airways and make it difficult to move air through (like breathing through a straw). During an asthma flare-up, kids may have coughing, wheezing (a breezy whistling sound in the chest when breathing), chest tightness, an increased heart rate, sweating, and shortness of breath.

How Is Asthma Diagnosed?[1]

Diagnosing asthma can be tricky and time-consuming because kids with asthma can have very different symptoms. For example, some kids cough constantly at night but seem fine during the day, while others seem to get a lot of chest colds that linger. It's common for kids to have symptoms like these for months before being seen by a doctor.

When considering a diagnosis of asthma, a doctor rules out other possible causes of the symptoms. He or she asks questions about the family's asthma and allergy history, performs a physical exam, and might order a chest X-rays or lung function tests.

During this process, parents will give the doctor such detailed information as:

- **symptoms:** how severe they are; when, where, and how often they happen; and how long they last

- **allergies:** the child's and the family's allergy history

- **illnesses:** how often the child gets colds, how severe they are, and how long they last

- **triggers:** exposure to allergens and things in the air that can irritate the airways, recent life changes or stressful events, or other things that seem to lead to a flare-up

This information helps the doctor understand the pattern of symptoms, which can help determine what type of asthma the child has and how best to treat it.

To confirm the diagnosis of asthma, a breathing test may be done with a spirometer, a machine that analyzes airflow through the airways. A spirometer also can be used to see if the child's breathing problems can be helped with medicine, which is a primary sign of asthma.

The doctor may take a spirometer reading, give the child an inhaled medication that opens the airways, and then take another reading to see if breathing improves. If the medicine eases airway narrowing significantly, then there's a strong possibility that the child has asthma.

If your child is diagnosed with asthma, it's important to learn how to manage asthma so it won't control your family. Educate yourself about asthma and learn to identify and eliminate triggers.

Help your child keep an asthma diary, develop and follow an asthma action plan, and take medicines as prescribed. Also, a **peak flow meter**—a handheld tool that measures breathing ability—can be used at home. When peak flow readings drop, it's a sign of increasing airway inflammation.

Exercise-Induced Asthma[2]

Up to 80% of kids with asthma have symptoms when they exercise. It makes sense that cigarette smoke and pollen could trigger asthma symptoms, but why exercise?

- Cold, dry air that's inhaled during exercise is believed to be the main cause of these symptoms. When kids exercise or play strenuously, they tend to breathe quickly, shallowly, and through the mouth. So the air reaching their lungs misses the warming and humidifying effects that happen when they breathe more slowly through the nose.

- The cool, dry air causes the airways in the lungs to become narrower, which blocks the flow of air and makes it harder to breathe. This narrowing, called bronchoconstriction, occurs in up to 20% of people who *don't* have asthma, which is why it's sometimes referred to as "exercise-induced bronchoconstriction (EIB)" rather than "exercise-induced asthma (EIA)."

Symptoms

Symptoms of exercise-induced asthma include wheezing, tightness or pain in the chest, coughing, and in some cases, prolonged shortness of breath. Some symptoms are more noticeable than others, which means exercise-induced asthma can sometimes go undiagnosed.

Someone may have exercise-induced asthma if he or she:

- gets winded or tired easily during or after exercise

- coughs after coming inside from being active outdoors

- can't run for more than a few minutes without stopping

Kids with exercise-induced asthma often begin having symptoms 5 to 10 minutes after starting to exercise. Symptoms usually peak 5 to 10 minutes after stopping the activity and may take an hour or longer to end. Some people with EIA even have symptoms for hours after exercise. Although symptoms often appear while kids are active, sometimes they can appear only after the activity has stopped.

Of course, there's a difference between someone with exercise-induced asthma and someone who's out of shape and is simply winded.

Out-of-shape people can catch their breath within minutes, whereas it takes much longer for someone with EIA to recover. And extremes of temperature, especially cold weather, can make it even worse.

Diagnosing EIA

A doctor who suspects exercise-induced asthma will ask about the family's asthma and allergy history and about the symptoms and what has triggered them in the past.

After taking a detailed history and performing a physical exam, the doctor may ask your child to perform a breathing test after exercising. This can be done in the office on a treadmill, after your child has run outside for 6 to 8 minutes, or after participating in whatever activity has triggered flare-ups in the past.

Treating EIA

Doctors sometimes recommend pretreatment, which means taking medication before exercise or strenuous activity, for kids with exercise-induced asthma. This medication is often the same short-term medication used during flare-ups, known as quick-relief medicine (also called rescue or fast-acting medicine), although in this case its function is preventative. By taking this medication before exercise, the airway narrowing triggered by exercise can be prevented.

If pretreatment isn't enough to control symptoms, the doctor may recommend that someone also use long-term control medicine (also called controller or maintenance medicine), which is usually taken regularly over time to reduce airway inflammation.

If, despite medication, your child still has breathing trouble during exercise, let the doctor know. The medication dosages may need to be adjusted for better control. Also, contact the doctor if there are any changes with your child's breathing problems.

Recommended Activities for Kids with EIA

Exercise is a great idea for everyone, including kids with exercise-induced asthma. Try to encourage your child to be active while also keeping asthma symptoms under control by following the doctor's instructions.

In addition to keeping kids fit, exercise can improve lung function by strengthening the breathing muscles in the chest. Ask your doctor about exercise and what kinds of precautions your child should take.

Of course, some sports are less likely to cause problems for kids with exercise-induced asthma, such as:

- Walking

- Jogging

- Hiking

- Golf

- Baseball

- Football

- Gymnastics

- Shorter track and field events

Endurance sports (like long-distance running and cycling) and those requiring extended energy output (like soccer and basketball) may be more challenging, as can cold-weather endurance sports like cross-country skiing or ice hockey.

But that doesn't mean your child can't participate in these sports if he or she truly enjoys them. In fact, many athletes with asthma have found that with proper training and medication, they can participate in any sport they choose.

Tips for Kids with Exercise-Induced Asthma

For the most part, kids with exercise-induced asthma can do anything their peers can do. But be sure to follow the suggestions given by your child's doctor.

Here are some of the tips often recommended:

- Warm up before exercise to prevent chest tightening. (Warm-up exercises can include 5 to 10 minutes of walking or any other light activity, in addition to stretching or flexibility exercises.)

- Take quick-relief medicine as close to the start of exercise as possible.

- Breathe through the nose during exercise.

- Take brief rests during exercise and use quick-relief medicine, as prescribed, if symptoms start.

- Cool down after exercise to help slow the change of air temperature in the lungs.

In addition, someone experiencing symptoms shouldn't start exercising until the symptoms stop.

It's also wise for kids with EIA to avoid exercising outside during very cold weather. If your child will be playing outside when it's cold, wearing a ski mask or a scarf over the mouth and nose should help.

If air pollution or pollen also trigger asthma symptoms, your child may want to exercise indoors when air quality is poor or pollen counts are high. And exercise should be avoided during any upper respiratory infection.

You can help by ensuring your child takes all medicine prescribed by the doctor, even on days when he or she feels fine. Skipping long-term control medicine can make symptoms worse, and forgetting to take quick-relief medicine before exercise can lead to severe flare-ups and even emergency department visits.

Kids should always have access to their quick-relief medicine. Keep extras on hand and be sure to regularly check all supplies so your child isn't carrying around an empty inhaler.

Allergy-Triggered Asthma[1]

About 75 percent to 85 percent of people with asthma have some type of allergy. Even if the main triggers are colds or exercise, allergies can sometimes play a minor role in making asthma worse.

How do allergies cause flare-ups in kids with asthma? Kids inherit the tendency to have allergies from their parents. With any kind of allergy, the immune system overreacts to normally harmless allergens. Those substances (such as pollen) can cause allergic reactions in some people. As part of this overreaction, the body produces an antibody— called immunoglobulin E (IgE)—that recognizes and attaches to the allergen when the body is exposed to it.

When this happens, it starts a process that ends in the release of certain substances in the body. One of them is histamine, which causes allergic symptoms that can affect the eyes, nose, throat, skin, gastro-intestinal tract, or lungs. When the airways in the lungs are affected, symptoms of asthma can happen.

The released histamine is what causes the familiar sneezing, runny nose, and itchy, watery eyes associated with some allergies— ways the body attempts to rid itself of the invading allergen. In kids with asthma, histamine also can trigger asthma symptoms and flare-ups.

An allergist can usually pinpoint allergies. Once they're identified, the best treatment is to avoid exposure to them whenever possible, such by taking environmental control measures inside the home.

When triggers can't be avoided, antihistamine medicines (to block the release of histamine in the body) or nasal steroids (to block allergic inflammation in the nose) might be prescribed. In some cases, an allergist can prescribe immunotherapy, a series of allergy shots that gradually make the body unresponsive to specific allergens.

Asthma Categories[1]

The severity of a child's asthma symptoms will fall into one of four main categories of asthma, each with different characteristics and requiring different treatment approaches:

1. **Intermittent asthma**

   A child who has brief episodes of wheezing, coughing, or shortness of breath no more than twice a week is said to have mild intermittent asthma. Symptoms between flare-ups are rare, with one or two instances per month of mild symptoms at night.

2. **Mild persistent asthma**

   Kids with episodes of wheezing, coughing, or shortness of breath more than twice a week but less than once a day are said to have mild persistent asthma. Symptoms usually happen at least twice a month at night and flare-ups may affect normal physical activity.

3. **Moderate persistent asthma**

   Kids with moderate persistent asthma have daily symptoms and need daily medicine. Nighttime symptoms happen more than once a week. Flare-ups occur more than twice a week, last for several days, and usually affect normal physical activity.

4. **Severe persistent asthma**

   Kids with severe persistent asthma have symptoms continuously. They tend to have frequent flare-ups that may require emergency treatment and even hospitalization. Many kids with severe persistent asthma have symptoms at night and can handle only limited physical activity.

Asthma severity can both worsen and improve over time, placing a child in a new asthma category that needs different treatment.

All kids with asthma should follow a custom asthma action plan to control symptoms. And even mild asthma should never be ignored because airway inflammation is present even in between flare-ups.

Chapter 41

Bronchopulmonary Dysplasia

What Is Bronchopulmonary Dysplasia?

Bronchopulmonary dysplasia, or BPD, is a serious lung condition that affects infants. BPD mostly affects premature infants who need oxygen therapy (oxygen given through nasal prongs, a mask, or a breathing tube).

Most infants who develop BPD are born more than 10 weeks before their due dates, weigh less than 2 pounds (about 1,000 grams) at birth, and have breathing problems. Infections that occur before or shortly after birth also can contribute to BPD.

Some infants who have BPD may need long-term breathing support from nasal continuous positive airway pressure (NCPAP) machines or ventilators.

Other Names for Bronchopulmonary Dysplasia

- Arrest of lung development
- Evolving chronic lung disease
- Neonatal chronic lung disease
- Respiratory insufficiency

This chapter includes text excerpted from "Bronchopulmonary Dysplasia," National Heart, Lung, and Blood Institute (NHLBI), January 12, 2012. Reviewed September 2016.

What Causes Bronchopulmonary Dysplasia?

Bronchopulmonary dysplasia (BPD) develops as a result of an infant's lungs becoming irritated or inflamed.

The lungs of premature infants are fragile and often aren't fully developed. They can easily be irritated or injured within hours or days of birth. Many factors can damage premature infants' lungs.

Ventilation

Newborns who have breathing problems or can't breathe on their own may need ventilator support. Ventilators are machines that use pressure to blow air into the airways and lungs.

Although ventilator support can help premature infants survive, the machine's pressure might irritate and harm the babies' lungs. For this reason, doctors only recommend ventilator support when necessary.

High Levels of Oxygen

Newborns who have breathing problems might need oxygen therapy (oxygen given through nasal prongs, a mask, or a breathing tube). This treatment helps the infants' organs get enough oxygen to work well.

However, high levels of oxygen can inflame the lining of the lungs and injure the airways. Also, high levels of oxygen can slow lung development in premature infants.

Infections

Infections can inflame the lungs. As a result, the airways narrow, which makes it harder for premature infants to breathe. Lung infections also increase the babies' need for extra oxygen and breathing support.

Heredity

Studies show that heredity may play a role in causing BPD. More studies are needed to confirm this finding.

Who Is at Risk for Bronchopulmonary Dysplasia?

The more premature an infant is and the lower his or her birth weight, the greater the risk of bronchopulmonary dysplasia (BPD).

Most infants who develop BPD are born more than 10 weeks before their due dates, weigh less than 2 pounds (about 1,000 grams) at birth, and have breathing problems. Infections that occur before or shortly after birth also can contribute to BPD.

The number of babies who have BPD is higher now than in the past. This is because of advances in care that help more premature infants survive.

Many babies who develop BPD are born with serious respiratory distress syndrome (RDS). However, some babies who have mild RDS or don't have RDS also develop BPD. These babies often have very low birth weights and one or more other conditions, such as patent ductus arteriosus (PDA) and sepsis.

PDA is a heart problem that occurs soon after birth in some babies. Sepsis is a serious bacterial infection in the bloodstream.

What Are the Signs and Symptoms of Bronchopulmonary Dysplasia?

Many babies who develop bronchopulmonary dysplasia (BPD) are born with serious respiratory distress syndrome (RDS). The signs and symptoms of RDS at birth are:

- rapid, shallow breathing
- sharp pulling in of the chest below and between the ribs with each breath
- grunting sounds
- flaring of the nostrils

Babies who have RDS are treated with surfactant replacement therapy. They also may need oxygen therapy (oxygen given through nasal prongs, a mask, or a breathing tube).

Shortly after birth, some babies who have RDS also are treated with nasal continuous positive airway pressure (NCPAP) or ventilators (machines that support breathing).

Often, the symptoms of RDS start to improve slowly after about a week. However, some babies get worse and need more oxygen or breathing support from NCPAP or a ventilator.

A first sign of BPD is when premature infants—usually those born more than 10 weeks early—still need oxygen therapy by the time they reach their original due dates. These babies are diagnosed with BPD.

Infants who have severe BPD may have trouble feeding, which can lead to delayed growth. These babies also may develop:

- **Pulmonary hypertension (PH).** PH is increased pressure in the pulmonary arteries. These arteries carry blood from the heart to the lungs to pick up oxygen.

- **Cor pulmonale.** Cor pulmonale is failure of the right side of the heart. Ongoing high blood pressure in the pulmonary arteries and the lower right chamber of the heart causes this condition.

How Is Bronchopulmonary Dysplasia Diagnosed?

Infants who are born early—usually more than 10 weeks before their due dates—and still need oxygen therapy by the time they reach their original due dates are diagnosed with bronchopulmonary dysplasia (BPD).

BPD can be mild, moderate, or severe. The diagnosis depends on how much extra oxygen a baby needs at the time of his or her original due date. It also depends on how long the baby needs oxygen therapy.

To help confirm a diagnosis of BPD, doctors may recommend tests, such as:

- **Chest X-ray.** A chest X-ray takes pictures of the structures inside the chest, such as the heart and lungs. In severe cases of BPD, this test may show large areas of air and signs of inflammation or infection in the lungs. A chest X-ray also can detect problems (such as a collapsed lung) and show whether the lungs aren't developing normally.

- **Blood tests.** Blood tests are used to see whether an infant has enough oxygen in his or her blood. Blood tests also can help determine whether an infection is causing an infant's breathing problems.

- **Echocardiography.** This test uses sound waves to create a moving picture of the heart. Echocardiography is used to rule out heart defects or pulmonary hypertension as the cause of an infant's breathing problems.

How Is Bronchopulmonary Dysplasia Treated?

Preventive Measures

If your doctor thinks you're going to give birth too early, he or she may give you injections of a corticosteroid medicine.

The medicine can speed up surfactant production in your baby. Surfactant is a liquid that coats the inside of the lungs. It helps keep the lungs open so your infant can breathe in air once he or she is born.

Corticosteroids also can help your baby's lungs, brain, and kidneys develop more quickly while he or she is in the womb.

Premature babies who have very low birth weights also might be given corticosteroids within the first few days of birth. Doctors sometimes prescribe inhaled nitric oxide shortly after birth for babies who have very low birth weights. This treatment can help improve the babies' lung function.

These preventive measures may help reduce infants' risk of respiratory distress syndrome (RDS), which can lead to BPD.

Treatment for Respiratory Distress Syndrome

The goals of treating infants who have RDS include:

- Reducing further injury to the lungs

- Providing nutrition and other support to help the lungs grow and recover

- Preventing lung infections by giving antibiotics

Treatment of RDS usually begins as soon as an infant is born, sometimes in the delivery room. Most infants who have signs of RDS are quickly moved to a neonatal intensive care unit (NICU). They receive around-the-clock treatment from healthcare professionals who specialize in treating premature infants.

Treatments for RDS include surfactant replacement therapy, breathing support with nasal continuous positive airway pressure (NCPAP) or a ventilator, oxygen therapy (oxygen given through nasal prongs, a mask, or a breathing tube), and medicines to treat fluid buildup in the lungs.

Treatment for Bronchopulmonary Dysplasia

Treatment in the NICU is designed to limit stress on infants and meet their basic needs of warmth, nutrition, and protection. Once doctors diagnose BPD, some or all of the treatments used for RDS will continue in the NICU.

Such treatment usually includes:

- Using radiant warmers or incubators to keep infants warm and reduce the risk of infection.

- Ongoing monitoring of blood pressure, heart rate, breathing, and temperature through sensors taped to the babies' bodies.

- Using sensors on fingers or toes to check the amount of oxygen in the infants' blood.

- Giving fluids and nutrients through needles or tubes inserted into the infants' veins. This helps prevent malnutrition and promotes growth. Nutrition is vital to the growth and development of the lungs. Later, babies may be given breast milk or infant formula through feeding tubes that are passed through their noses or mouths and into their throats.

- Checking fluid intake to make sure that fluid doesn't build up in the babies' lungs.

As BPD improves, babies are slowly weaned off NCPAP or ventilators until they can breathe on their own. These infants will likely need oxygen therapy for some time.

If your infant has moderate or severe BPD, echocardiography might be done every few weeks to months to check his or her pulmonary artery pressure.

If your child needs long-term ventilator support, he or she will likely get a tracheostomy. A tracheostomy is a surgically made hole. It goes through the front of the neck and into the trachea, or windpipe. Your child's doctor will put the breathing tube from the ventilator through the hole.

Using a tracheostomy instead of an endotracheal tube has some advantages. (An endotracheal tube is a breathing tube inserted through the nose or mouth and into the windpipe.)

Long-term use of an endotracheal tube can damage the trachea. This damage may need to be corrected with surgery later. A tracheostomy can allow your baby to interact more with you and the NICU staff, start talking, and develop other skills.

While your baby is in the NICU, he or she also may need physical therapy. Physical therapy can help strengthen your child's muscles and clear mucus out of his or her lungs.

Infants who have BPD may spend several weeks or months in the hospital. This allows them to get the care they need.

Before your baby goes home, learn as much as you can about your child's condition and how it's treated. Your baby may continue to have some breathing symptoms after he or she leaves the hospital.

Your child will likely continue on all or some of the treatments that were started at the hospital, including:

- Medicines, such as bronchodilators, steroids, and diuretics.

- Oxygen therapy or breathing support from NCPAP or a ventilator.

- Extra nutrition and calories, which may be given through a feeding tube.

- Preventive treatment with a medicine called palivizumab for severe respiratory syncytial virus (RSV). This common virus leads to mild, cold-like symptoms in adults and older, healthy children. However, in infants—especially those in high-risk groups—RSV can lead to severe breathing problems.

Your child also should have regular checkups with and timely vaccinations from a pediatrician. This is a doctor who specializes in treating children. If your child needs oxygen therapy or a ventilator at home, a pulmonary specialist might be involved in his or her care.

Seek out support from family, friends, and hospital staff. Ask the case manager or social worker at the hospital about what you'll need after your baby leaves the hospital.

The doctors and nurses can assist with questions about your infant's care. Also, you may want to ask whether your community has a support group for parents of premature infants.

How Can Bronchopulmonary Dysplasia Be Prevented?

Taking steps to ensure a healthy pregnancy might prevent your infant from being born before his or her lungs have fully developed. These steps include:

- seeing your doctor regularly during your pregnancy

- following a healthy diet

- not smoking and avoiding tobacco smoke, alcohol, and illegal drugs

- controlling any ongoing medical conditions you have

- preventing infection

If your doctor thinks that you're going to give birth too early, he or she may give you injections of a corticosteroid medicine.

The medicine can speed up surfactant production in your baby. Surfactant is a liquid that coats the inside of the lungs. It helps keep them open so your infant can breathe in air once he or she is born.

Usually, within about 24 hours of your taking this medicine, the baby's lungs start making enough surfactant. This will reduce the infant's risk of RDS, which can lead to BPD.

Corticosteroids also can help your baby's lungs, brain, and kidneys develop more quickly while he or she is in the womb.

If your baby does develop RDS, it will probably be fairly mild. If the RDS isn't mild, BPD will likely develop.

Chapter 42

Croup

About Croup

Croup is a condition that causes swelling and irritation of the upper airways—the voice box (larynx) and windpipe (trachea). It's caused by the same viruses that cause the common cold. Kids with croup have a "barky" cough or hoarseness, especially when crying.

Croup is most common in kids 6 months to 3 years old, but some older children also get croup. Most cases happen in the fall and early winter.

There are two types of croup: viral croup and spasmodic croup. Both types cause a barking cough.

- **Viral croup** always includes other signs of a cold, such as a runny nose, fever, and fatigue. The virus goes away within 3 to 7 days after it began.

- **Spasmodic croup** may happen in a child with a mild cold. The barking cough usually begins at night and isn't accompanied by fever. Spasmodic croup has a tendency to come back again.

Most cases of croup are mild and can be treated at home. Rarely, croup can be severe and even life-threatening.

Text in this chapter is excerpted from "Croup," © 1995–2016. The Nemours Foundation/KidsHealth®. Reprinted with permission.

Signs and Symptoms

At first, a child may have cold symptoms, like a stuffy or runny nose and a fever. As the upper airways become inflamed and swollen, the child may become hoarse, with a harsh, barking cough. This loud cough often sounds like a seal barking.

If the upper airway continues to swell, it becomes hard for a child to breathe. The child may make a high-pitched or squeaking noise while breathing in—this is called **stridor**. A child also might breathe very fast or have **retractions** (when the skin between the ribs pulls in during breathing). In the most serious cases, a child may appear pale or have a bluish color around the mouth due to a lack of oxygen.

Symptoms of croup are often worse at night and when a child is upset or crying.

Diagnosis

Doctors usually diagnose croup by listening for the telltale barking cough and stridor. They will also ask questions, for example whether your child has had any recent illnesses with a fever, runny nose, and congestion, and if your child has a history of croup or upper airway problems.

If the child's croup is severe and slow to get better after treatment, the child may be sent to an emergency room (ER). A neck X-ray may be done to rule out other reasons for the breathing problems, such as:

- an object stuck in the throat

- a peritonsillar abscess (collection of pus at the back of the mouth)

- epiglottitis (swelling of the epiglottis, the flap of tissue that covers the windpipe)

An X-ray of a child with croup usually will show the top of the airway narrowing to a point, which doctors call a "steeple sign."

Treatment

Most cases of viral croup are mild and can be treated at home. Breathing in moist air may help kids feel better, and pain medicine (ibuprofen or acetaminophen) may make them more comfortable. Kids should drink plenty of fluids to prevent dehydration, and rest often.

The best way to expose a child to moist air is to use a **cool-mist humidifier** or run a hot shower to create a **steam-filled bathroom** where the child can sit with an adult for 10 minutes. Breathing in the mist will sometimes stop a child from severe coughing. In the cooler weather, taking the child outside for a few minutes to breath in the cool air may ease symptoms. You also can try taking your child for a drive with the car windows slightly lowered.

In certain kids, doctors will prescribe steroids to decrease airway swelling. For severe cases, kids will be put on a breathing treatment that contains a medicine called epinephrine. This medicine quickly reduces swelling in the airways. Sometimes kids with croup will need to stay in a hospital until they're breathing better.

Chapter 43

Human Metapneumovirus

About HMPV

Human metapneumovirus (HMPV) can cause upper and lower respiratory disease in people of all ages, especially among young children, older adults, and people with weakened immune systems. HMPV was discovered in 2001 and is in the paramyxovirus family along with measles and respiratory syncytial virus (RSV). Broader use of molecular diagnostic testing has increased identification and awareness of HMPV as an important cause of upper and lower respiratory infection.

Symptoms

Symptoms commonly associated with HMPV include cough, fever, nasal congestion, and shortness of breath. Clinical symptoms of HMPV infection may progress to bronchiolitis or pneumonia and are similar to other viruses that cause upper and lower respiratory infections. The incubation period is estimated to be 3 to 6 days, and the median duration of illness can vary depending upon severity but is similar to other respiratory infections caused by viruses.

This chapter includes text excerpted from "Human Metapneumovirus (HMPV) Clinical Features," Centers for Disease Control and Prevention (CDC), February 2, 2016.

Surveillance and Seasonality

Surveillance data from Centers for Disease Control and Prevention's (CDC) the National Respiratory and Enteric Virus Surveillance System (NREVSS) shows HMPV to be most active during late winter or early spring in temperate climates.

Transmission

HMPV is most likely spread from an infected person to others through—

- secretions from coughing and sneezing,
- close personal contact, such as touching or shaking hands, and
- touching objects or surfaces that have the viruses on them then touching the mouth, nose, or eyes

In the United States, HMPV circulates in distinct annual seasons. HMPV circulation begins in winter and lasts until or through spring. HMPV, RSV, and influenza can circulate simultaneously during the respiratory virus season.

Prevention and Treatment

There are steps that can be taken to help prevent the spread of HMPV and other respiratory viruses. Specifically, people who have cold-like symptoms should

- cover their coughs and sneezes
- wash their hands frequently and correctly (with soap and water for 20 seconds)
- avoid sharing their cups and eating utensils with others
- refrain from kissing others

In addition, cleaning possible contaminated surfaces (such as doorknobs, shared toys) may potentially help stop the spread of HMPV.

There is no specific antiviral therapy for HMPV. Medical care is supportive.

Since HMPV is a recently recognized respiratory virus, healthcare professionals may not routinely consider or test for HMPV. However, healthcare professionals should consider HMPV testing during winter and spring, especially when HMPV is commonly circulating.

Chapter 44

Interstitial Lung Disease in Children

What Is Childhood Interstitial Lung Disease?

Childhood interstitial lung disease, or chILD, is a broad term for a group of rare lung diseases that can affect babies, children, and teens. These diseases have some similar symptoms, such as chronic cough, rapid breathing, and shortness of breath.

These diseases also harm the lungs in similar ways. For example, they damage the tissues that surround the lungs' alveoli and bronchial tubes (airways). Sometimes these diseases directly damage the air sacs and airways.

The various types of chILD can decrease lung function, reduce blood oxygen levels, and disturb the breathing process.

Types of Childhood Interstitial Lung Disease

The broad term "childhood interstitial lung disease" (chILD) refers to a group of rare lung diseases that can affect babies, children, and teens. Some of these diseases are more common in certain age groups. Diseases more common in infancy include:

- Surfactant dysfunction mutations

This chapter includes text excerpted from "Childhood Interstitial Lung Disease," National Heart, Lung, and Blood Institute (NHLBI), March 21, 2014.

- Developmental disorders, such as alveolar capillary dysplasia
- Lung growth abnormalities
- Neuroendocrine cell hyperplasia of infancy (NEHI)
- Pulmonary interstitial glycogenosis (PIG)

Diseases more common in children older than 2 years of age and teens include:

- Idiopathic interstitial pneumonias:
  - Nonspecific interstitial pneumonia
  - Cryptogenic organizing pneumonia
  - Acute interstitial pneumonia
  - Desquamative interstitial pneumonia
  - Lymphocytic interstitial pneumonia
- Other primary disorders:
  - Alveolar hemorrhage syndromes
  - Aspiration syndromes
  - Hypersensitivity pneumonitis
  - Infectious or postinfectious disease (bronchiolitis obliterans)
  - Eosinophilic pneumonia
  - Pulmonary alveolar proteinosis
  - Pulmonary infiltrates with eosinophilia
  - Pulmonary lymphatic disorders (lymphangiomatosis, lymphangiectasis)
  - Pulmonary vascular disorders (haemangiomatosis)
- ILD associated with systemic disease processes:
  - Connective tissue diseases
  - Histiocytosis
  - Malignancy-related lung disease
  - Sarcoidosis
  - Storage diseases

- Disorders of the compromised immune system:

  - Opportunistic infection

  - Disorders related to therapeutic intervention

  - Lung and bone marrow transplant-associated lung diseases

  - Diffuse alveolar damage of unknown cause

The various types of chILD can affect many parts of the lungs, including the alveoli (air sacs), bronchial tubes (airways), and capillaries. (Capillaries are the tiny blood vessels that surround the air sacs.) The structures of the lung that chILD may affect are shown in the illustration below.

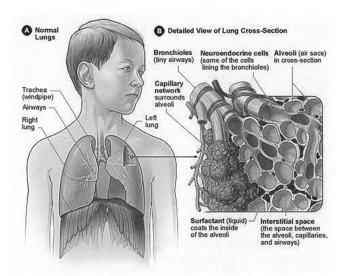

Figure 44.1. *Normal Lungs and Lung Structures*

Figure A shows the location of the lungs and airways in the body. Figure B is a detailed view of the lung structures that childhood interstitial lung disease may affect, such as the bronchioles, neuroendocrine cells, alveoli, capillary network, surfactant, and interstitial space.

Other Names for Childhood Interstitial Lung Disease

- Chronic lung disease

- Diffuse infiltrative lung disease

- Diffuse lung disease

- Diffuse parenchyma lung disease

- Interstitial pneumonitis

- The chILD syndrome

What Causes Childhood Interstitial Lung Disease?

Many times, these diseases have no clear cause.

Some conditions and factors that may cause or lead to chILD include:

- **Inherited conditions,** such as surfactant disorders. Surfactant is a liquid that coats the inside of the lungs. It helps with breathing and may help protect the lungs from bacterial and viral infections.

- **Birth defects** that cause problems with the structure or function of the lungs.

- **Aspiration.** This term refers to inhaling substance—such as food, liquid, or vomit—into the lungs. Inhaling these substances can injure the lungs. Aspiration may occur in children who have swallowing problems or gastroesophageal reflux disease (GERD). GERD occurs if acid from the stomach backs up into the throat.

- **Immune system disorders.** The immune system protects the body against bacteria, viruses, and toxins. Children who have immune system disorders aren't able to fight illness and disease as well as children who have healthy immune systems.

- Exposure to substances in the environment that can irritate the lungs, such as molds and chemicals.

- Some cancer treatments, such as radiation and chemotherapy.

- **Systemic or autoimmune diseases,** such as collagen vascular disease or inflammatory bowel disease. Systemic diseases are diseases that involve many of the body's organs. Autoimmune diseases occur if the body's immune system mistakenly attacks the body's tissues and cells.

- A bone marrow transplant or a lung transplant.

Who Is at Risk for Childhood Interstitial Lung Disease?

Childhood interstitial lung disease (chILD) is rare. Most children are not at risk for chILD. However, some factors increase the risk of developing chILD. These risk factors include:

- Having a family history of interstitial lung disease or chILD.

- Having an inherited surfactant disorder or a family history of this type of disorder. Surfactant is a liquid that coats the inside of the lungs. It helps with breathing and may help protect the lungs from bacterial and viral infections.

- Having problems with aspiration. This term "aspiration" refers to inhaling substances—such as food, liquid, or vomit—into the lungs.

- Having an immune system disorder. The immune system protects the body against bacteria, viruses, and toxins. Children who have immune system disorders aren't able to fight illness and disease as well as children who have healthy immune systems.

- Being exposed to substances in the environment that can irritate the lungs, such as molds and chemicals.

- Having a systemic or autoimmune disease, such as collagen vascular disease or inflammatory bowel disease. Systemic diseases are diseases that involve many of the body's organs. Autoimmune diseases occur if the body's immune system mistakenly attacks the body's tissues and cells.

- Undergoing some cancer treatments, such as radiation and chemotherapy.

- Having a bone marrow transplant or a lung transplant.

Certain types of chILD are more common in infants and young children, while others can occur in children of any age.

The risk of death seems to be higher for children who have chILD and pulmonary hypertension, developmental or growth disorders, bone marrow transplants, or certain surfactant problems.

What Are the Signs and Symptoms of Childhood Interstitial Lung Disease?

Childhood interstitial lung disease (chILD) has many signs and symptoms because the disease has many forms. Signs and symptoms may include:

- fast breathing, which also is called tachypnea

- labored breathing, which also is called respiratory distress

- low oxygen levels in the blood, which also is called hypoxemia

- recurrent coughing, wheezing, or crackling sounds in the chest

- shortness of breath during exercise (in older children) or while eating (in infants), which also is called dyspnea

- poor growth or failure to gain weight

- recurrent pneumonia or bronchiolitis

If your child has any of these signs and symptoms, contact his or her doctor. The doctor may refer you to a pediatric pulmonologist. This is a doctor who specializes in diagnosing and treating children who have lung diseases and conditions.

How Is Childhood Interstitial Lung Disease Diagnosed?

Doctors diagnose childhood interstitial lung disease (chILD) based on a child's medical and family histories and the results from tests and procedures. To diagnose chILD, doctors may first need to rule out other diseases as the cause of a child's symptoms.

Early diagnosis of chILD may help doctors stop or even reverse lung function problems. Often though, doctors find chILD hard to diagnose because:

- There are many types of the disease and a range of underlying causes

- The disease's signs and symptoms are the same as those for many other diseases

- The disease may coexist with other diseases

Going to a pediatric pulmonologist who has experience with chILD is helpful. A pediatric pulmonologist is a doctor who specializes in diagnosing and treating children who have lung diseases and conditions.

Medical and Family Histories

Your child's medical history can help his or her doctor diagnose chILD. The doctor may ask whether your child:

- Has severe breathing problems that occur often.

- Has had severe lung infections.

- Had serious lung problems as a newborn.

- Has been exposed to possible lung irritants in the environment, such as birds, molds, dusts, or chemicals.

- Has ever had radiation or chemotherapy treatment.

- Has an autoimmune disease, certain birth defects, or other medical conditions. (Autoimmune diseases occur if the body's immune system mistakenly attacks the body's tissues and cells.)

The doctor also may ask how old your child was when symptoms began, and whether other family members have or have had severe lung diseases. If they have, your child may have an inherited form of chILD.

Diagnostic Tests and Procedures

No single test can diagnose the many types of chILD. Thus, your child's doctor may recommend one or more of the following tests. For some of these tests, infants and young children may be given medicine to help them relax or sleep.

- A **chest X-ray**. This painless test creates pictures of the structures inside your child's chest, such as the heart, lungs, and blood vessels. A chest X-ray can help rule out other lung diseases as the cause of your child's symptoms.

- A **high-resolution CT scan (HRCT)**. An HRCT scan uses X-rays to create detailed pictures of your child's lungs. This test can show the location, extent, and severity of lung disease.

- **Lung function tests**. These tests measure how much air your child can breathe in and out, how fast he or she can breathe air out, and how well your child's lungs deliver oxygen to the blood. Lung function tests can assess the severity of lung disease. Infants and young children may need to have these tests at a center that has special equipment for children.

- **Bronchoalveolar lavage**. For this procedure, the doctor injects a small amount of saline (salt water) through a tube inserted in the child's lungs. The fluid helps bring up cells from the tissues around the air sacs. The doctor can then look at these cells under a microscope. This procedure can help detect an infection, lung injury, bleeding, aspiration, or an airway problem.

- Various tests to rule out conditions such as asthma, cystic fibrosis, acid reflux, heart disease, neuromuscular disease, and immune deficiency.

- Various tests for systemic diseases linked to chILD. Systemic diseases are diseases that involve many of the body's organs.

- Blood tests to check for inherited (genetic) diseases and disorders.

If these tests don't provide enough information, your child's doctor may recommend a lung biopsy. A lung biopsy is the most reliable way to diagnose chILD and the specific disease involved.

A lung biopsy is a surgical procedure that's done in a hospital. Before the biopsy, your child will receive medicine to make him or her sleep.

During the biopsy, the doctor will take small samples of lung tissue from several places in your child's lungs. This often is done using video-assisted thoracoscopy.

For this procedure, the doctor inserts a small tube with a light and camera (endoscope) into your child's chest through small cuts between the ribs. The endoscope provides a video image of the lungs and allows the doctor to collect tissue samples.

After the biopsy, the doctor will look at these samples under a microscope.

How Is Childhood Interstitial Lung Disease Treated?

Childhood interstitial lung disease (chILD) is rare, and little research has been done on how to treat it. At this time, chILD has no cure. However, some children who have certain diseases, such as neuroendocrine cell hyperplasia of infancy, may slowly improve over time.

Current treatment approaches include supportive therapy, medicines, and, in the most serious cases, lung transplants.

Supportive Therapy

Supportive therapy refers to treatments that help relieve symptoms or improve quality of life. Supportive approaches used to relieve common chILD symptoms include:

- **Oxygen therapy.** If your child's blood oxygen level is low, he or she may need oxygen therapy. This treatment can improve breathing, support growth, and reduce strain on the heart.

- **Bronchodilators.** These medications relax the muscles around your child's airways, which helps open the airways and makes breathing easier.

- Breathing devices. Children who have severe disease may need ventilators or other devices to help them breathe easier.

- **Extra nutrition.** This treatment can help improve your child's growth and help him or her gain weight. Close monitoring of growth is especially important.

- **Techniques and devices to help relieve lung congestion.** These may include chest physical therapy (CPT) or wearing a vest that helps move mucus (a sticky substance) to the upper airways so it can be coughed up. CPT may involve pounding the chest and back over and over with your hands or a device to loosen mucus in the lungs so that your child can cough it up.

- **Supervised pulmonary rehabilitation (PR).** PR is a broad program that helps improve the well-being of people who have chronic (ongoing) breathing problems.

Medicines

Corticosteroids are a common treatment for many children who have chILD. These medicines help reduce lung inflammation.

Other medicines can help treat specific types or causes of chILD. For example, antimicrobial medicines can treat a lung infection. Acid-blocking medicines can prevent acid reflux, which can lead to aspiration.

Lung Transplant

A lung transplant may be an option for children who have severe chILD if other treatments haven't worked.

Currently, lung transplants are the only effective treatment for some types of chILD that have a high risk of death, such as alveolar capillary dysplasia and certain surfactant dysfunction mutations.

Early diagnosis of these diseases gives children the chance to receive lung transplants. So far, chILD doesn't appear to come back in patients' transplanted lungs.

How Can Childhood Interstitial Lung Disease Be Prevented?

At this time, most types of chILD can't be prevented. People who have a family history of inherited (genetic) interstitial lung disease may want to consider genetic counseling. A counselor can explain the risk of children inheriting chILD.

You and your child can take steps to help prevent infections and other illnesses that worsen chILD and its symptoms. For example:

• Make hand washing a family habit to avoid germs and prevent illnesses.

• Try to keep your child away from people who are sick. Even a common cold can cause problems for someone who has chILD.

• Talk with your child's doctor about vaccines that your child needs, such as an annual flu shot. Make sure everyone in your household gets all of the vaccines that their doctors recommend.

• Talk with your child's doctor about how to prevent your child from getting respiratory syncytial virus. This common virus leads to cold and flu symptoms for most people. However, it can make children who have lung diseases very sick.

• Avoid exposing your child to air pollution, tobacco smoke, and other substances that can irritate his or her lungs. Strongly advise your child not to smoke now or in the future.

Chapter 45

Meconium Aspiration

About Meconium Aspiration

Every parent-to-be hopes for an uncomplicated birth and a healthy baby. But some babies do face delivery room complications. One that may affect a newborn's health is meconium aspiration, also referred to as meconium aspiration syndrome (MAS). Although it can be serious, most cases of MAS are *not*.

MAS can happen before, during, or after labor and delivery when a newborn inhales (or aspirates) a mixture of meconium and amniotic fluid (the fluid in which the baby floats inside the amniotic sac). Meconium is the baby's first feces, or poop, which is sticky, thick, and dark green and is typically passed in the womb during early pregnancy and again in the first few days after birth.

The inhaled meconium can partially or completely block the baby's airways. Although air can flow past the meconium as the baby breathes in, the meconium becomes trapped in the airways when the baby breathes out. The meconium irritates the baby's airways and makes it difficult to breathe.

MAS can affect the baby's breathing in a number of ways, including chemical irritation to the lung tissue, airway obstruction by a meconium plug, infection, and the inactivation of surfactant by the meconium (surfactant is a natural substance that helps the lungs expand properly).

The severity of MAS depends on the amount of meconium the baby inhales as well as underlying conditions, such as infections within the uterus or postmaturity (when a baby is overdue, or more than 40 weeks gestational age). Generally, the more meconium a baby inhales, the more serious the condition.

Although 6 percent to 25 percent of newborns have meconium-stained amniotic fluid, only about 11 percent of them will have some degree of MAS.

Causes

Before a baby is born, fluid usually moves in and out of the trachea (the upper part of the airway) only. Meconium can be inhaled into the lungs if the baby gasps while still in the womb or during the initial gasping breaths after delivery. This gasping usually happens because a problem (such as an infection or compression of the umbilical cord) made it hard for the baby to get enough oxygen before birth.

MAS is often related to fetal stress. This can be caused by problems in the womb, such as infections, or by difficulties during the birth. A distressed baby may have hypoxia (decreased oxygen), which can make the baby's intestinal activity increase and cause relaxation of the anal sphincter (the muscular valve that controls the passage of feces out of the anus). This relaxation then moves meconium into the amniotic fluid that envelops the baby.

But meconium passage during labor and delivery isn't always associated with fetal distress. Sometimes, babies who aren't distressed during labor pass meconium before birth. In either case, a baby that gasps or inhales meconium can develop MAS.

Other risk factors for MAS include:

- a long or difficult delivery

- advanced gestational age (or postmaturity)

- a mother who smokes cigarettes heavily or who has diabetes, high blood pressure (hypertension), or chronic respiratory or cardiovascular disease

- umbilical cord complications

- poor intrauterine growth (poor growth of the baby while in the uterus)

Prematurity is *not* a risk factor. In fact, MAS is rare in babies born before 34 weeks.

Signs and Symptoms

Before or at birth, the doctor will likely notice one or more symptoms of MAS, including:

- meconium or dark green streaks or stains in the amniotic fluid
- discoloration of the baby's skin—either blue (cyanosis) or green (from being stained by the meconium)
- problems with breathing—including rapid breathing (tachypnea), labored (difficulty) breathing, or suspension of breathing (apnea)
- low heart rate in the baby before birth
- low Apgar score (given to newborns just after birth to quickly evaluate color, heartbeat, reflexes, muscle tone, and breathing)
- limpness in the baby
- postmaturity (signs that a baby is overdue, such as long nails)

Diagnosis

If a baby is thought to have inhaled meconium, treatment will begin during delivery. If the baby has trouble breathing, the doctor will insert a laryngoscope into the trachea to remove any meconium. The doctor also will listen to the baby's lungs to check for sounds that are common with MAS.

The doctor might order tests, such as a blood test (called a blood gas analysis) that helps determine if the baby is getting enough oxygen and a chest X-ray that can show patches or streaks on the lungs that are found in babies with MAS.

Treatment

Current guidelines say that if a newborn has inhaled meconium but is active, looks well, and has a strong heartbeat (>100 bpm), the delivery team can watch the baby for MAS symptoms (such as increased respiratory rate, grunting, or cyanosis), which usually appear within the first 24 hours.

For a newborn that has inhaled meconium and is not very active, has a lower heart rate (<100 bpm), is limp, and has poor muscle tone, the goal is to clear the airway as much as possible to decrease the amount of meconium the baby inhales. This is done by using an endotracheal tube (a plastic tube that's placed into the baby's windpipe through the mouth or nose) and applying suction as the tube is slowly removed. This allows suctioning of both the upper and lower airways. The doctor will continue trying to clear the airway until there's no meconium in the suctioned fluids.

Most babies with MAS improve within a few days or weeks, depending on the severity of the aspiration. Although a baby's rapid breathing may continue for days after the birth, there's usually no permanent lung damage. Some studies, however, suggest that babies born with MAS are at a higher risk for reactive airway disease (an asthma-like narrowing of the airways that can cause wheezing, coughing, and shortness of breath).

Babies with MAS may be sent to a special care nursery or a neonatal intensive care unit (NICU) to be closely watched for the next few days. Treatments might include:

- oxygen therapy

- antibiotics to treat infection

- use of surfactant

- nitric oxide inhalation

- frequent blood tests to see if the baby is getting enough oxygen

Severe Aspiration

Babies who have severe aspiration and need mechanical ventilation are at a higher risk for bronchopulmonary dysplasia, a lung condition that can be treated with medication or oxygen.

Another complication associated with MAS is a collapsed lung. Also known as pneumothorax, a collapsed lung is treated by reinflating the lung (inserting a tube between the ribs, allowing the lung to gradually re-expand).

Although rare, a small percentage of babies with severe MAS develop aspiration pneumonia. If this happens, the doctor may recommend advanced lung rescue therapy. Three therapies are used to treat aspiration pneumonia and severe forms of MAS:

1. **Surfactant therapy:** An artificial surfactant is put into the baby's lungs to help keep the air sacs open.

2. **High-frequency oscillation:** This special ventilator vibrates air enriched with extra oxygen into the baby's lungs.

3. **Rescue therapy:** Nitric oxide is added to the oxygen in the ventilator. It dilates the blood vessels and allows more blood flow and oxygen to reach the baby's lungs.

If one of these therapies (or a combination of them) doesn't work, there is another alternative. Extra corporeal membrane oxygenation (ECMO) is a form of cardiopulmonary bypass, meaning that an artificial heart and lung will temporarily take over to supply blood flow to the baby's body. ECMO lowers the fatality rate for these severely distressed babies from 80 percent to 10 percent. Not all hospitals are ECMO centers, so babies that need ECMO might need to be moved to another hospital.

Babies with severe cases of MAS may come home from the hospital on oxygen. They may be more likely to have wheezing and lung infections during their first year, but lungs can regenerate new air sacs, so the long-term outlook for their lungs is excellent.

Possible Long-Term Complications

Severely affected babies are at risk for chronic lung disease and also may have developmental abnormalities and hearing loss. Babies diagnosed with MAS will be screened at the hospital for hearing problems or neurological damage.

Although very rare, severe cases of MAS can be fatal. But deaths from MAS have decreased greatly thanks to treatments such as suctioning and a reduction in the number of post-term births.

Prevention

It's important for a pregnant woman to tell her doctor immediately if she sees meconium in the amniotic fluid when her water breaks, or if the fluid has dark green stains or streaks. Doctors also use a fetal monitor during labor to watch the baby's heart rate for any signs of fetal distress.

In some cases, doctors may recommend amnioinfusion (diluting the amniotic fluid with saline) to wash meconium out of the amniotic sac before the baby has a chance to inhale it at birth.

Although MAS is a frightening complication for parents to face during the birth of their child, most cases are *not* severe. Babies are monitored for fetal distress during labor, and doctors pay careful attention for any signs of meconium aspiration. If it does happen, treatment will begin immediately.

For most infants who have inhaled meconium, early treatment can prevent further complications and help reassure anxious new parents.

Chapter 46

Respiratory Distress Syndrome of the Newborn

What Is Respiratory Distress Syndrome?

Respiratory distress syndrome (RDS) is a breathing disorder that affects newborns. RDS rarely occurs in full-term infants. The disorder is more common in premature infants born about 6 weeks or more before their due dates.

RDS is more common in premature infants because their lungs aren't able to make enough surfactant. Surfactant is a liquid that coats the inside of the lungs. It helps keep them open so that infants can breathe in air once they're born.

Without enough surfactant, the lungs collapse and the infant has to work hard to breathe. He or she might not be able to breathe in enough oxygen to support the body's organs. The lack of oxygen can damage the baby's brain and other organs if proper treatment isn't given.

Most babies who develop RDS show signs of breathing problems and a lack of oxygen at birth or within the first few hours that follow.

Other Names for Respiratory Distress Syndrome

- Hyaline membrane disease

This chapter includes text excerpted from "Respiratory Distress Syndrome," National Heart, Lung, and Blood Institute (NHLBI), January 24, 2012. Reviewed September 2016.

- Neonatal respiratory distress syndrome

- Infant respiratory distress syndrome

- Surfactant deficiency

What Causes Respiratory Distress Syndrome?

The main cause of RDS is a lack of surfactant in the lungs. Surfactant is a liquid that coats the inside of the lungs.

A fetus's lungs start making surfactant during the third trimester of pregnancy (weeks 26 through labor and delivery). The substance coats the insides of the air sacs in the lungs. This helps keep the lungs open so breathing can occur after birth.

Without enough surfactant, the lungs will likely collapse when the infant exhales (breathes out). The infant then has to work harder to breathe. He or she might not be able to get enough oxygen to support the body's organs.

Some full-term infants develop RDS because they have faulty genes that affect how their bodies make surfactant.

Who Is at Risk for Respiratory Distress Syndrome?

Certain factors may increase the risk that your infant will have RDS. These factors include:

- Premature delivery. The earlier your baby is born, the greater his or her risk for RDS. Most cases of RDS occur in babies born before 28 weeks of pregnancy.

- Stress during your baby's delivery, especially if you lose a lot of blood.

- Infection.

- Your having diabetes.

Your baby also is at greater risk for RDS if you require an emergency Cesarean delivery (C-section) before your baby is full term. You may need an emergency C-section because of a condition, such as a detached placenta, that puts you or your infant at risk.

Planned C-sections that occur before a baby's lungs have fully matured also can increase the risk of RDS. Your doctor can do tests before delivery that show whether it's likely that your baby's lungs are fully developed. These tests assess the age of the fetus or lung maturity.

What Are the Signs and Symptoms of Respiratory Distress Syndrome?

Signs and symptoms of RDS usually occur at birth or within the first few hours that follow. They include:

- rapid, shallow breathing
- sharp pulling in of the chest below and between the ribs with each breath
- grunting sounds
- flaring of the nostrils

The infant also may have pauses in breathing that last for a few seconds. This condition is called apnea.

Respiratory Distress Syndrome Complications

Depending on the severity of an infant's RDS, he or she may develop other medical problems.

Lung Complications

Lung complications may include a collapsed lung (atelectasis), leakage of air from the lung into the chest cavity (pneumothorax), and bleeding in the lung (hemorrhage).

Some of the life-saving treatments used for RDS may cause bronchopulmonary dysplasia, another breathing disorder.

Blood and Blood Vessel Complications

Infants who have RDS may develop sepsis, an infection of the bloodstream. This infection can be life threatening.

Lack of oxygen may prevent a fetal blood vessel called the ductus arteriosus from closing after birth as it should. This condition is called patent ductus arteriosus, or PDA.

The ductus arteriosus connects a lung artery to a heart artery. If it remains open, it can strain the heart and increase blood pressure in the lung arteries.

Other Complications

Complications of RDS also may include blindness and other eye problems and a bowel disease called necrotizing enterocolitis. Infants who have severe RDS can develop kidney failure.

Some infants who have RDS develop bleeding in the brain. This bleeding can delay mental development. It also can cause mental retardation or cerebral palsy.

How Is Respiratory Distress Syndrome Diagnosed?

RDS is common in premature infants. Thus, doctors usually recognize and begin treating the disorder as soon as babies are born.

Doctors also do several tests to rule out other conditions that could be causing an infant's breathing problems. The tests also can confirm that the doctors have diagnosed the condition correctly.

The tests include:

- **Chest X-ray.** A chest X-ray creates a of the structures inside the chest, such as the heart and lungs. This test can show whether your infant has signs of RDS. A chest X-ray also can detect problems, such as a collapsed lung, that may require urgent treatment.

- **Blood tests.** Blood tests are used to see whether an infant has enough oxygen in his or her blood. Blood tests also can help find out whether an infection is causing the infant's breathing problems.

- **Echocardiography (echo).** This test uses sound waves to create a moving picture of the heart. Echo is used to rule out heart defects as the cause of an infant's breathing problems.

How Is Respiratory Distress Syndrome Treated?

Treatment for respiratory distress syndrome (RDS) usually begins as soon as an infant is born, sometimes in the delivery room.

Most infants who show signs of RDS are quickly moved to a neonatal intensive care unit (NICU). There they receive around-the-clock treatment from healthcare professionals who specialize in treating premature infants.

The most important treatments for RDS are:

- Surfactant replacement therapy

- Breathing support from a ventilator or nasal continuous positive airway pressure (NCPAP) machine. These machines help premature infants breathe better.

- Oxygen therapy

Other Treatments

Other treatments for RDS include medicines, supportive therapy, and treatment for patent ductus arteriosus (PDA). PDA is a condition that affects some premature infants.

How Can Respiratory Distress Syndrome Be Prevented?

Taking steps to ensure a healthy pregnancy might prevent your infant from being born before his or her lungs have fully developed. These steps include:

- seeing your doctor regularly during your pregnancy
- following a healthy diet
- avoiding tobacco smoke, alcohol, and illegal drugs
- managing any medical conditions you have
- preventing infections

If you're having a planned Cesarean delivery (C-section), your doctor can do tests before delivery to show whether it's likely that your baby's lungs are fully developed. These tests assess the age of the fetus or lung maturity.

Your doctor may give you injections of a corticosteroid medicine if he or she thinks you may give birth too early. This medicine can speed up surfactant production and development of the lungs, brain, and kidneys in your baby.

Treatment with corticosteroids can reduce your baby's risk of RDS. If the baby does develop RDS, it will probably be fairly mild.

Corticosteroid treatment also can reduce the chances that your baby will have bleeding in the brain.

Chapter 47

Respiratory Syncytial Virus (Bronchiolitis)

Infection and Incidence

Respiratory syncytial virus (RSV) can cause upper respiratory infections (such as colds) and lower respiratory tract infections (such as bronchiolitis and pneumonia). In children younger than 1 year of age, RSV is the most common cause of bronchiolitis, an inflammation of the small airways in the lung, and pneumonia, an infection of the lungs.

Almost all children will have had an RSV infection by their second birthday. When infants and children are exposed to RSV for the first time,

- 25 to 40 out of 100 of them have signs or symptoms of bronchiolitis or pneumonia, and

- 5 to 20 out of 1,000 will require hospitalization. Most children hospitalized for RSV infection are younger than 6 months of age.

Infants and children infected with RSV usually show symptoms within 4 to 6 days of infection. Most will recover in 1 to 2 weeks. However, even after recovery, very young infants and children with weakened immune systems can continue to spread the virus for 1 to 3 weeks.

This chapter includes text excerpted from "Respiratory Syncytial Virus (RSV)," Centers for Disease Control and Prevention (CDC), November 4, 2014.

People of any age can get another RSV infection, but infections later in life are generally less severe. Premature infants, children younger than 2 years of age with congenital heart or chronic lung disease, and children with compromised (weakened) immune systems due to a medical condition or medical treatment are at highest risk for severe disease. Adults with compromised immune systems and those 65 and older are also at increased risk of severe disease.

In the United States and other areas with similar climates, RSV infections generally occur during fall, winter, and spring. The timing and severity of RSV circulation in a given community can vary from year to year.

Symptoms and Care

Symptoms of RSV infection are similar to other respiratory infections. Illness usually begins 4 to 6 days after exposure (range: 2 to 8 days) with a runny nose and decrease in appetite. Coughing, sneezing, and fever typically develop 1 to 3 days later. Wheezing may also occur. In very young infants, irritability, decreased activity, and breathing difficulties may be the only symptoms of infection. Most otherwise healthy infants infected with RSV do not need to be hospitalized. In most cases, even among those who need to be hospitalized, hospitalization usually only lasts a few days, and full recovery from illness occurs in about 1 to 2 weeks.

Visits to a healthcare provider for an RSV infection are very common. During such visits, the healthcare provider will assess the severity of disease to determine if the patient should be hospitalized. In the most severe cases of disease, infants may require supplemental oxygen, suctioning of mucus from the airways, or intubation (have breathing tubes inserted) with mechanical ventilation.

There is no specific treatment for RSV infection.

Transmission and Prevention

Transmission

People infected with RSV are usually contagious for 3 to 8 days. However, some infants and people with weakened immune systems can be contagious for as long as 4 weeks. Children are often exposed to and infected with RSV outside the home, such as in school or childcare. They can then transmit the virus to other members of the family.

RSV can be spread when an infected person coughs or sneezes into the air, creating virus-containing droplets that can linger briefly in the air. Other people can become infected if the droplet particles contact their nose, mouth, or eye.

Infection can also result from direct and indirect contact with nasal or oral secretions from infected people. Direct contact with the virus can occur, for example, by kissing the face of a child with RSV. Indirect contact can occur if the virus gets on an environmental surface, such as a doorknob, that is then touched by other people. Direct and indirect transmissions of virus usually occur when people touch an infectious secretion and then rub their eyes or nose.

RSV can survive on hard surfaces such as tables and crib rails for many hours. RSV typically lives on soft surfaces such as tissues and hands for shorter amounts of time.

Prevention

There are steps that can be taken to help prevent the spread of RSV. Specifically, people who have cold-like symptoms should

- cover their coughs and sneezes

- wash their hands frequently and correctly (with soap and water for 20 seconds)

- avoid sharing their cups and eating utensils with others

- refrain from kissing others

In addition, cleaning contaminated surfaces (such as doorknobs) may help stop the spread of RSV.

Parents should pay special attention to protecting children at high risk for developing severe disease if infected with RSV. Such children include premature infants, children younger than 2 years of age with chronic lung or heart conditions, and children with weakened immune systems.

Ideally, people with cold-like symptoms should not interact with children at high risk for severe disease. If this is not possible, these people should carefully follow the prevention steps mentioned above and wash their hands before interacting with children at high risk. They should also refrain from kissing high-risk children while they have cold-like symptoms. When possible, limiting the time that high-risk children spend in child-care centers or other potentially contagious settings may help prevent infection and spread of the virus during the RSV season.

Chapter 48

Sudden Infant Death Syndrome (SIDS)

What Is Sudden Infant Death Syndrome (SIDS)?

Sudden infant death syndrome (SIDS) is the sudden, unexplained death of a baby younger than 1 year of age that doesn't have a known cause even after a complete investigation. This investigation includes performing a complete autopsy, examining the death scene, and reviewing the clinical history.

When a baby dies, healthcare providers, law enforcement personnel, and communities try to find out why. They ask questions, examine the baby, gather information, and run tests. If they can't find a cause for the death, and if the baby was younger than 1 year old, the medical examiner or coroner will call the death SIDS.

If there is still some uncertainty as to the cause after it is determined to be fully unexplained, then the medical examiner or corner might leave the cause of death as "unknown."

Fast Facts about SIDS

- SIDS is the leading cause of death among babies between 1 month and 1 year of age.

This chapter includes text excerpted from "What Is SIDS?" *Eunice Kennedy Shriver* National Institute of Child Health and Human Development (NICHD), October 29, 2015.

- More than 2,000 babies died of SIDS in 2010, the last year for which such statistics are available.

- Most SIDS deaths occur when in babies between 1 month and 4 months of age, and the majority (90%) of SIDS deaths occur before a baby reaches 6 months of age. However SIDS deaths can occur anytime during a baby's first year.

- SIDS is a sudden and silent medical disorder that can happen to an infant who seems healthy.

- SIDS is sometimes called "crib death" or "cot death" because it is associated with the timeframe when the baby is sleeping. Cribs themselves don't cause SIDS, but the baby's sleep environment can influence sleep-related causes of death.

- Slightly more boys die of SIDS than do girls.

- In the past, the number of SIDS deaths seemed to increase during the colder months of the year. But today, the numbers are more evenly spread throughout the calendar year.

- SIDS rates for the United States have dropped steadily since 1994 in all racial and ethnic groups. Thousands of infant lives have been saved, but some ethnic groups are still at higher risk for SIDS.

SIDS Is Not

SIDS is **not** the cause of every sudden infant death.

Each year in the United States, thousands of babies die suddenly and unexpectedly. These deaths are called SUID, which stands for "Sudden Unexpected Infant Death."

SUID includes all unexpected deaths: those without a clear cause, such as SIDS, and those from a known cause, such as suffocation. One-half of all SUID cases are SIDS. Many unexpected infant deaths are accidents, but a disease or something done on purpose can also cause a baby to die suddenly and unexpectedly.

"Sleep-related causes of infant death" are those linked to how or where a baby sleeps or slept. These deaths are due to accidental causes, such as suffocation, entrapment, or strangulation. Entrapment is when the baby gets trapped between two objects, such as a mattress and a wall, and can't breathe. Strangulation is when something presses on or wraps around the baby's neck, blocking the baby's airway. These deaths are not SIDS.

Other things that SIDS is **not**:

- SIDS is not the same as suffocation and is not caused by suffocation.
- SIDS is not caused by vaccines, immunizations, or shots.
- SIDS is not contagious.
- SIDS is not the result of neglect or child abuse.
- SIDS is not caused by cribs.
- SIDS is not caused by vomiting or choking.
- SIDS is not completely preventable, but there are ways to reduce the risk.

What Causes SIDS?

We don't know exactly what causes SIDS at this time.

Scientists and healthcare providers are working very hard to find the cause or causes of SIDS. If we know the cause or causes, someday we might be able to prevent SIDS from happening at all.

More and more research evidence suggests that infants who die from SIDS are born with brain abnormalities or defects. These defects are typically found within a network of nerve cells that send signals to other nerve cells. The cells are located in the part of the brain that probably controls breathing, heart rate, blood pressure, temperature, and waking from sleep. At the present time, there is no way to identify babies who have these abnormalities, but researchers are working to develop specific screening tests.

But scientists believe that brain defects alone may not be enough to cause a SIDS death. Evidence suggests that other events must also occur for an infant to die from SIDS. Researchers use the Triple-Risk Model to explain this concept. In this model, all three factors have to occur at the same time for an infant to die from SIDS. Having only one of these factors may not be enough to cause death from SIDS, but when all three combine, the chances of SIDS are high.

Even though the exact cause of SIDS is unknown, there are ways to reduce the risk of SIDS and other sleep-related causes of infant death.

What Do We Know about Risk for SIDS and Other Sleep-Related Causes of Infant Death?

Even though we don't know the exact cause of SIDS, we do know that some things can increase a baby's risk for SIDS and other sleep-related causes of infant death. The good news is that there are ways to reduce the risk.

Known Risk Factors for SIDS and Other Sleep-Related Causes of Infant Death

Babies who usually sleep on their backs but who are then placed to sleep on their stomachs, such as for a nap, are at very high risk for SIDS.

Babies are at higher risk for SIDS if they:

- Sleep on their stomachs.

- Sleep on soft surfaces, such as an adult mattress, couch, or chair or under soft coverings.

- Sleep on or under soft or loose bedding.

- Get too hot during sleep.

- Are exposed to cigarette smoke in the womb or in their environment, such as at home, in the car, in the bedroom, or other areas.

- Sleep in an adult bed with parents, other children, or pets; this situation is especially dangerous if:

  - The adult smokes, has recently had alcohol, or is tired.

  - The baby is covered by a blanket or quilt.

  - The baby sleeps with more than one bed-sharer.

  - The baby is younger than 11 to 14 weeks of age.

Ways to Reduce the Risk of SIDS and Other Sleep-Related Causes of Infant Death

Research shows that there are several ways to reduce the risk of SIDS and other sleep-related causes of infant death:

- Always place your baby on his or her back to sleep, for naps and at night, to reduce the risk of SIDS.

- Use a firm sleep surface, such as a mattress in a safety-approved* crib, covered by a fitted sheet, to reduce the risk of SIDS and other sleep-related causes of infant death.

  Visit the U.S. Consumer Product Safety Commission website for more information about crib safety: www.cpsc.gov/en/ Safety-Education/Safety-Education-Centers/cribs

- Room sharing—keeping baby's sleep area separate from your sleep area in the same room where you sleep—reduces the risk of SIDS and other sleep-related causes of infant death.

- Keep soft objects, toys, crib bumpers, and loose bedding out of your baby's sleep area to reduce the risk of SIDS and other sleep-related causes of infant death.

- To reduce the risk of SIDS, do not smoke during pregnancy, and do not smoke or allow smoking around your baby.

- Breastfeed your baby to reduce the risk of SIDS.

- Give your baby a dry pacifier that is not attached to a string for naps and at night to reduce the risk of SIDS.

- Do not let your baby get too hot during sleep.

- Follow healthcare provider guidance on your baby's vaccines and regular health checkups.

- Avoid products that claim to reduce the risk of SIDS and other sleep-related causes of infant death

- Do not use home heart or breathing monitors to reduce the risk of SIDS.

- Give your baby plenty of tummy time when he or she is awake and when someone is watching.

Chapter 49

Transient Tachypnea of the Newborn

Some newborns have very fast or labored breathing in the first few hours of life because of a lung condition called transient tachypnea of the newborn (TTN).

Babies with TTN will be closely watched in the hospital and some might need extra oxygen for a few days. Most babies make a full recovery. TTN usually does not have any lasting effects on a child's growth or development.

About TTN

While inside the mother, a developing fetus does not use the lungs to breathe—all oxygen comes from the blood vessels of the placenta. During this time, the baby's lungs are filled with fluid.

As the baby's due date nears, the lungs begin to absorb the fluid. Some fluid also may be squeezed out during birth as the baby passes through the birth canal. After delivery, as a newborn takes those first breaths, the lungs fill with air and more fluid is pushed out. Any remaining fluid is then coughed out or slowly absorbed through the bloodstream and lymphatic system.

In babies with TTN, though, extra fluid stays in the lungs or is cleared out too slowly. This makes it harder for a baby to breathe in oxygen properly. As a result, the baby must breathe faster and harder to get enough oxygen into the lungs.

Causes of TTN

Transient tachypnea of the newborn is often diagnosed in the first few hours after a baby is born. **Transient** means it does not last long (usually, less than 24 hours) and **tachypnea** refers to the baby's very fast breathing (more than 60 breaths per minute).

TTN can happen in babies of all ages, but is more common in:

- preemies because their lungs are not fully developed

- babies born via rapid vaginal deliveries or C-sections without labor. They don't undergo the usual hormonal changes of labor, so their lungs don't have time to absorb much fluid.

- babies whose mothers have asthma or diabetes

Signs and Symptoms of TTN

Symptoms of TTN include:

- very fast, labored breathing of more than 60 breaths a minute

- grunting or moaning sounds when the baby breathes out (exhales)

- flaring nostrils or head bobbing

- skin pulling in between the ribs or under the ribcage with each breath (known as retractions)

- bluish skin around the mouth and nose (this is called cyanosis)

Diagnosis

To diagnose a baby with TTN, the doctor will do a physical examination, and also might order one or all of the following:

Chest X-ray. In a baby with TTN, an X-ray of the lungs will appear streaky and fluid may be seen. The X-ray will otherwise appear normal.

Pulse-oximetry monitoring. This sort of monitoring can tell doctors how well the lungs are sending oxygen to the blood. A small piece of tape with an oxygen sensor is placed around a baby's foot or hand, then connected to a monitor. Sometimes oxygen levels are checked with a blood test. If oxygen levels are low, extra oxygen may be given to the baby.

Complete blood count (CBC). Blood may be drawn from one of the baby's veins or a heel to check for signs of infection.

Treating TTN

Babies with TTN are watched closely. Doctors check their heart rate, breathing rate, and oxygen levels to make sure breathing slows down and the oxygen level is normal. Sometimes, babies are admitted to the neonatal intensive care unit (NICU) for extra care.

Breathing Help

Some babies with TTN need extra oxygen. They get this through a small tube under the nose called a **nasal cannula**.

A baby who gets extra oxygen but still struggles to breathe might need **continuous positive airway pressure** (CPAP) to keep air flowing through the lungs. With CPAP, a baby wears a special nasal cannula or a mask around the nose while a machine continuously pushes a stream of pressurized air into the nose to help keep the lungs open during breathing. Rarely, a baby will need support with a ventilator (a machine that pumps air in and out of the lungs).

Nutrition

Nutrition can be a problem when a baby is breathing so fast that he or she can't suck, swallow, and breathe at the same time. In that case, intravenous (IV) fluids will keep the baby hydrated while preventing blood sugar from dipping too low.

If your baby has TTN and you want to breastfeed, talk to your doctor or a nurse about maintaining your milk supply by using a breast pump while your newborn receives IV fluids. Sometimes babies can take breast milk or formula through a nasogastric (NG) or orogastric (OG) tube—a tube placed through the nose or mouth to deliver food directly to the stomach. If your baby has one of these tubes, ask the doctor about providing breast milk for your baby.

Symptoms of TTN usually improve within 24 to 72 hours. A baby can be sent home from the hospital once the breathing is normal and he or she has been feeding well for at least 24 hours.

Bringing Your Baby Home

Babies with TTN usually recover fully. But even after TTN goes away, watch for signs of breathing problems and call your doctor right away if you see any.

Call 911 if your baby:

- has trouble breathing
- breathes rapidly
- has skin that looks blue
- has skin in between the ribs or under the ribcage that pulls in during breathing

Part Six

Diagnosing and Treating Respiratory Disorders

Chapter 50

Overview of Pulmonary Function Tests and Spirometry

What Are Lung Function Tests?

Lung function tests, also called pulmonary function tests, measure how well your lungs work. These tests are used to look for the cause of breathing problems, such as shortness of breath.

Lung function tests measure:

- How much air you can take into your lungs. This amount is compared with that of other people your age, height, and sex. This allows your doctor to see whether you're in the normal range.

- How much air you can blow out of your lungs and how fast you can do it.

- How well your lungs deliver oxygen to your blood.

- The strength of your breathing muscles.

Doctors use lung function tests to help diagnose conditions such as asthma, pulmonary fibrosis (scarring of the lung tissue), and COPD (chronic obstructive pulmonary disease).

This chapter includes text excerpted from "Lung Function Tests," National Heart, Lung, and Blood Institute (NHLBI), September 17, 2012. Reviewed September 2016.

Lung function tests also are used to check the extent of damage caused by conditions such as pulmonary fibrosis and sarcoidosis. Also, these tests might be used to check how well treatments, such as asthma medicines, are working.

Types of Lung Function Tests

Breathing Tests

Spirometry

Spirometry measures how much air you breathe in and out and how fast you blow it out. This is measured two ways: peak expiratory flow rate (PEFR) and forced expiratory volume in 1 second (FEV1).

PEFR is the fastest rate at which you can blow air out of your lungs. FEV1 refers to the amount of air you can blow out in 1 second.

During the test, a technician will ask you to take a deep breath in. Then, you'll blow as hard as you can into a tube connected to a small machine. The machine is called a spirometer.

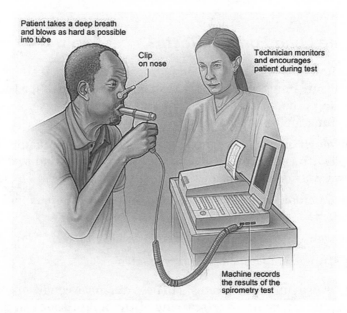

Figure 50.1. *Spirometry*

The image shows how spirometry is done. The patient takes a deep breath and blows as hard as possible into a tube connected to a spirometer. The spirometer measures the amount of air breathed out. It also measures how fast the air was blown out.

Your doctor may have you inhale a medicine that helps open your airways. He or she will want to see whether the medicine changes or improves the test results.

Spirometry helps check for conditions that affect how much air you can breathe in, such as pulmonary fibrosis (scarring of the lung tissue). The test also helps detect diseases that affect how fast you can breathe air out, like asthma and COPD (chronic obstructive pulmonary disease).

Lung Volume Measurement

Body plethysmography is a test that measures how much air is present in your lungs when you take a deep breath. It also measures how much air remains in your lungs after you breathe out fully.

During the test, you sit inside a glass booth and breathe into a tube that's attached to a computer.

For other lung function tests, you might breathe in nitrogen or helium gas and then blow it out. The gas you breathe out is measured to show how much air your lungs can hold.

Lung volume measurement can help diagnose pulmonary fibrosis or a stiff or weak chest wall.

Lung Diffusion Capacity

This test measures how well oxygen passes from your lungs to your bloodstream. During this test, you breathe in a type of gas through a tube. You hold your breath for a brief moment and then blow out the gas.

Abnormal test results may suggest loss of lung tissue, emphysema (a type of COPD), very bad scarring of the lung tissue, or problems with blood flow through the body's arteries.

Tests to Measure Oxygen Level

Pulse oximetry and arterial blood gas tests show how much oxygen is in your blood. During pulse oximetry, a small sensor is attached to your finger or ear. The sensor uses light to estimate how much oxygen is in your blood. This test is painless and no needles are used.

For an arterial blood gas test, a blood sample is taken from an artery, usually in your wrist. The sample is sent to a laboratory, where its oxygen level is measured. You may feel some discomfort during an arterial blood gas test because a needle is used to take the blood sample.

Testing in Infants and Young Children

Spirometry and other measures of lung function usually can be done for children older than 6 years, if they can follow directions well. Spirometry might be tried in children as young as 5 years. However, technicians who have special training with young children may need to do the testing.

Instead of spirometry, a growing number of medical centers measure respiratory system resistance. This is another way to test lung function in young children.

The child wears nose clips and has his or her cheeks supported with an adult's hands. The child breathes in and out quietly on a mouthpiece, while the technician measures changes in pressure at the mouth. During these lung function tests, parents can help comfort their children and encourage them to cooperate.

Very young children (younger than 2 years) may need an infant lung function test. This requires special equipment and medical staff. This type of test is available only at a few medical centers.

The doctor gives the child medicine to help him or her sleep through the test. A technician places a mask over the child's nose and mouth and a vest around the child's chest.

The mask and vest are attached to a lung function machine. The machine gently pushes air into the child's lungs through the mask. As the child exhales, the vest slightly squeezes his or her chest. This helps push more air out of the lungs. The exhaled air is then measured.

In children younger than 5 years, doctors likely will use signs and symptoms, medical history, and a physical exam to diagnose lung problems.

Doctors can use pulse oximetry and arterial blood gas tests for children of all ages.

Other Names for Lung Function Tests

- Lung diffusion testing; also called diffusing capacity and diffusing capacity of the lung for carbon monoxide, or DLCO.

- Pulmonary function tests, or PFTs.

Arterial blood gas tests also are called blood gas analyses or ABGs.

Who Needs Lung Function Tests?

People who have breathing problems, such as shortness of breath, may need lung function tests. These tests help find the cause of breathing problems.

Doctors use lung function tests to help diagnose conditions such as asthma, pulmonary fibrosis (scarring of the lung tissue), and COPD (chronic obstructive pulmonary disease).

Lung function tests also are used to check the extent of damage caused by conditions such as pulmonary fibrosis and sarcoidosis. Also, these tests might be used to check how well treatments, such as asthma medicines, are working.

Diagnosing Lung Conditions

Your doctor will diagnose a lung condition based on your medical and family histories, a physical exam, and test results.

Medical and Family Histories

Your doctor will ask you questions, such as:

- Do you ever feel like you can't get enough air?
- Does your chest feel tight sometimes?
- Do you have periods of coughing or wheezing (a whistling sound when you breathe)?
- Do you ever have chest pain?
- Can you walk or run as fast as other people your age?

Your doctor also will ask whether you or anyone in your family has ever:

- had asthma or allergies
- had heart disease
- smoked
- traveled to places where they may have been exposed to tuberculosis
- had a job that exposed them to dust, fumes, or particles (like asbestos)

Physical Exam

Your doctor will check your heart rate, breathing rate, and blood pressure. He or she also will listen to your heart and lungs with a stethoscope and feel your abdomen and limbs.

517

Your doctor will look for signs of heart or lung disease, or another disease that might be causing your symptoms.

Lung and Heart Tests

Based on your medical history and physical exam, your doctor will recommend tests. A chest X-ray usually is the first test done to find the cause of a breathing problem. This test takes pictures of the organs and structures inside your chest.

Your doctor may do lung function tests to find out even more about how well your lungs work.

Your doctor also may do tests to check your heart, such as an EKG (electrocardiogram) or an exercise stress test. An EKG detects and records your heart's electrical activity. A stress test shows how well your heart works during physical activity.

What to Expect before Lung Function Tests

If you take breathing medicines, your doctor may ask you to stop them for a short time before spirometry, lung volume measurement, or lung diffusion capacity tests.

No special preparation is needed before pulse oximetry and arterial blood gas tests. If you're getting oxygen therapy, your doctor may ask you to stop using it for a short time before the tests. This allows your doctor to check your blood oxygen level without the added oxygen.

What to Expect during Lung Function Tests

Breathing Tests

Spirometry might be done in your doctor's office or in a special lung function laboratory (lab). Lung volume measurement and lung diffusion capacity tests are done in a special lab or clinic. For these tests, you sit in a chair next to a machine that measures your breathing. For spirometry, you sit or stand next to the machine.

Before the tests, a technician places soft clips on your nose. This allows you to breathe only through a tube that's attached to the testing machine. The technician will tell you how to breathe into the tube. For example, you might be asked to breathe normally, slowly, or rapidly.

Some tests require deep breathing, which might make you feel short of breath, dizzy, or light-headed, or it might make you cough.

Spirometry

For this test, you take a deep breath and then exhale as fast and as hard as you can into the tube. With spirometry, your doctor may give you medicine to help open your airways. Your doctor will want to see whether the medicine changes or improves the test results.

Lung Volume Measurement

For body plethysmography, you sit in a clear glass booth and breathe through the tube attached to the testing machine. The changes in pressure inside the booth are measured to show how much air you can breathe into your lungs.

For other tests, you breathe in nitrogen or helium gas and then exhale. The gas that you breathe out is measured.

Lung Diffusion Capacity

During this test, you breathe in gas through the tube, hold your breath for 10 seconds, and then rapidly blow it out. The gas contains a small amount of carbon monoxide, which won't harm you.

Tests to Measure Oxygen Level

Pulse oximetry is done in a doctor's office or hospital. An arterial blood gas test is done in a lab or hospital.

Pulse Oximetry

For this test, a small sensor is attached to your finger or ear using a clip or flexible tape. The sensor is then attached to a cable that leads to a small machine called an oximeter. The oximeter shows the amount of oxygen in your blood. This test is painless and no needles are used.

Arterial Blood Gas

During this test, your doctor or technician inserts a needle into an artery, usually in your wrist, and takes a sample of blood. You may feel some discomfort when the needle is inserted. The sample is then sent to a lab where its oxygen level is measured.

After the needle is removed, you may feel mild pressure or throbbing at the needle site. Applying pressure to the area for 5 to 10 minutes should stop the bleeding. You'll be given a small bandage to place on the area.

What to Expect after Lung Function Tests

You can return to your normal activities and restart your medicines after lung function tests. Talk with your doctor about when you'll get the test results.

What Do Lung Function Tests Show?

Breathing Tests

Spirometry

Spirometry can show whether you have:

- A blockage (obstruction) in your airways. This may be a sign of asthma, COPD (chronic obstructive pulmonary disease), or another obstructive lung disorder.

- Smaller than normal lungs (restriction). This may be a sign of heart failure, pulmonary fibrosis (scarring of the lung tissue), or another restrictive lung disorder.

Lung Volume Measurement

These tests measure how much air your lungs can hold when you breathe in and how much air is left in your lungs when you breathe out. Abnormal test results may show that you have pulmonary fibrosis or a stiff or weak chest wall.

Lung Diffusion Capacity

This test can show a problem with oxygen moving from your lungs into your bloodstream. This might be a sign of loss of lung tissue, emphysema (a type of COPD), or problems with blood flow through the body's arteries.

Tests to Measure Oxygen Level

Pulse oximetry and arterial blood gas tests measure the oxygen level in your blood. These tests show how well your lungs are taking in oxygen and moving it into the bloodstream. A low level of oxygen in the blood might be a sign of a lung or heart disorder.

What Are the Risks of Lung Function Tests?

Spirometry, lung volume measurement, and lung diffusion capacity tests usually are safe. These tests rarely cause problems.

Pulse oximetry has no risks. Side effects from arterial blood gas tests are rare.

Chapter 51

Bronchoscopy

What Is Bronchoscopy?

Bronchoscopy is a procedure used to look inside the lungs' airways, called the bronchi and bronchioles. The airways carry air from the trachea, or windpipe, to the lungs.

During the procedure, your doctor passes a thin, flexible tube called a bronchoscope through your nose (or sometimes your mouth), down your throat, and into your airways. If you have a breathing tube, the bronchoscope can be passed through the tube to your airways.

The bronchoscope has a light and small camera that allow your doctor to see your windpipe and airways and take pictures. You'll be given medicine to make you relaxed and sleepy during the procedure.

If there's a lot of bleeding in your lungs or a large object stuck in your throat, your doctor may use a bronchoscope with a rigid tube. The rigid tube, which is passed through the mouth, is wider. This allows your doctor to see inside it more easily, treat bleeding, and remove stuck objects.

A rigid bronchoscopy usually is done in a hospital operating room using general anesthesia. The term "anesthesia" refers to a loss of feeling and awareness. General anesthesia temporarily puts you to sleep.

This chapter includes text excerpted from "Bronchoscopy," National Heart, Lung, and Blood Institute (NHLBI), February 8, 2012. Reviewed September 2016.

Who Needs Bronchoscopy?

The most common reason why your doctor may decide to do a bronchoscopy is if you have an abnormal chest X-ray or chest computed tomography (CT) scan. These tests may show a tumor, a pneumothorax (collapsed lung), or signs of an infection.

A chest X-ray takes a picture of your heart and lungs. A chest CT scan uses special X-rays to take pictures of the inside of your body.

Other reasons for bronchoscopy include if you're coughing up blood or if you have a cough that has lasted more than a few weeks.

The procedure also can be done to remove something that's stuck in an airway (like a piece of food), to place medicine in a lung to treat a lung problem, or to insert a stent (small tube) in an airway to hold it open when a tumor or other condition causes a blockage.

Bronchoscopy also can be used to check for swelling in the upper airways and vocal cords of people who were burned around the throat area or who inhaled smoke from a fire.

In children, the procedure most often is used to remove something blocking an airway. In some cases, it's used to find out what's causing a cough that has lasted for at least a few weeks.

What to Expect before Bronchoscopy

Your doctor will do the bronchoscopy in a special clinic or in a hospital. To prepare for the procedure, tell your doctor:

- What medicines you're taking, including prescription and over-the-counter medicines. It's helpful to give your doctor a list of the medicines you take.

- About any previous bleeding problems.

- About any allergies to medicines or latex.

The medicine you'll get before the procedure will make you sleepy, so you should arrange for a ride home from the clinic or hospital.

Avoid eating or drinking for 4 to 8 hours before the procedure. Your doctor will let you know the right amount of time.

What to Expect during Bronchoscopy

Your doctor will do the bronchoscopy in an exam room at a special clinic or in a hospital. The bronchoscopy itself usually lasts about 30 minutes. But the entire procedure, including preparation and recovery time, takes about 4 hours.

Your doctor will give you medicine through an intravenous (IV) line in your bloodstream or by mouth to make you sleepy and relaxed.

Your doctor also will squirt or spray a liquid medicine into your nose and throat to make them numb. This helps prevent coughing and gagging when the bronchoscope (long, thin tube) is inserted.

Then, your doctor will insert the bronchoscope through your nose or mouth and into your airways. As the tube enters your mouth, you may gag a little. Once it enters your throat, that feeling will go away.

Your doctor will look at your vocal cords and airways through the bronchoscope (which has a light and a small camera).

During the procedure, your doctor may take a sample of lung fluid or tissue for further testing. Samples can be taken using:

- **Bronchoalveolar lavage.** For this method, your doctor passes a small amount of salt water (a saline solution) through the bronchoscope and into part of your lung. He or she then suctions the salt water back out. The fluid picks up cells and bacteria from the airway, which your doctor can study.

- **Transbronchial lung biopsy.** For this method, your doctor inserts forceps into the bronchoscope and takes a small sample of tissue from inside the lung.

- **Transbronchial needle aspiration.** For this method, your doctor inserts a needle into the bronchoscope and removes cells from the lymph nodes in your lungs. These nodes are small, bean-shaped masses. They trap bacteria and cancer cells and help fight infection.

You may feel short of breath during bronchoscopy, but enough air is getting to your lungs. Your doctor will check your oxygen level. If the level drops, you'll be given oxygen.

If you have a lot of bleeding in your lungs or a large object stuck in your throat, your doctor may use a bronchoscope with a rigid tube. The rigid tube, which is passed through the mouth, is wider. This allows your doctor to see inside it more easily, treat bleeding, and remove stuck objects.

A rigid bronchoscopy usually is done in a hospital operating room using general anesthesia. The term "anesthesia" refers to a loss of feeling and awareness. General anesthesia temporarily puts you to sleep.

After the procedure is done, your doctor will remove the bronchoscope.

What to Expect before Bronchoscopy

After bronchoscopy, you'll need to stay at the clinic or hospital for up to a few hours. If your doctor uses a bronchoscope with a rigid tube, the recovery time is longer. While you're at the clinic or hospital:

- You may have a chest X-ray if your doctor took a sample of lung tissue. This test will check for a pneumothorax and bleeding. A pneumothorax is a condition in which air or gas collects in the space around the lungs. This can cause one or both lungs to collapse. Usually, this condition is easily treated.

- A nurse will check your breathing and blood pressure.

- You can't eat or drink until the numbness in your throat wears off. This takes 1 to 2 hours.

After recovery, you'll need to have someone take you home. You'll be too sleepy to drive.

If samples of tissue or fluid were taken during the procedure, they'll be tested in a lab. Talk to your doctor about when you'll get the lab results.

Recovery and Recuperation

Your doctor will let you know when you can return to your normal activities, such as driving, working, and physical activity. For the first few days, you may have a sore throat, cough, and hoarseness. Call your doctor right away if you:

- develop a fever

- have chest pain

- have trouble breathing

- cough up more than a few tablespoons of blood

What Does Bronchoscopy Show?

Bronchoscopy may show a tumor, signs of an infection, excess mucus in the airways, the site of bleeding, or something blocking your airway.

Your doctor will use the procedure results to decide how to treat any lung problems that were found. Other tests may be needed.

What Are the Risks of Bronchoscopy?

Bronchoscopy usually is a safe procedure. However, there's a small risk for problems, such as:

- A drop in your oxygen level during the procedure. Your doctor will give you oxygen if this happens.

- Minor bleeding and developing a fever or pneumonia.

A rare, but more serious side effect is a pneumothorax. A pneumothorax is a condition in which air or gas collects in the space around the lungs. This can cause one or both lungs to collapse.

Usually, this condition is easily treated or may go away on its own. If it interferes with breathing, a tube may need to be placed in the space around the lungs to remove the air.

Chapter 52

Chest CT Scan

What Is a Chest CT Scan?

A chest computed tomography scan, or chest CT scan, is a painless, noninvasive test. It creates precise pictures of the structures in your chest, such as your lungs. "Noninvasive" means that no surgery is done and no instruments are inserted into your body.

A chest CT scan is a type of X-ray. However, a CT scan's pictures show more detail than pictures from a standard chest X-ray.

Like other X-ray tests, chest CT scans use a form of energy called ionizing radiation. This energy helps create pictures of the inside of your chest.

Types of Chest CT Scans

A CT scanner is a large, tunnel-like machine with a hole in the center. During a chest CT scan, you lie on a table as it moves small distances at a time through the hole.

An X-ray beam rotates around your body as you move through the hole. A computer takes data from the X-rays and creates a series of pictures, called slices, of the inside of your chest.

Different types of chest CT scans have different diagnostic uses.

This chapter includes text excerpted from "Chest CT Scan," National Heart, Lung, and Blood Institute (NHLBI), February 29, 2012. Reviewed September 2016.

High-Resolution Chest CT Scan

High-resolution CT (HRCT) scans provide more than one slice in a single rotation of the X-ray tube. Each slice is very thin and provides a lot of details about the organs and other structures in your chest.

Spiral Chest CT Scan

For this scan, the table moves continuously through the tunnel-like hole as the X-ray tube rotates around you. This allows the X-ray beam to follow a spiral path.

The machine's computer can process the many slices into a very detailed, three-dimensional (3D) picture of the lungs and other structures in the chest.

Other Names for Chest CT Scans

- Lung imaging test

- Computed axial tomography (CAT) scan

- Helical CT scan (another name for spiral CT scan)

Who Needs a Chest CT Scan?

Your doctor may recommend a chest CT scan if you have symptoms of lung problems, such as chest pain or trouble breathing. The scan can help find the cause of the symptoms.

A chest CT scan looks for problems such as tumors, excess fluid around the lungs, and pulmonary embolism (a blood clot in the lungs). The scan also checks for other conditions, such as tuberculosis, emphysema, and pneumonia.

Your doctor may recommend a chest CT scan if a standard chest X-ray doesn't help diagnose the problem. The chest CT scan can:

- provide more detailed pictures of your lungs and other chest structures than a standard chest X-ray

- find the exact location of a tumor or other problem

- show something that isn't visible on a chest X-ray

What to Expect before a Chest CT Scan

What to Wear

Wear loose-fitting, comfortable clothing for the test. Sometimes the CT scan technician (a person specially trained to do CT scans) may ask you to wear a hospital gown.

You also may want to avoid wearing jewelry and other metal objects. You'll be asked to take off any jewelry, eyeglasses, and metal objects that might interfere with the test.

You may be asked to remove hearing aids and dentures as well. Let the technician know if you have any body piercing on your chest.

Pregnancy and Other Conditions

Tell your doctor whether you're pregnant or may be pregnant. If possible, you should avoid unnecessary radiation exposure during pregnancy. This is because of the concern that radiation may harm the fetus.

You and your doctor will decide whether the benefits of a chest CT scan outweigh the possible risks to the fetus, or whether another test might be better. If you do have the chest CT scan, the technician will take extra steps to reduce the fetus' exposure to radiation.

You also should tell your doctor whether:

- you're taking any medicines

- you have any allergies

- you've recently been ill

- you have any medical conditions (for example, heart disease, asthma, diabetes, kidney disease, or thyroid problems)

These factors or conditions may raise your risk of having a bad reaction to the test.

The CT Scanner

The CT scanner is a large, tunnel-like machine with a hole in the center. You'll lie on a table that goes through the hole.

Tell your doctor if you're afraid of tight or closed spaces. He or she may give you medicine to help you relax. This medicine may make you sleepy, so you'll need to arrange for a ride home after the test.

Contrast Dye

Your doctor may inject a substance called contrast dye into a vein in your arm for the test. You may feel some discomfort when the needle is inserted. As the dye is injected, you also may feel warm and have a metallic taste in your mouth. These feelings last only a few minutes.

The contrast dye highlights areas inside your chest, which helps create clearer pictures.

Your doctor may ask you to not eat or drink for a few hours before the test, especially if contrast dye is part of the test.

Some people are allergic to the contrast dye. If you have allergic symptoms, such as itching or hives, tell the technician or doctor right away. He or she can give you medicine to relieve the symptoms.

The most common type of contrast dye used in CT scans contains iodine. Let your doctor know if you're allergic to iodine.

If you're breastfeeding, ask your doctor how long you should wait after the test before you breastfeed. The contrast dye can be passed to your baby through your breast milk.

You may want to prepare for the test by pumping and saving milk for 24 to 48 hours in advance. You can bottle-feed your baby in the hours after the CT scan.

What to Expect during a Chest CT Scan

A chest CT scan takes about 30 minutes, which includes preparation time. The actual scanning time is much shorter, only a few minutes or less.

The CT scanner is a large, tunnel-like machine that has a hole in the middle. You'll lie on a narrow table that moves through the hole.

While you're inside the scanner, an X-ray tube moves around your body. You'll hear soft buzzing, clicking, or whirring noises as the scanner takes pictures.

The CT scan technician who controls the machine will be in the next room. He or she can see you through a glass window and talk to you through a speaker.

Moving your body can cause the pictures to blur. The technician will ask you to lie still and hold your breath for short periods. This will help make the pictures as clear as possible.

The scan itself doesn't hurt, but you may feel anxious if you get nervous in tight or closed spaces. Your doctor may give you medicine to help you relax.

What to Expect after a Chest CT Scan

You usually can return to your normal routine right after a chest CT scan.

If you got medicine to help you relax during the CT scan, your doctor will tell you when you can return to your normal routine. The medicine may make you sleepy, so you'll need someone to drive you home.

If contrast dye was used during the test, you may have a bruise where the needle was inserted. Your doctor may give you special instructions, such as drinking plenty of liquids to flush out the contrast dye.

What Does a Chest CT Scan Show?

A chest CT scan provides detailed pictures of the size, shape, and position of your lungs and other structures in your chest. Doctors use this test to:

- Follow up on abnormal results from standard chest X-rays.

- Find the cause of lung symptoms, such as shortness of breath or chest pain.

- Find out whether you have a lung problem, such as a tumor, excess fluid around the lungs, or a pulmonary embolism (a blood clot in the lungs). The test also is used to check for other conditions, such as tuberculosis, emphysema, and pneumonia.

What Are the Risks of a Chest CT Scan?

Chest CT scans use radiation. The amount of radiation will vary based on the type of CT scan. On average, though, the amount of radiation will not exceed the amount you're naturally exposed to over 3 years. The radiation from the test is gone from the body within a few days.

Children are more sensitive to radiation because they're smaller than adults and still growing.

Exposure to radiation is associated with a risk of cancer. However, it's not known whether the amount of radiation from a chest CT scan increases your risk of cancer.

You and your doctor will decide whether the benefits of the CT scan outweigh any possible risks. Your doctor also will try to avoid ordering repeated CT scans over a short period.

Chapter 53

Chest MRI

What Is Chest MRI?

Chest MRI (magnetic resonance imaging) is a safe, noninvasive test. "Noninvasive" means that no surgery is done and no instruments are inserted into your body. This test creates detailed pictures of the structures in your chest, such as your chest wall, heart, and blood vessels.

Chest MRI uses radio waves, magnets, and a computer to create these pictures. The test is used to:

- look for tumors in the chest

- look at blood vessels, lymph nodes, and other structures in the chest

- help explain the results of other tests, such as a chest X-ray or chest computed tomography scan, also called a chest CT scan

As part of some chest MRIs, a substance called contrast dye is injected into a vein in your arm. This dye allows the MRI to take more detailed pictures of the structures in your chest.

Chest MRI has few risks. Unlike a CT scan or standard X-ray, MRI doesn't use radiation or pose any risk of cancer. Rarely, the contrast dye used for some chest MRIs may cause an allergic reaction or worsen kidney function in people who have kidney disease.

This chapter includes text excerpted from "Chest MRI," National Heart, Lung, and Blood Institute (NHLBI), October 1, 2010. Reviewed September 2016.

Other Names for Chest MRI

Chest MRI also may be called chest nuclear magnetic resonance.

Who Needs Chest MRI?

Your doctor may recommend chest MRI if he or she thinks you have a chest condition, such as:

- a tumor

- problems in the blood vessels, such as an aneurysm or blood clot

- abnormal lymph nodes

- another chest condition, such as a pleural disorder

Chest MRI also may be used to help explain the results of other tests, such as chest X-ray and chest CT scan.

Researchers are exploring ways to use chest MRI to study blood flow in the lungs. The test may help detect early signs of pulmonary hypertension (PH). PH is increased pressure in the pulmonary arteries. These arteries carry blood from your heart to your lungs to pick up oxygen.

What to Expect before Chest MRI

Your doctor or an MRI technician will ask you some questions before the test, such as:

- Are you pregnant or do you think you could be? Generally, you shouldn't have a chest MRI if you're pregnant, especially during the first trimester. Sometimes, though, an MRI is needed to help diagnose a serious condition that may harm you or your baby. If you're pregnant, discuss the risks and benefits of an MRI with your doctor.

- Have you had any surgery? If so, what kind?

- Do you use transdermal patches (patches that stick to the skin) to take any of your medicines? Some medicine patches contain aluminum and other metals. These metals can cause skin burns during an MRI. Examples of transdermal patches are nicotine and fentanyl (medicine used for pain) patches.

- Do you have any metal objects in your body, like metal screws or pins in a bone?

- Do you have any medical devices in your body, such as a pacemaker, an implantable cardioverter defibrillator, cochlear (inner-ear) implants, or brain aneurysm clips? The strong magnets in the MRI machine can damage these devices.

Your answers will help your doctor decide whether you should have chest MRI.

Items Not Allowed in the MRI Room

Your doctor or technician will ask you to not wear or bring metal, electronic, or magnetic objects into the MRI room. Examples include:

- cell phones

- hearing aids

- credit cards

- jewelry and watches

- eyeglasses

- pens

- removable dental work

- any other magnetic objects

MRI magnets can damage these objects, or the objects may interfere with the MRI machine.

The MRI Machine

The MRI machine looks like a long, narrow tunnel. During the MRI, you lie on your back on a sliding table. The table passes through the scanner as it takes pictures of your chest. Newer machines are shorter and wider and don't completely surround you; others are open on all sides.

Tell your doctor if you're afraid of tight or closed spaces. He or she may give you medicine to help you relax, or find you a place that has an open MRI machine.

If you receive medicine to relax you, your doctor may ask you to stop eating about 6 hours before you take it. This medicine may make you tired, so you'll need someone to drive you home.

Contrast Dye

Your doctor may inject a substance called contrast dye into a vein in your arm before the MRI. You may feel some discomfort where the needle is inserted. You also may have a cool feeling as the dye is injected.

Contrast dye allows the MRI to take more detailed pictures of the structures in your chest. The dye used for chest MRIs doesn't contain iodine, so it won't create problems for people who are allergic to iodine. Rarely, people develop allergic symptoms from the dye, such as hives and itchy eyes. If this happens, your doctor can give you medicine to relieve your symptoms.

If you're breastfeeding, ask your doctor how long you need to wait after the test before you breastfeed. The contrast dye can be passed to your baby through your breast milk.

You may want to prepare for the test by pumping and saving milk for 24 to 48 hours in advance. You can bottle-feed your baby in the hours after the test.

What to Expect during Chest MRI

Chest MRI usually is done at a hospital or at a special medical imaging facility. A radiologist or other doctor with special training in this type of test oversees the testing.

Chest MRI usually takes 45 to 90 minutes, depending on how many pictures are needed. The test may take less time with some newer MRI machines.

How the Test Is Done

Chest MRI is painless and has few risks. During the test, you lie on your back on a sliding table as it passes through the MRI machine. A technician will control the machine from the next room. He or she will be able to see you through a glass window and talk to you through a speaker. Tell the technician if you have a hearing problem.

What to Expect after Chest MRI

You usually can return to your normal routine right after chest MRI.

If you got medicine to help you relax during the test, your doctor will tell you when you can return to your normal routine. The medicine may make you tired, so you'll need someone to drive you home.

If contrast dye was used during the test, you may have a bruise where the dye was injected.

What Does Chest MRI Show?

The pictures from chest MRI may show a tumor, problems in the blood vessels (such as an aneurysm or blood clot), abnormal lymph nodes, or another chest condition (such as a pleural disorder).

What Are the Risks of Chest MRI?

The magnetic fields and radio waves used during chest MRI pose no risk.

Serious reactions to the contrast dye used for some MRI tests are very rare. However, side effects are possible and include the following:

- headache
- nausea (feeling sick to your stomach)
- dizziness
- changes in taste
- allergic reactions, such as hives and itchy eyes

Rarely, contrast dye is harmful to people who have moderate to severe kidney disease.

Chapter 54

Chest X-Ray

What Is a Chest X-Ray?

A chest X-ray is a painless, noninvasive test that creates pictures of the structures inside your chest, such as your heart, lungs, and blood vessels. "Noninvasive" means that no surgery is done and no instruments are inserted into your body.

This test is done to find the cause of symptoms such as shortness of breath, chest pain, chronic cough (a cough that lasts a long time), and fever.

Other Names for a Chest X-Ray

- Chest radiography

- CXR

Who Needs a Chest X-Ray?

Doctors may recommend chest X-rays for people who have symptoms such as shortness of breath, chest pain, chronic cough (a cough that lasts a long time), or fever. The test can help find the cause of these symptoms.

This chapter includes text excerpted from "Chest X-ray," National Heart, Lung, and Blood Institute (NHLBI), August 1, 2010. Reviewed September 2016.

Chest X-rays look for conditions such as pneumonia, heart failure, lung cancer, lung tissue scarring, or sarcoidosis. The test also is used to check how well treatments for certain conditions are working.

Chest X-rays also are used to evaluate people who test positive for tuberculosis exposure on skin tests.

Sometimes, doctors recommend more chest X-rays within hours, days, or months of an earlier chest X-ray. This allows them to follow up on a condition.

People who are having certain types of surgery also may need chest X-rays. Doctors often use the test before surgery to look at the structures inside the chest.

What to Expect before a Chest X-Ray

You don't have to do anything special to prepare for a chest X-ray. However, you may want to wear a shirt that's easy to take off. Before the test, you'll be asked to undress from the waist up and wear a gown.

You also may want to avoid wearing jewelry and other metal objects. You'll be asked to take off any jewelry, eyeglasses, and metal objects that might interfere with the X-ray picture. Let the X-ray technician (a person specially trained to do X-ray tests) know if you have any body piercings on your chest.

Let your doctor know if you're pregnant or may be pregnant. In general, women should avoid all X-ray tests during pregnancy. Sometimes, though, having an X-ray is important to the health of the mother and fetus. If an X-ray is needed, the technician will take extra steps to protect the fetus from radiation.

What to Expect during a Chest X-Ray

Chest X-rays are done at doctors' offices, clinics, hospitals, and other healthcare facilities. The location depends on the situation. An X-ray technician oversees the test. This person is specially trained to do X-ray tests.

The entire test usually takes about 15 minutes.

During the Test

Depending on your doctor's request, you'll stand, sit, or lie for the chest X-ray. The technician will help position you correctly. He or she may cover you with a heavy lead apron to protect certain parts of your body from the radiation.

The X-ray equipment usually consists of two parts. One part, a box-like machine, holds the X-ray film or a special plate that records the picture digitally. You'll sit or stand next to this machine. The second part is the X-ray tube, which is located about 6 feet away.

Before the pictures are taken, the technician will walk behind a wall or into the next room to turn on the X-ray machine. This helps reduce his or her exposure to the radiation.

Usually, two views of the chest are taken. The first is a view from the back. The second is a view from the side.

For a view from the back, you'll sit or stand so that your chest rests against the image plate. The X-ray tube will be behind you. For the side view, you'll turn to your side and raise your arms above your head.

If you need to lie down for the test, you'll lie on a table that contains the X-ray film or plate. The X-ray tube will be over the table.

You'll need to hold very still while the pictures are taken. The technician may ask you to hold your breath for a few seconds. These steps help prevent a blurry picture.

Although the test is painless, you may feel some discomfort from the coolness of the exam room and the X-ray plate. If you have arthritis or injuries to the chest wall, shoulders, or arms, you may feel discomfort holding a position during the test. The technician may be able to help you find a more comfortable position.

When the test is done, you'll need to wait while the technician checks the quality of the X-ray pictures. He or she needs to make sure that the pictures are good enough for the doctor to use.

What to Expect after a Chest X-Ray

You usually can go back to your normal routine right after a chest X-ray.

A radiologist will analyze, or "read," your X-ray images. This doctor is specially trained to supervise X-ray tests and look at the X-ray pictures.

The radiologist will send a report to your doctor (who requested the X-ray test). Your doctor will discuss the results with you.

In an emergency, you'll get the X-ray results right away. Otherwise, it may take 24 hours or more. Talk with your doctor about when you should expect the results.

What Does a Chest X-Ray Show?

Chest X-rays show the structures in and around the chest. The test is used to look for and track conditions of the heart, lungs, bones, and chest cavity. For example, chest X-ray pictures may show signs of pneumonia, heart failure, lung cancer, lung tissue scarring, or sarcoidosis.

Chest X-rays do have limits. They only show conditions that change the size of tissues in the chest or how the tissues absorb radiation. Also, chest X-rays create two-dimensional pictures. This means that denser structures, like bone or the heart, may hide some signs of disease. Very small areas of cancer and blood clots in the lungs usually don't show up on chest X-rays.

For these reasons, your doctor may recommend other tests to confirm a diagnosis.

What Are the Risks of a Chest X-Ray?

Chest X-rays have few risks. The amount of radiation used in a chest X-ray is very small. A lead apron may be used to protect certain parts of your body from the radiation.

The test gives out a radiation dose similar to the amount of radiation you're naturally exposed to over 10 days.

Chapter 55

Lung Ventilation/ Perfusion Scan

What Is a Lung Ventilation/Perfusion Scan?

A lung ventilation/perfusion scan, or VQ scan, is a test that measures air and blood flow in your lungs. A VQ scan most often is used to help diagnose or rule out a pulmonary embolism, or PE.

A PE is a sudden blockage in a lung artery. The blockage usually is caused by a blood clot that travels to the lung from a vein in the leg. PE is a serious condition that can cause low blood oxygen levels, damage to the lungs, or even death.

A VQ scan also can detect poor blood flow in the lungs' blood vessels and uneven air distribution, and it can provide pictures that help doctors prepare for some types of lung surgery.

Other Names for Lung Ventilation/Perfusion Scans

Lung ventilation/perfusion scans also are called VQ scans, pulmonary ventilation/perfusion scans, and nuclear medicine tests.

This chapter includes text excerpted from "Lung Ventilation/Perfusion Scan," National Heart, Lung, and Blood Institute (NHLBI), July 25, 2014.

Who Needs a Lung Ventilation/Perfusion Scan?

You may need a VQ scan if you have signs or symptoms of a PE. A PE is a sudden blockage in a lung artery. A blood clot usually causes the blockage.

Signs and symptoms of a PE include chest pain, trouble breathing, rapid breathing, coughing, and coughing up blood. An irregular heartbeat called an arrhythmia also may suggest a PE.

Some blood clots that can cause a PE travel to the lungs from veins deep in the legs. This can cause pain and swelling in the affected limb.

Doctors use VQ scans to help find out whether a PE is causing these signs and symptoms. A VQ scan alone, however, won't confirm whether you have a PE. Your doctor also will consider other factors when making a diagnosis.

Doctors also use VQ scans to detect poor blood flow in the lungs' blood vessels, air trapping or uneven air distribution, and to examine the lungs before some types of surgery.

What to Expect before a Lung Ventilation/Perfusion Scan?

A VQ scan may be done during an emergency to help diagnose or rule out a PE. A PE is a sudden blockage in a lung artery. This serious condition can cause low blood oxygen levels, damage to the lungs, or even death.

If your VQ scan isn't done during an emergency, your doctor will tell you how to prepare for the test. Most people don't need to take any special steps to prepare for a VQ scan.

Your doctor may ask you to wear clothing that has no metal hooks or snaps. These materials can block the scanner's view. Or, you may be asked to wear a hospital gown for the test.

Tell your doctor whether you're pregnant or may be pregnant. If possible, you should avoid radiation exposure during pregnancy, as it may harm the fetus.

You and your doctor will decide whether the benefits of a VQ scan outweigh the small risk to the fetus, or whether another test might be better.

If you're breastfeeding, ask your doctor how long you should wait after the test before you breastfeed. The radioisotopes used for VQ scans can pass through your breast milk to your baby.

You may want to prepare for the scan by pumping and saving milk for 24 to 48 hours in advance. You can bottle-feed your baby in the hours after the VQ scan.

What to Expect during a Lung Ventilation/Perfusion Scan

VQ scans are done at radiology clinics or hospitals.

For the test, you lie on a table for about 1 hour and have two types of scans: ventilation and perfusion. The ventilation scan shows the pattern of air flow in your lungs. The perfusion scan shows the pattern of blood flow in your lungs.

You must lie very still during the tests or the pictures may blur. If you're having trouble staying still, your doctor may give you medicine to help you relax.

Both scans use radioisotopes (a low-risk radioactive substance). This substance releases energy inside your body. Special scanners outside of your body use the energy to create images of air and blood flow in your lungs.

The radioisotopes used in VQ scans can cause an allergic reaction, including itching and hives. Medicines can relieve these symptoms.

Ventilation

For this scan, you lie on a table that moves under the arm of the scanner. You wear a breathing mask over your nose and mouth and inhale a small amount of radioisotope gas mixed with oxygen.

As you breathe, the scanner takes pictures that show air going into your lungs. You'll need to hold your breath for a few seconds at the start of each picture.

The scan is painless, and each picture takes only a few minutes. However, wearing the mask can make some people feel anxious. If this happens, your doctor may give you medicine to help you relax.

Perfusion

For this scan, a small amount of radioisotope is injected into a vein in your arm. The scanner then takes pictures of blood flow through your lungs.

The scan itself doesn't hurt, but you may feel some discomfort from the radioisotope injection.

What to Expect after a Lung Ventilation/Perfusion Scan

Most people can return to their normal activities right after a VQ scan.

If you got medicine to help you relax during the scan, your doctor will tell you when you can return to your normal activities.

The medicine may make you tired, so you'll need someone to drive you home.

You may have a bruise on your arm where the radioisotopes were injected. You'll need to drink plenty of fluids to flush the radioisotopes out of your body. Your doctor can advise you about how much fluid to drink.

What Does a Lung Ventilation/Perfusion Scan Show?

A VQ scan shows how well air and blood are flowing through your lungs. Normal results show full air and blood flow to all parts of your lungs.

If air flow is normal but blood flow isn't, you may have a PE. A PE is a sudden blockage in a lung artery. The blockage usually is caused by a blood clot that travels to the lung from a vein in the leg.

The results of the scan show whether you're at high, medium, or low risk for a PE. However, a VQ scan alone won't confirm whether you have a PE. A scan showing low blood flow in spots may reflect other lung problems, such as lung damage from COPD (chronic obstructive pulmonary disease).

Your doctor uses the VQ scan results—along with results from a physical exam, chest X-ray, and other tests—to make a diagnosis.

What Are the Risks of a Lung Ventilation/Perfusion Scan?

VQ scans involve little risk for most people. The radioisotopes used for both tests expose you to a small amount of radiation. The amount of radiation in the gas and injection together are about the same as the amount a person is naturally exposed to in 1 year.

If you're pregnant or breastfeeding, talk with your doctor about the risk of radiation to your baby. He or she will consider whether another test can be used instead.

Very rarely, the radioisotopes used in VQ scans can cause an allergic reaction. Hives or a rash may result. Medicines can relieve this reaction.

Chapter 56

Sweat Test for Cystic Fibrosis

What It Is

A chloride sweat test helps diagnose cystic fibrosis (CF), an inherited disorder that makes kids sick by disrupting the normal function of epithelial cells. These cells make up the sweat glands in the skin and also line passageways inside the lungs, liver, pancreas, and digestive and reproductive systems. Kids who have CF are at risk for repeated lung infections.

The sweat test measures the amount of chloride in sweat. Kids with cystic fibrosis can have two to five times the normal amount of chloride in their sweat. In a sweat test, the skin is stimulated to produce enough sweat to be absorbed into a special collector and then analyzed.

Doctors may test an infant suspected of having cystic fibrosis as early as 48 hours after birth, though any test done during a baby's first month might need to be repeated because newborns may not produce enough sweat to ensure reliable results.

Why It's Done

Doctors will order a chloride sweat test for kids with positive newborn screen for cystic fibrosis, a family history of cystic fibrosis, or

Text in this chapter is excerpted from "Cystic Fibrosis (CF) Chloride Sweat Test," © 1995–2016. The Nemours Foundation/KidsHealth®. Reprinted with permission.

symptoms of the disorder. Symptoms and signs include failure to grow, repeated lung infections, and digestive problems.

Preparation

No special preparation is necessary for this test. Before having this test, your child may eat, drink, and exercise as usual, and continue to take any current medicines. Creams and lotions should not be applied to the skin 24 hours before the procedure. A sweat test usually takes about an hour, so you may want to bring books or toys to help your child pass the time.

There are no needles used in this procedure.

The Procedure

An area of skin on the arm will be washed and dried. Next, two electrodes are attached with straps. One of these contains a disc with pilocarpine gel, a medicine that makes the sweat glands produce sweat. A weak electric current pushes the medicine through the skin. After this is done, the electrodes are removed and the skin is cleansed.

A special sweat collection device is then attached to the clean skin surface in the area where the sweat glands were stimulated. It's taped to the skin to keep it from moving. The sweat is collected for 30 minutes. The sweat that's collected turns blue when it comes into contact with blue dye within the collector, making it visible to the technician.

After enough sweat is in the tubing inside the collector, it's removed and placed in the sweat analyzer. The collector is removed and the arm is cleaned again. Your child's skin may remain red and continue sweating for several hours after the test.

What to Expect

This test shouldn't be painful, though some kids do feel a slight tingling or tickling sensation when the electrodes apply current to the skin.

Getting the Results

Results are usually available in 1–2 days.

If your child has a sweat chloride level of more than 60 millimoles per liter, it's considered abnormal and indicates a high likelihood of cystic fibrosis, though some children with CF do have borderline or even normal sweat chloride levels. If more sweat is needed, the test might be repeated. If results are positive or unclear, a blood test may be done, especially for babies.

Risks

This test poses very little risk of complications. The electrical current may cause your child's skin to be red or to sweat excessively for a short period of time. In rare cases, the skin may look slightly sunburned.

Helping Your Child

You may choose to stay with your child to help keep him or her distracted during the test.

Chapter 57

Tuberculin Tests

Tuberculosis (TB) is caused by a bacterium called *Mycobacterium tuberculosis*. The bacteria usually attack the lungs, but TB bacteria can attack any part of the body such as the kidney, spine, and brain. Not everyone infected with TB bacteria becomes sick. As a result, two TB-related conditions exist: latent TB infection (LTBI) and TB disease. If not treated properly, TB disease can be fatal.

There are two kinds of tests that are used to detect TB bacteria in the body: the TB skin test (TST) and TB blood tests. A positive TB skin test or TB blood test only tells that a person has been infected with TB bacteria. It does not tell whether the person has latent TB infection (LTBI) or has progressed to TB disease. Other tests, such as a chest X-ray and a sample of sputum, are needed to see whether the person has TB disease.

Tuberculin Skin Testing

What Is It?

The **Mantoux tuberculin skin test** (TST) is the standard method of determining whether a person is infected with *Mycobacterium tuberculosis*. Reliable administration and reading of the TST requires standardization of procedures, training, supervision, and practice.

This chapter includes text excerpted from "Tuberculosis (TB)," Centers for Disease Control and Prevention (CDC), May 4, 2016.

How Is the TST Administered?

The TST is performed by injecting 0.1 ml of tuberculin purified protein derivative (PPD) into the inner surface of the forearm. The injection should be made with a tuberculin syringe, with the needle bevel facing upward. The TST is an intradermal injection. When placed correctly, the injection should produce a pale elevation of the skin (a wheal) 6 to 10 mm in diameter.

How Is the TST Read?

The skin test reaction should be read between 48 and 72 hours after administration. A patient who does not return within 72 hours will need to be rescheduled for another skin test.

The reaction should be measured in millimeters of the induration (palpable, raised, hardened area or swelling). The reader should not measure erythema (redness). The diameter of the indurated area should be measured across the forearm (perpendicular to the long axis).

How Are TST Reactions Interpreted?

Skin test interpretation depends on two factors:

- measurement in millimeters of the induration

- person's risk of being infected with tuberculosis (TB) and of progression to disease if infected

Classification of the Tuberculin Skin Test Reaction

- An **induration of 5 or more millimeters** is considered positive in

  - HIV-infected persons

  - a recent contact of a person with TB disease

  - persons with fibrotic changes on chest radiograph consistent with prior TB

  - patients with organ transplants

  - persons who are immunosuppressed for other reasons (e.g., taking the equivalent of >15 mg/day of prednisone for 1 month or longer, taking tumor necrosis factor (TNF)-antagonists)

- An **induration of 10 or more millimeters** is considered positive in

  - recent immigrants (< 5 years) from high-prevalence countries

  - injection drug users

  - residents and employees of high-risk congregate settings

  - mycobacteriology laboratory personnel

  - persons with clinical conditions that place them at high risk

  - children < 4 years of age

  - infants, children, and adolescents exposed to adults in high-risk categories

- An **induration of 15 or more millimeters** is considered positive in

  - Any person, including persons with no known risk factors for TB. However, targeted skin testing programs should only be conducted among high-risk groups.

Who Can Receive a TST?

Most persons can receive a TST. TST is contraindicated only for persons who have had a severe reaction (e.g., necrosis, blistering, anaphylactic shock, or ulcerations) to a previous TST. It is not contraindicated for any other persons, including infants, children, pregnant women, persons who are HIV-infected, or persons who have been vaccinated with BCG.

How Often Can TSTs Be Repeated?

In general, there is no risk associated with repeated tuberculin skin test placements. If a person does not return within 48–72 hours for a tuberculin skin test reading, a second test can be placed as soon as possible. There is no contraindication to repeating the TST, unless a previous TST was associated with a severe reaction.

What Is a Boosted Reaction?

In some persons who are infected with *M. tuberculosis*, the ability to react to tuberculin may wane over time. When given a TST years after infection, these persons may have a false-negative reaction. However, the TST may stimulate the immune system, causing a positive, or boosted reaction to subsequent tests. Giving a second TST after an initial negative TST reaction is called two-step testing.

Why Is Two-Step Testing Conducted?

Two-step testing is useful for the initial skin testing of adults who are going to be retested periodically, such as healthcare workers or nursing home residents. This two-step approach can reduce the likelihood that a boosted reaction to a subsequent TST will be misinterpreted as a recent infection.

Can TSTs Be given to Persons Receiving Vaccinations?

Vaccination with live viruses may interfere with TST reactions. For persons scheduled to receive a TST, testing should be done as follows:

- either on the same day as vaccination with live-virus vaccine or 4–6 weeks after the administration of the live-virus vaccine

- at least one month after smallpox vaccination

Chapter 58

Other Respiratory Disorder Tests

Gallium Scan

A gallium scan is a safe, effective, and painless scan. It uses a compound that gives off a small amount of radiation (radioisotope). The compound is received by injection. The compound is used only for diagnostic purposes and helps the doctor locate specific sites of tumor, abscess, inflammation, or other abnormalities within a patient's body. The scan takes place in the Nuclear Medicine Department.

Preparation

- No preparation is required before the injection is received. The patient may eat and drink anything.

Procedure

- After the injection is received and before the pictures are taken, the patient must have a good bowel movement. If a laxative is needed to do this, the patient can ask for one.

This chapter contains text excerpted from the following sources: Text beginning with the heading "Gallium Scan" is excerpted from "Gallium Scan," National Institutes of Health (NIH). Reviewed September 2016; Text under the heading "Mediastinoscopy" is excerpted from "NCI Dictionary of Cancer Terms," National Cancer Institute (NCI). Reviewed September 2016; Text under the heading "Pleural Needle Biopsy," is © 2017 Omnigraphics. Reviewed September 2016.

- A small amount of the radioisotope will be injected into a vein. A pinprick will be felt as the injection is given.

- Depending on the purpose of the scan, it may be done 24 or 48 hours after the injection. Sometimes the scan is repeated daily, over 3 to 4 days, but no additional injection will be given. If the test takes place over several days, the patient may return to the diagnostic imaging section at the time scheduled by the appointment clerk.

- During the scan, the patient lies on the back on a firm table with the head flat. A very sensitive machine (scanner) that receives and records radiation, will move over the body from the head to the toes. Many pictures will be taken as the scanner moves.

- The patient stays very still while these pictures are being taken.

- The scan lasts 1 to 2 hours.

After the Procedure

- There are no side effects, but a small amount of radioisotope may still be present in the body for up to 4 weeks.

- The patient may urinate in the toilet as usual. Urine and blood will be labeled "Radioactive" if sent to the laboratory during the first 4 weeks after the injection. The body rids itself of the compound as it does with food that is eaten.

Patients may ask questions about the procedure to the nurse and doctor who are ready to assist them at all times.

Special Instructions

- Because it uses radioactivity, this scan is not performed in pregnant women. Someone who is pregnant or thinks she is pregnant should inform the doctor immediately so that a decision can be made about this scan.

- Also, breast-feeding patients must inform their doctor immediately. Some scans can be performed in breast-feeding women if they are willing to stop breast-feeding for a while.

Mediastinoscopy

Mediastinoscopy is a procedure in which a mediastinoscope is used to examine the organs in the area between the lungs and nearby lymph nodes. A mediastinoscope is a thin, tube-like instrument with a light and a lens for viewing. It may also have a tool to remove tissue to be checked under a microscope for signs of disease. The mediastinoscope is inserted into the chest through an incision above the breastbone. This procedure is usually done to get a tissue sample from the lymph nodes on the right side of the chest.

Pleural Needle Biopsy

Pleural needle biopsy, also known as closed pleural biopsy, is a medical procedure that is usually performed to identify the cause of fluid accumulation in and around the lungs. This procedure is also used to check for diseases and infections in the chest, such as tuberculosis or cancer. During a pleural needle biopsy, a surgeon or other medical professional collects samples of the lungs, the tissue linings of the lungs, and the inside of the chest wall (also known as the pleural cavity).

Procedure

Blood tests and chest X-rays are typically ordered prior to a pleural needle biopsy. Pleural needle biopsies are performed at a hospital, doctor's office, or other medical center. The person receiving the biopsy will typically be in a sitting position. The healthcare provider cleans the skin at the biopsy site and administers anesthetic to numb the skin, the lining of the lungs, and the chest wall. A hollow needle is inserted through the skin into the chest cavity. In some cases, an ultrasound or other medical imaging system is used to guide the needle. A smaller needle is then inserted through the hollow needle. Tissue samples are collected using the smaller needle. Because samples are taken from the lungs, the person receiving the biopsy is often asked to sing, hum, or make the sound "eee" during the procedure, to minimize the risk of air entering the chest cavity and to keep the lungs inflated. After the tissue samples are collected, a bandage is placed over the biopsy site. Post-biopsy chest X-rays may also be ordered.

Results

The results of a pleural needle biopsy can indicate the presence of a variety of health conditions including cancer, tumor, mesothelioma, tuberculosis or other infection, or vascular disease. A surgical pleural biopsy may be required if the results of a pleural needle biopsy are inconclusive.

Risks

During a pleural needle biopsy, there is a small risk that the needle used for sample collection may puncture the wall of the lung. This can result in a collapsed lung. There is also a small risk of air entering the chest cavity during the procedure, which can also result in a collapsed lung. In most cases, a punctured or collapsed lung will heal without intervention. In some cases, the collapsed lung will need to be re-inflated and any accumulated fluid will need to be drained.

Reference

1. "Pleural Needle Biopsy," MedlinePlus, August 11, 2015.

2. Manzoor, Kamran. "Pleural Biopsy," Medscape, WebMD LLC, December 16, 2015.

Chapter 59

Medicines for Respiratory Symptoms

Chapter Contents

Section 59.1

Antibiotics for Respiratory Infections

This section includes text excerpted from "Get Smart: Know When Antibiotics Work," Centers for Disease Control and Prevention (CDC), March 4, 2016.

Adult Treatment Recommendations

The table below summarizes the most recent recommendations for appropriate antibiotic prescribing for adults seeking care in an outpatient setting. Antibiotic prescribing guidelines establish standards of care and focus quality improvement efforts.

The table also offers information related to over-the-counter (OTC) medication for symptomatic therapy. OTC medications can provide symptom relief, but have not been shown to shorten the duration of illness. They also have a low incidence of minor adverse effects. Providers and patients should weigh the potential for benefits and minor adverse effects when considering symptomatic therapy.

Table 59.1. Most Recent Recommendations for Adult Antibiotic Treatment

Condition	Epidemiology	Diagnosis	Management

Acute rhinosinusitis	• About 1 out of 8 adults (12%) in 2012 reported receiving a diagnosis of rhinosinusitis in the previous 12 months, resulting in more than 30 million diagnoses
	• Ninety–98 percent of rhinosinusitis cases are viral, and antibiotics are not guaranteed to help even if the causative agent is bacterial.
		• Diagnose acute bacterial rhinosinusitis based on symptoms that are:
		  • **Severe (>3–4 days)**, such as a fever ≥39°C (102°F) and purulent nasal discharge or facial pain;
		  • **Persistent (>10 days)** without improvement, such as nasal discharge or daytime cough; or
		  • **Worsening (3–4 days)** such as worsening or new onset fever, daytime cough, or nasal discharge after initial improvement of a viral upper respiratory infections (URI) lasting 5–6 days.
		• Sinus radiographs are not routinely recommended.
			• If a bacterial infection is established:
			  • Watchful waiting is encouraged for uncomplicated cases for which reliable follow-up is available.
			  • Amoxicillin or amoxicillin/clavulanate is the recommended first-line therapy.
			  • Macrolides such as azithromycin are not recommended due to high levels of Streptococcus pneumoniae antibiotic resistance (~40%).
			  • For penicillin-allergic patients, doxycycline or a respiratory fluoroquinolone (levofloxacin or moxifloxacin) are recommended as alternative agents.

Table 59.1. Continued

Condition	Epidemiology	Diagnosis	Management

Acute uncomplicated bronchitis	• Cough is the most common symptom for which adult patients visit their primary care provider, and acute bronchitis is the most common diagnosis in these patients.	• Evaluation should focus on ruling out pneumonia, which is rare among otherwise healthy adults in the absence of abnormal vital signs (heart rate ≥ 100 beats/min, respiratory rate ≥ 24 breaths/min, or oral temperature $\geq 38°C$) and abnormal lung examination findings (focal consolidation, egophony, fremitus).
		• Colored sputum does not indicate bacterial infection.
		• For most cases, chest radiography is not indicated.
			• Routine treatment of uncomplicated acute bronchitis with antibiotics is not recommended, regardless of cough duration.
			• Options for symptomatic therapy include:
			  • Cough suppressants (codeine, dextromethorphan);
			  • First-generation antihistamines (diphenhydramine);
			  • Decongestants (phenylephrine); and
			  • Beta-agonists (albuterol).

Common cold or non-specific upper respiratory tract infection (URI)	• The common cold is the third most frequent diagnosis in office visits, and most adults experience two to four colds annually. • At least 200 viruses can cause the common cold.	• Prominent cold symptoms include fever, cough, rhinorrhea, nasal congestion, postnasal drip, sore throat, headache, and myalgias.	• Decongestants (pseudoephedrine and phenylephrine) combined with a first-generation antihistamine may provide short-term symptom relief of nasal symptoms and cough. • Non-steroidal anti-inflammatory drugs can be given to relieve symptoms.

Table 59.1. Continued

Condition	Epidemiology	Diagnosis	Management
			• Evidence is lacking to support antihistamines (as monotherapy), opioids, intranasal corticosteroids, and nasal saline irrigation as effective treatments for cold symptom relief. • Providers and patients must weigh the benefits and harms of symptomatic therapy.
Pharyngitis	• Group A beta-hemolytic streptococcal (GAS) infection is the only common indication for antibiotic therapy for sore throat cases. • Only 5–10 percent of adult sore throat cases are caused by GAS.	• Clinical features alone do not distinguish between GAS and viral pharyngitis; a rapid antigen detection test (RADT) is necessary to establish a GAS pharyngitis diagnosis. • Those who meet two or more Centor criteria (e.g., fever, tonsillar exudates, tender cervical lymphadenopathy, absence of cough) should receive a RADT. Throat cultures are not routinely recommended for adults.	• Antibiotic treatment is NOT recommended for patients with negative RADT results. • Amoxicillin and penicillin V remain first-line therapy due to their reliable antibiotic activity against GAS. • For penicillin-allergic patients, cephalexin, cefadroxil, clindamycin, or macrolides are recommended. • GAS antibiotic resistance to azithromycin and clindamycin are increasingly common. • Recommended treatment course for all oral beta-lactams is 10 days.

Table 59.1. Continued

Condition	Epidemiology	Diagnosis	Management
Acute uncomplicated cystitis	• Cystitis is among the most common infections in women and is usually caused by *E. coli.*	• Classic symptoms include dysuria, frequent voiding of small volumes, and urinary urgency. Hematuria and suprapubic discomfort are less common. • Nitrites and leukocyte esterase are the most accurate indicators of acute uncomplicated cystitis	• For acute uncomplicated cystitis in healthy adult non-pregnant, premenopausal women: • Nitrofurantoin, trimethoprim/ sulfamethoxazole (TMP-SMX, where local resistance is <20%), and fosfomycin are appropriate first-line agents. • Fluoroquinolones (e.g., ciprofloxacin) should be reserved for situations in which other agents are not appropriate.

Section 59.2

Antihistamines

This section includes text excerpted from "Antihistamines,"
National Institutes of Health (NIH), June 9, 2014.

Histamine is an important mediator of immediate hypersensitivity reactions acting locally and causing smooth muscle contraction, vasodilation, increased vascular permeability, edema and inflammation. Histamine acts through specific cellular receptors which have been categorized into four types, H1 through H4. Antihistamines represent a class of medications that block the histamine type 1 (H1) receptors. Importantly, antihistamines do not block or decrease the release of histamine, but rather ameliorate its local actions. Agents that specially block other H2 receptors are generally referred to as H2 blockers rather than antihistamines.

H1 receptors are widely distributed and are particularly common on smooth muscle of the bronchi, gastrointestinal tract, uterus and large blood vessels. H1 receptors are also found in the central nervous system. The antihistamines are widely used to treat symptoms of allergic conditions including itching, nasal stuffiness, runny nose, teary eyes, urticaria, dizziness, nausea and cough. Their most common use alone or in combination with other agents is for symptoms of upper respiratory illnesses such as the common cold. The central nervous system effects of antihistamines include sedation and decrease in anxiety, tension and adventitious movements.

Antihistamines are typically separated into sedating (first generation) and nonsedating (second generation) forms, based upon their central nervous system effects, the nonsedating agents being less likely to cross the blood-brain barrier. In addition, some antihistamines have additional anticholinergic, antimuscarinic or other actions. The antihistamines are some of the most commonly used drugs in medicine, and most are available in multiple forms, both by prescription and in over-the-counter products, alone or combined with analgesics or sympathomimetic agents. Common uses include short term treatment of symptoms of the common cold, seasonal allergic rhinitis (hay fever), motion sickness, nausea, vertigo, cough, urticaria, pruritus and anaphylaxis. The sedating antihistamines are also used as mild sleeping aids and to alleviate tension and anxiety. Many antihistamines are also available in topical forms, as creams, nasal sprays and eye drops for local use in alleviating allergic symptoms. The nonsedating antihistamines are typically used in extended or long term treatment of allergic disorders, including allergic rhinitis (hay fever), sinusitis, atopic dermatitis, and chronic urticaria.

The antihistamines have several adverse side effects which are related to their antihistaminic actions. Side effects are, however, usually mild and rapidly reversed with stopping therapy or decreasing the dose. These common side effects include sedation, impaired motor function, dizziness, dry mouth and throat, blurred vision, urinary retention and constipation. Antihistamines can worsen urinary retention and narrow angle glaucoma.

The antihistamines rarely cause liver injury. Their relative safety probably relates to their use in low doses for a short time only. The nonsedating antihistamines, however, are often used for an extended period and several forms have been linked to rare instances of clinically apparent acute liver injury which has generally been mild and self-limiting; the antihistamines most commonly linked to liver injury have been cyproheptadine, cetirizine and terfenadine (which is no longer in clinical use).

Section 59.3

Cough and Cold Medicines for Respiratory Symptoms

This section includes text excerpted from "Symptom Relief," Centers for Disease Control and Prevention (CDC), April 17, 2015.

While antibiotics cannot treat infections caused by viruses, there are still a number of things you or your child can do to relieve some symptoms and feel better while a viral illness runs its course. Over-the-counter medicines may also help relieve some symptoms.

How to Feel Better

General Advice

For upper respiratory infections, such as sore throats, ear infections, sinus infections, colds, and bronchitis, try the following:

- Get plenty of rest.
- Drink plenty of fluids.
- Use a clean humidifier or cool mist vaporizer.
- Avoid smoking, secondhand smoke, and other pollutants (airborne chemicals or irritants).
- Take acetaminophen, ibuprofen or naproxen to relieve pain or fever.
- Use saline nasal spray or drops.

Sore Throat

Try the following tips if you or your child has a sore throat:

- Soothe a sore throat with ice chips, sore throat spray, popsicles, or lozenges (do not give lozenges to young children).
- Use a clean humidifier or cool mist vaporizer.
- Gargle with salt water.
- Drink warm beverages.
- Take acetaminophen, ibuprofen or naproxen to relieve pain or fever.

Ear Pain

The following tips can be used to help ease the pain from earaches:

- Put a warm moist cloth over the ear that hurts.
- Take acetaminophen, ibuprofen or naproxen to relieve pain or fever (read about what is safe to give your child).

Runny Nose

Stop a runny nose in its tracks by trying the following tips:

- Get plenty of rest.

- Increase fluid intake.

- Use a decongestant or saline nasal spray to help relieve nasal symptoms.

Cough

The following tips can be used to help with coughing:

- Use a clean humidifier or cool mist vaporizer.

- Breathe in steam from a bowl of hot water or shower.

- Use non-medicated lozenges (do not give lozenges to young children).

- Use honey if your child is at least 1 year old.

Over-the-Counter Medicines

For children and adults, over-the-counter (OTC) pain relievers, decongestants and saline nasal sprays may help relieve some symptoms, such as runny nose, congestion, fever, and aches, but they do not shorten the length of time you or your child is sick. Remember to always use OTC products as directed. Not all products are recommended for children of certain ages.

Pain Relievers for Children

For babies 6 months of age or younger, parents should only give acetaminophen for pain relief. For a child 6 months of age or older, either acetaminophen or ibuprofen can be given for pain relief. Be sure to ask your child's healthcare professional for the right dosage for your child's age and size. Do not give aspirin to your child because of Reye syndrome, a rare but very serious illness that harms the liver and brain.

Cough and Cold Medicines for Children Younger than 4 Years of Age

Do not use cough and cold products in children younger than 4 years of age unless specifically told to do so by a healthcare professional. Overuse and misuse of OTC cough and cold medicines in young children can result in serious and potentially life-threatening side effects. Instead, parents can clear nasal congestion (snot) in infants with a rubber suction bulb. A stuff nose can also be relieved with saline nose drops or a clean humidifier or cool-mist vaporizer.

Cough and Cold Medicines for Children Older than 4 Years of Age

OTC cough and cold medicines may give your child some temporary relief of symptoms even though they will not cure your child's illness. Parents should talk with their child's healthcare professional if they have any concerns or questions about giving their child an OTC medication. Parents should always tell their child's healthcare professional about all prescription and OTC medicines they are giving their child.

Chapter 60

Asthma Medications: Long-Term Control and Quick-Relief

Your Asthma Medicines: How They Work and How to Take Them

Most people who have asthma need two kinds of medicines: longterm control medicines and quick-relief medicines.

Long-Term Control Medicines

These are medicines that you take every day for a long time, to stop and control the inflammation in your airways and thereby prevent symptoms and attacks from coming on in the first place.

These medicines work slowly, and you may need to take them for several weeks or longer before you feel better. If your asthma is not

---

This chapter contains text excerpted from the following sources: Text beginning with the heading "Your Asthma Medicines: How They Work and How to Take Them" is excerpted from "So You Have Asthma," National Heart, Lung, and Blood Institute (NHLBI), March 2013; Text under the heading "Basic Facts about Asthma Medications" is excerpted from "Management of Asthma," Federal Bureau of Prisons (BOP), May 2013.

well controlled, your doctor may increase the dose or add another medicine to your treatment. Once your asthma is under control, your doctor may be able to reduce some of these medicines.

The most effective long-term control medicines are anti-inflammatory medicines. They reduce the inflammation in your airways, making the airways less sensitive and less likely to react to your asthma triggers.

Anti-inflammatory medicines are most effective when you take them every day, even when you don't have any symptoms.

The most effective anti-inflammatory medicines for most people who have asthma are inhaled corticosteroids.

Some people don't like the idea of taking steroids. But the inhaled corticosteroids used to treat asthma are very different from the illegal anabolic steroids taken by some athletes. They are not habit-forming—even if you take them every day for many years. And, because they are inhaled, the medicine goes right to your lungs where it is needed. Also, they have been studied for many years in large groups of adults and children as young as 2 years old and, in general, have been found to be well tolerated and safe when taken as directed by your doctor.

Like many other medicines, inhaled corticosteroids can have side effects. But most doctors agree that the benefits of taking them and preventing attacks far outweigh the risks of side effects. Take inhaled corticosteroids as your doctor prescribes and use a spacer or holding chamber with your inhaler to make sure the medicine goes directly to your lungs. Be sure to rinse your mouth out with water, and don't swallow the water, after taking these medicines. Rinsing helps prevent an infection in the mouth.

Other long-term control medicines used to treat asthma include:

- **Inhaled long-acting beta$_2$-agonists**—These bronchodilators can help prevent symptoms when taken *with* inhaled corticosteroids by helping to keep airway muscles relaxed.

  These medicines should *not* be used alone. They also should not be used to treat symptoms or an attack.

  Two-in-one medicines that contain both corticosteroids and long-acting beta$_2$-agonists are available.

- **Cromolyn sodium**—This nonsteroidal anti-inflammatory medicine can be used to treat mild persistent asthma, especially in children. It's not as effective as inhaled corticosteroids.

- **Leukotriene modifiers**—These antileukotriene medicines are a newer class of long-term control medicines that block the action of chemicals in your airways. If not blocked, these chemicals, called leukotrienes, increase the inflammation in your lungs during an asthma attack.

- Anti-leukotriene medicines, which are available in pill form, are used alone to treat mild persistent asthma or with inhaled corticosteroids to treat moderate persistent asthma. They are not as effective as inhaled corticosteroids for most patients.

- **Theophylline**—This medicine, also available in pill form, acts as a bronchodilator to relax and open the airways. It can help prevent nighttime symptoms. It is sometimes used alone to treat mild persistent asthma, but most of the time it is used with inhaled corticosteroids.

If you take theophylline, you need to have your blood levels checked regularly to make sure the dose is right for you.

With long-term control medicines, it's important to take them every day, as your doctor prescribes.

Quick-Relief Medicines

You take these medicines when you need immediate relief of your symptoms. Everyone who has asthma needs a quick-relief medicine—usually taken by inhaler—to stop asthma symptoms before they get worse.

The preferred quick-relief medicine is an inhaled short-acting beta$_2$-agonist. It acts quickly to relax tightened muscles around your airways so that your airways can open up and allow more air to flow through.

You should take your quick-relief medicine at the first sign of any asthma symptoms. Your doctor may recommend that you take this medicine at other times, as well—for example, before exercise.

Short-acting beta$_2$-agonists include albuterol, levalbuterol, and pirbuterol. They are also called by their brand names.

Other quick-relief medicines are:

- **Anticholinergics**—These medicines are used primarily in the emergency department, but if you have moderate to severe asthma, your doctor may recommend that you use them with a short-acting beta$_2$-agonist to relieve symptoms. Or, if you can't tolerate a short-acting beta$_2$-agonist, this may be the treatment of choice for you.

- **Systemic corticosteroids**—Usually taken in the form of a pill or syrup, systemic corticosteroids may be used to speed your recovery after an asthma attack and to prevent more attacks. You would take them for 3–10 days. People who have severe asthma may need to take systemic corticosteroids for longer periods of time.

Quick-relief medicine is very good at stopping asthma symptoms, but it does nothing to control the inflammation in your airways that produces these symptoms. If you need to use your quick-relief inhaler more often than usual, or if you need to use it more than 2 days a week, it may be a sign that you also need to take a long-term control medicine to reduce the inflammation in your airways. Discuss this with your doctor as soon as possible.

Basic Facts about Asthma Medications

For optimal self-management, patients need to be educated about their medication, especially how and when to use them. Regardless of the delivery device selected, detailed education on the use and maintenance of the device is necessary. The package inserts provided with these products often include detailed diagrams explaining proper technique. The patient should be able to demonstrate good technique initially and with each follow-up visit. Reinforcement of proper technique ensures proper delivery of medication.

Although numerous patients utilize metered dose inhalers (MDI) each day, many do not operate them correctly. As a result, both the provider and the patient may be unaware of improper usage and incorrectly assume a medication is ineffective. This may lead prescribers to unnecessarily change or step up therapy.

In order to promote the effective use of an inhaler, providers should:

- At each routine encounter, have the patient demonstrate using the MDI by performing an actual inhalation.

- Prescribe inhalers with valved holding chambers or require the use of a spacer with the prescribed MDI for those patients who cannot demonstrate adequate technique.

- Educate the patient on how many inhalations should be used at one time. For example, if the instructions say to utilize two puffs, how long should the patient wait after each puff?

- Educate the patient on the order in which inhalers should be used. For example, should the patient use a beta-agonist before using a corticosteroid?

Chapter 61

Corticosteroids for Asthma Treatment

Inhaled corticosteroids are the most effective medications for long-term management of persistent asthma and should be utilized by patients and clinicians as is recommended in the guidelines for treatment of asthma.

Use Inhaled Corticosteroids for Better Asthma Control and Fewer Flare-UpS

Because asthma is a chronic inflammatory disorder, persistent asthma is most effectively controlled with daily long-term control medication directed toward suppressing inflammation. Inhaled corticosteroids (ICS) are the most effective long-term therapy available for mild, moderate, or severe persistent asthma. ICS are anti-inflammatory medications that reduce airway hyperresponsiveness, inhibit inflammatory cell migration and activation, and block late phase reaction to allergen. In general, ICS are well tolerated and safe at the recommended dosages.

This chapter contains text excerpted from the following sources: Text in this chapter begins with excerpts from "Inhaled Corticosteroids: Keep Airways Open," National Asthma Control Initiative (NACI), National Heart, Lung, and Blood Institute (NHLBI), January 2013; Text beginning with the heading "Systemic Corticosteroids" is excerpted from "Management of Asthma," Federal Bureau of Prisons (BOP), May 2013.

Generally, ICS improve asthma control more effectively, in both children and adults, than any other single long-term control medication. However, alternative options for medications are available to tailor treatment to individual patient circumstances, needs, and preferences. The benefits of ICS outweigh the concerns about the potential risk of a small, non-progressive reduction in growth velocity in children, or other possible adverse effects.

Systemic Corticosteroids

Systemic corticosteroids are indicated for moderate-to-severe exacerbations to speed recovery and prevent recurrence of exacerbations. During an asthma exacerbation, doubling the dose of an inhaled corticosteroid is not effective. Hydrocortisone sodium succinate or dexamethasone, given either intramuscular or intravenously, are the most rapid-acting agents; however, their onset of action is several hours. Short-term therapy should continue until the inmate achieves 80 percent of his/her personal best objective measures, usually 3–10 days.

Note: *Tapering systemic steroids following clinical improvement after a short treatment course does not prevent relapse and is not recommended.*

Long-Term Control Medications

Corticosteroids

Inhaled corticosteroid (ICS) formulations such as beclomethasone, mometasone, budesonide, and fluticasone are used for long-term control of asthma; their regular use, when medically indicated for asthma, is associated with improved asthma control, reduced risk of exacerbations, and decreased risk of death. Although the benefits of ICSs outweigh the risk of systemic adverse effects, they should be titrated to as low a dose as needed to maintain control. The National Asthma Education and Prevention Program (NAEPP) Expert Panel reported that most patients were able to maintain asthma control with a 50 percent reduction in dose of their ICS, if the patient had been well-controlled on a high dose of an ICS alone for at least 60 days. Systemic corticosteroids such as methylprednisolone, prednisolone, and prednisone may be used long-term for the prevention of symptoms associated with severe persistent asthma.

Table 61.1. Inhaled Corticosteroids Dosing Chart

Inhaled Steroid	Low Dose	Medium Dose	High Dose
Beclomethasone HFA 40 mcg or 80 mcg	80–240 mcg **Initial**: 80 mcg BID	240–480 mcg **Initial**: 160 mcg BID	>480 mcg **Max**: 320 mcg BID
Budesonide 90 mcg or 180 mcg	180–600 mcg **Initial**: 180 mcg BID	600–1200 mcg **Initial**: 360 mcg BID	>1200 mcg **Max**: 720 mcg BID
Fluticasone HFA 44 mcg, 110 mcg, or 220 mcg	88–264 mcg **Initial**: 88 mcg BID	>264–440 mcg **Initail**:220 mcg BID (110 mcg 2 puffs BID)	>440 mcg **Max**: 880 mcg BID
Mometasone Furoate 110 mcg or 220 mcg	220 mcg **Initial**: 220 mcg daily	440 mcg **Initial**: 440 mcg daily or 220 mcg BID	>440 mcg **Max**: 440 mcg BID
Fluticasone/ Salmeterol 100/50 mcg, 250/50 mcg, or 500/50 mcg	100–300 mcg* **Initial**: 100/50 mcg BID	>300–500 mcg* **Initial**: 250/50 mcg BID	>500 mcg* **Max**: 500/50 mcg BID
Budesonide/ Formoterol 80/4.5 mcg or 160/4.5 mcg		320–640 mcg** **Initial**: 80/4.5 mcg two puffs BID	640 mcg** **Max**: 160/4.5 mcg two puffs BID
Flunisolide 250 mcg	500–1000 mcg **Initial**: 500 mcg BID	1000–2000 mcg	2000mcg **Max**: 1000 mcg BID

* Low, medium, and high dosing of fluticasone/salmeterol is determined by the dose of fluticasone administered.

** Medium, high, and max dosing of budesonide/formoterol is determined by the dose of budesonide administered.

Step Therapy for Asthma

The approach to treating asthma is a stepwise approach based on the NAEPP expert panel report. Clinicians should individualize treatment plans, as well as develop an individual action plan. Since the course of the disease is variable, once asthma control is achieved, monitoring is essential. At times it may be necessary to step up or down therapy. Stepping therapy down is necessary for identifying the minimum medication necessary to maintain control and minimizing the risk of adverse events.

Once the provider assesses the patient's impairment and risk, the provider should determine the level of care for the corresponding treatment level. This can be accomplished both at initiation of therapy and during follow-up care.

Step 1: Intermittent Asthma

At this stage in asthma therapy, a detailed asthma management plan should be in place. This plan should ensure that the inmate understands when and how a medication should be taken, how much to take, how to evaluate the response to therapy, when to seek medical care, and what to do when the desired effect is not achieved or side effects are encountered.

For certain persons with intermittent asthma, severe life-threatening exacerbations may occur, separated by lengthy periods of normal pulmonary function without symptoms. For an exacerbation that is precipitated by a viral respiratory infection, the following is recommended:

- History of severe exacerbations with viral respiratory infections: Systemic corticosteroids at the first sign of infection.

Step 2: Mild Persistent Asthma

Persistent asthma should be treated with a daily "maintenance" medication. The most effective medications and the mainstay of asthma therapy are the ICSs. At this stage of asthma severity, an ICS should be initiated at a low dose. Although some studies have looked at the usefulness of PRN ICS use in mild persistent asthma, there is no clear evidence of positive long-term outcomes. Therefore, intermittent usage of an ICS in asthma treatment is not recommended.

Step 3: Severe Persistent Asthma

At this step, consult with a pulmonary specialist is advised. An oral corticosteroid should be added to high-dose ICS and LABA on a trial basis. This trial is to assess reversibility; hence the need for long-term corticosteroid therapy. If corticosteroids need to be used for a longer period of time, then the lowest possible dose (single dose daily or on alternate days) should be utilized. Once asthma control is achieved, attempts should be made to reduce the systemic corticosteroids. Alternatively, a trial of a leukotriene receptor antagonist (LTRA), theophylline, or zileuton can be added to high-dose ICS and LABA.

Chapter 62

Oxygen Therapy

What Is Oxygen Therapy?

Oxygen therapy is a treatment that provides you with extra oxygen, a gas that your body needs to work well. Normally, your lungs absorb oxygen from the air. However, some diseases and conditions can prevent you from getting enough oxygen.

Oxygen therapy may help you function better and be more active. Oxygen is supplied in a metal cylinder or other container. It flows through a tube and is delivered to your lungs in one of the following ways:

- Through a nasal cannula, which consists of two small plastic tubes, or prongs, that are placed in both nostrils.

- Through a face mask, which fits over your nose and mouth.

- Through a small tube inserted into your windpipe through the front of your neck. Your doctor will use a needle or small incision (cut) to place the tube. Oxygen delivered this way is called transtracheal oxygen therapy.

Oxygen therapy can be done in a hospital, another medical setting, or at home. If you need oxygen therapy for a chronic (ongoing) disease or condition, you might receive home oxygen therapy.

This chapter includes text excerpted from "Oxygen Therapy," National Heart, Lung, and Blood Institute (NHLBI), February 24, 2012. Reviewed September 2016.

Other Names for Oxygen Therapy

- Oxygen

- Supplemental oxygen

Who Needs Oxygen Therapy?

Your doctor may recommend oxygen therapy if you have a low blood oxygen level. Normally, your lungs absorb oxygen from the air and transfer it into your bloodstream.

Some acute (short-term) and chronic (ongoing) diseases and conditions can prevent you from getting enough oxygen.

Acute Diseases and Conditions

You may receive oxygen therapy if you're in the hospital for a serious condition that prevents you from getting enough oxygen. Once you've recovered from the condition, the oxygen will likely be stopped.

Some diseases and conditions that may require short-term oxygen therapy are:

- **Severe pneumonia.** Pneumonia is an infection in one or both of the lungs. If severe, the infection causes your lungs' air sacs to become very inflamed. This prevents the air sacs from moving enough oxygen into your blood.

- **Severe asthma attack.** Asthma is a lung disease that inflames and narrows the airways. Most people who have asthma, including many children, can safely manage their symptoms. But if you have a severe asthma attack, you may need hospital care that includes oxygen therapy.

- **Respiratory distress syndrome (RDS) or bronchopulmonary dysplasia (BPD) in premature babies.** Premature babies may develop one or both of these serious lung conditions. As part of their treatment, they may receive extra oxygen through a nasal continuous positive airway pressure (NCPAP) machine or a ventilator, or through a tube in the nose.

Chronic Diseases and Conditions

Long-term home oxygen therapy might be used to treat some diseases and conditions, such as:

- **COPD (chronic obstructive pulmonary disease).** This is a progressive disease in which damage to the air sacs prevents them from moving enough oxygen into the bloodstream. "Progressive" means the disease gets worse over time.

- **Late-stage heart failure.** This is a condition in which the heart can't pump enough oxygen-rich blood to meet the body's needs.

- **Cystic fibrosis (CF).** CF is an inherited disease of the secretory glands, including the glands that make mucus and sweat. People who have CF have thick, sticky mucus that collects in their airways. The mucus makes it easy for bacteria to grow. This leads to repeated, serious lung infections. Over time, these infections can severely damage the lungs.

- **Sleep-related breathing disorders** that lead to low levels of oxygen in the blood during sleep, such as sleep apnea.

How Does Oxygen Therapy Work?

Oxygen therapy provides you with extra oxygen, a gas that your body needs to work well. Oxygen comes in different forms and can be delivered to your lungs in several ways.

Oxygen Therapy Systems

Oxygen is supplied in three forms: as compressed gas, as liquid, or as a concentrated form taken from the air.

Compressed oxygen gas is stored under pressure in metal cylinders. The cylinders come in many sizes. Some of the cylinders are small enough to carry around. You can put one on a small wheeled cart or in a shoulder bag or backpack.

Liquid oxygen is very cold. When released from its container, the liquid becomes gas. Liquid oxygen is delivered to your home in a large container. From this container, smaller, portable units can be filled.

The advantage of liquid oxygen is that the storage units need less space than compressed or concentrated oxygen. However, liquid oxygen costs more than the other forms of oxygen. Also, it evaporates easily, so it doesn't last for a long time.

Oxygen concentrators filter out other gases in the air and store only oxygen. Oxygen concentrators come in several sizes, including portable units.

Oxygen concentrators cost less than the other oxygen therapy systems. One reason is because they don't require oxygen refills. However, oxygen concentrators are powered by electricity. Thus, you'll need a backup supply of oxygen in case of a power outage.

Delivery Devices

Most often, oxygen is given through a nasal cannula. A nasal cannula consists of two small plastic tubes, or prongs, that are placed in both nostrils.

To help hold the cannula in place, you can put the longer ends of it over your ears or attach them to a special kind of eyeglass frame that helps hide the tubing. The tubing then comes around the back of your ears and under your chin, where it joins together. From there, it's attached to the tube from the oxygen container.

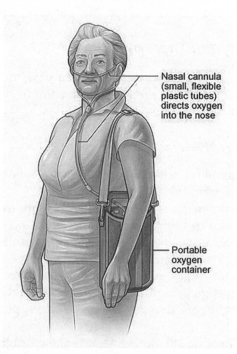

Nasal cannula (small, flexible plastic tubes) directs oxygen into the nose

Portable oxygen container

Figure 62.1. *Nasal Cannula and Portable Oxygen Container*

The image shows how a nasal cannula and portable oxygen container are attached to a patient.

You might use a face mask instead of a nasal cannula. The mask fits over your mouth and nose. This method mainly is used if you need a high flow rate of oxygen or if your nose is clogged from a cold.

The face mask is held in place with a strap that goes around your head or with tubes that fit around your ears. The oxygen is delivered through a tube that attaches to the front of the mask.

Oxygen also can be delivered through a small tube inserted into your windpipe through the front of your neck. Your doctor will use a needle or small incision (cut) to place the tube. Oxygen delivered this way is called transtracheal oxygen therapy.

If you're getting transtracheal oxygen therapy, you'll need to have a humidifier attached to your oxygen system. This is because the oxygen doesn't pass through your nose or mouth like it does with the other delivery systems. A humidifier adds moisture to the oxygen and prevents your airways from getting too dry.

Oxygen also can be delivered through machines that support breathing, such as CPAP (continuous positive airway pressure) devices or ventilators.

What to Expect before Oxygen Therapy

During an emergency—such as a serious accident, possible heart attack, or other life-threatening event—you might be started on oxygen therapy right away.

Otherwise, your doctor will decide whether you need oxygen therapy based on test results. An arterial blood gas test and a pulse oximetry test can measure the amount of oxygen in your blood.

For an arterial blood gas test, a small needle is inserted into an artery, usually in your wrist. A sample of blood is taken from the artery. The sample is then sent to a laboratory, where its oxygen level is measured.

For a pulse oximetry test, a small sensor is attached to your fingertip or toe. The sensor uses light to estimate how much oxygen is in your blood.

If the tests show that your blood oxygen level is low, your doctor may prescribe oxygen therapy. In the prescription, your doctor will include the number of liters of oxygen per minute that you need (oxygen flow rate). He or she also will include how often you need to use the oxygen (frequency of use).

Frequency of use includes when and for how long you should use the oxygen. Depending on your condition and blood oxygen level, you may need oxygen only at certain times, such as during sleep or while exercising.

If your doctor prescribes home oxygen therapy, he or she can help you find a home equipment provider. The provider will give you the equipment and other supplies you need.

What to Expect during Oxygen Therapy

During an emergency—such as a serious accident, possible heart attack, or other life-threatening event—you might be started on oxygen therapy right away.

While you're in the hospital, your doctor will check on you to make sure you're getting the right amount of oxygen. Nurses or respiratory therapists also may assist with the oxygen therapy.

If you're having oxygen therapy at home, a home equipment provider will help you set up the oxygen therapy equipment at your house.

Trained staff will show you how to use and take care of the equipment. They'll supply the oxygen and teach you how to safely handle it.

Your home equipment provider will give you a complete list of safety steps that you'll need to follow at home and in public. For example, while on oxygen, you should:

- never smoke or be around people who are smoking

- never use paint thinners, cleaning fluids, gasoline, aerosol sprays, and other flammable materials

- stay at least 5 feet away from gas stoves, candles, and other heat sources

What Are the Risks of Oxygen Therapy?

Oxygen therapy can cause complications and side effects. These problems might include a dry or bloody nose, skin irritation from the nasal cannula or face mask, fatigue (tiredness), and morning headaches.

If these problems persist, tell your doctor and home equipment provider. Depending on the problem, your doctor may need to change your oxygen flow rate or the length of time you're using the oxygen.

If nose dryness is a problem, your doctor may recommend a nasal spray or have a humidifier added to your oxygen equipment.

If you have an uncomfortable nasal cannula or face mask, your home equipment provider can help you find a device that fits better. Your provider also can recommend over-the-counter gels and devices that are designed to lessen skin irritation.

Complications from transtracheal oxygen therapy can be more serious. With this type of oxygen therapy, oxygen is delivered through a tube inserted into your windpipe through the front of your neck.

With transtracheal oxygen therapy:

- Mucus balls might develop on the tube inside the windpipe. Mucus balls tend to form as a result of the oxygen drying out the airways. Mucus balls can cause coughing and clog the windpipe or tube.

- Problems with the tube slipping or breaking.

- Infection.

- Injury to the lining of the windpipe.

Proper medical care and correct handling of the tube and other supplies may reduce the risk of complications.

Other Risks

In certain people, oxygen therapy may suppress the drive to breathe, affecting how well the respiratory system works. This is managed by adjusting the oxygen flow rate.

Oxygen poses a fire risk, so you'll need to take certain safety steps. Oxygen itself isn't explosive, but it can worsen a fire. In the presence of oxygen, a small fire can quickly get out of control. Also, the cylinder that compressed oxygen gas comes in might explode if exposed to heat.

Your home equipment provider will give you a complete list of safety steps you'll need to take at home and when out in public.

For example, when you're not using the oxygen, keep it in an airy room. Never store compressed oxygen gas cylinders and liquid oxygen containers in small, enclosed places, such as in closets, behind curtains, or under clothes.

Oxygen containers let off small amounts of oxygen. These small amounts can build up to harmful levels if they're allowed to escape into small spaces.

Chapter 63

Pulmonary Rehabilitation

What Is Pulmonary Rehabilitation?

Pulmonary rehabilitation, also called pulmonary rehab or PR, is a broad program that helps improve the well-being of people who have chronic (ongoing) breathing problems.

For example, PR may benefit people who have COPD (chronic obstructive pulmonary disease), sarcoidosis, idiopathic pulmonary fibrosis, or cystic fibrosis.

PR also can benefit people who need lung surgery, both before and after the surgery.

PR doesn't replace medical therapy. Instead, it's used with medical therapy and may include:

- exercise training

- nutritional counseling

- education on your lung disease or condition and how to manage it

- energy-conserving techniques

- breathing strategies

- psychological counseling and/or group support

This chapter includes text excerpted from "Pulmonary Rehabilitation," National Heart, Lung, and Blood Institute (NHLBI), August 1, 2010. Reviewed September 2016.

PR involves a long-term commitment from the patient and a team of healthcare providers. The PR team may include doctors, nurses, and specialists. Examples of specialists include respiratory therapists, physical and occupational therapists, dietitians or nutritionists, and psychologists or social workers.

PR often is an outpatient program based in a hospital or clinic. Some patients also can receive PR in their homes.

When you start PR, your rehab team will create a plan that's tailored to your abilities and needs. You'll likely attend your PR program weekly. Your team also will expect you to follow your plan, including exercises and lifestyle changes, at home.

PR has many benefits. It can improve your ability to function and your quality of life. The program also may help relieve your breathing problems. Even if you have advanced lung disease, you can still benefit from PR.

Who Needs Pulmonary Rehabilitation?

Your doctor may recommend PR if you have a chronic (ongoing) lung disease. He or she also may suggest PR if you have a condition that makes it hard for you to breathe and limits your activities.

For example, you may benefit from PR if you have:

- **COPD (chronic obstructive pulmonary disease)**. COPD includes emphysema and chronic bronchitis. The symptoms of COPD include coughing (either a dry cough or a cough that expels phlegm or mucus from your airways), wheezing, shortness of breath, chest tightness, and other symptoms.

- **An interstitial lung disease**. This type of disease causes scarring of the lung tissue over time. This can lead to coughing, shortness of breath, and other symptoms. Examples of interstitial lung diseases include sarcoidosis and idiopathic pulmonary fibrosis.

- **Cystic fibrosis (CF)**. CF is an inherited disease that causes thick, sticky mucus to collect in the lungs and block the airways. CF can cause coughing and frequent respiratory infections.

Your doctor also may recommend PR before and after lung surgery to help you prepare for and recover from the surgery. For example, people who have surgery for lung cancer or COPD may benefit from PR.

PR also can help people who have muscle-wasting disorders that may affect the muscles used for breathing. One example of this type of disorder is muscular dystrophy.

PR works best if you start it when your disease is in a moderate stage. However, even people who have advanced lung disease can benefit from PR.

What to Expect before Pulmonary Rehabilitation

When you first start PR, your team of healthcare providers will want to learn more about your health.

For example, they'll want to know how well you're able to breathe and exercise. You'll have lung function tests to check your breathing. These tests measure how much air you can breathe in and out, how fast you can breathe air out, and how well your lungs deliver oxygen to your blood.

Your team can check your ability to exercise several ways. They may measure how far you can walk in 6 minutes (called a 6-minute walk test). Or, they may ask you to exercise on a treadmill while your oxygen level, blood pressure, and heart rate are measured.

Your PR team also will review your medical therapy to see whether it needs to be changed during the PR program. For example, you may need to start using, or increase the use of, inhaled bronchodilators. These medicines can help you breathe easier during exercise. You also may need oxygen therapy to help you get the most out of your exercise plan.

Your PR team may assess your mental health. If you have anxiety or are very depressed, they may refer you to a specialist who can treat these issues.

In addition, the team may measure your weight and height, ask about your food intake and general nutrition, and recommend a blood test to assess loss of muscle mass.

The data your PR team gathers at the start of your program will help them create a plan that's tailored to your abilities and needs.

What to Expect during Pulmonary Rehabilitation

PR can have many parts, and not all programs offer every part.

Exercise Training

Your PR team will give you a physical activity plan tailored to your needs. They'll design the plan to improve your endurance and muscle strength, so you're better able to carry out daily activities.

The plan will likely include exercises for both your arms and legs. You might use a treadmill, stationary bike, or weights to do your exercises.

If you can't handle long exercise sessions, your plan may involve several short sessions with rest breaks in between. While you exercise, your team may check your blood oxygen levels with a device that's attached to your finger.

You'll probably have to do your exercises at least three times a week to get the most benefits from them.

Nutritional Counseling

The data your PR team gathers when you start the PR program will show whether you're overweight or underweight. Both of these conditions can make it hard for you to breathe.

If you're overweight, fat around your waist can push up against your diaphragm (a muscle that helps you breathe). This will give your lungs less room to expand during breathing. Your team may recommend a healthy eating plan to help you lose weight.

You also can have breathing problems if you're underweight. Some people who have chronic (ongoing) lung diseases have trouble maintaining weight. If you lose too much weight, you can lose muscle mass. This can weaken the muscles used for breathing.

If you're underweight, your team may recommend a healthy eating plan to help you gain weight. They also may give you calorie and protein supplements to help you avoid weight loss and loss of muscle mass.

Education

Part of PR involves learning about your disease or condition and how to manage it (including how to avoid situations that worsen symptoms). Your symptoms may get worse if you have a respiratory infection or breathe in lung irritants, such as cigarette smoke or air pollution.

Your PR team will teach you about the importance of vaccinations and other ways to prevent infections. If you smoke, you'll be offered a program to help you quit.

Part of PR education is making sure you know when and how to take your medicines. Your PR team will teach you how to use inhalers and nebulizers if you need them to take your medicine. They also will show you how to use oxygen if you're getting oxygen therapy.

In addition, your PR team will help you create a self-management plan. This plan will explain what you should do if your symptoms get worse or you have signs of a respiratory infection.

The self-management plan will describe what you can do on your own to relieve symptoms. It also will explain when you should contact your doctor or seek emergency care.

Most PR programs last a few months. To fully benefit from your program, you'll be taught how to use the exercises, breathing strategies, and other lifestyle changes you learn in PR at home. This also will be part of your self-management plan.

Energy-Conserving Techniques

One way to help prevent symptoms like shortness of breath is to find easier ways to do daily tasks. PR programs often give you tips on how you can conserve your energy and breathe easier.

These tips include ways to avoid reaching, lifting, and bending. Such movements use energy and tighten your abdominal muscles, making it harder for you to breathe.

Stress also can use up energy and make you short of breath. Many PR programs teach relaxation skills and ways to avoid or relieve stress.

Breathing Strategies

While in PR, you'll learn strategies that can improve your breathing. For example, you may learn how to take longer, deeper, less frequent breaths. One example of this type of exercise is pursed-lip breathing.

Pursed-lip breathing decreases how often you take breaths and keeps your airways open longer. This allows more air to flow in and out of your lungs so you can be more physically active.

To do pursed-lip breathing, you breathe in through your nostrils. Then you slowly breathe out through slightly pursed lips, as if you're blowing out a candle. You exhale two to three times longer than you inhale. Some people find it helpful to count to two while inhaling and to four or six while exhaling.

Psychological Counseling and Support

People who have chronic lung diseases are more prone to depression, anxiety, and other emotional problems. Thus, many PR programs offer counseling or support groups. If your program doesn't, your PR team can refer you to such services.

What to Expect after Pulmonary Rehabilitation

Most PR programs last a few months. At the end of your program, you'll undergo tests and answer questions. Some of these tests, such as exercise tests, will be the same ones you had at the start of your program.

The data gathered at the end of the program will show whether your symptoms, physical activity level, and quality of life have improved. If they have, your team will encourage you to continue your exercises, breathing strategies, and other prescribed changes on your own.

If you have little to no improvement, talk with your doctor. He or she might want to change your medical therapy. Or, your doctor might recommend more tests. These tests can show whether you have another condition that also may have to be treated to improve your breathing.

What Are the Benefits and Risks of Pulmonary Rehabilitation?

Benefits

PR can't cure your lung disease or completely relieve your breathing problems. However, PR does have many benefits. For example, it may:

- improve your quality of life

- help you function better in your daily life

- increase your ability to exercise

- decrease the symptoms of your disease or condition

- help you manage anxiety and depression

You also may have fewer breathing problems as a result of PR. Although PR doesn't improve your lung function, it allows you to make the most of the limited lung function you have.

Risks

PR usually is safe. The only risks are related to the exercise part of the program. For example, physical activity may cause injuries to your muscles or bones.

If you have another disorder, such as heart disease, physical activity may increase your risk of having a heart attack or arrhythmia. An arrhythmia is a problem with the rate or rhythm of your heartbeat.

The health data that your PR team collects at the start of your program and during the program can help prevent these problems.

Chapter 64

Thoracentesis

What Is Thoracentesis?

Thoracentesis is a procedure to remove excess fluid in the space between the lungs and the chest wall. This space is called the pleural space.

Normally, the pleural space is filled with a small amount of fluid— about 4 teaspoons full. Some conditions—such as heart failure, lung infections, and tumors—can cause more fluid to build up. When this happens, it's called a pleural effusion. A lot of extra fluid can press on the lungs, making it hard to breathe.

Who Needs Thoracentesis?

Your doctor may recommend thoracentesis if you have a pleural effusion.

Doctors use thoracentesis to find the cause of a pleural effusion. The procedure also might be done to remove excess fluid from the pleural space and help you breathe easier.

The most common cause of a pleural effusion is heart failure. This is a condition in which the heart can't pump enough blood to the body.

Other causes include lung cancer, tumors, pneumonia, tuberculosis, pulmonary embolism, and other lung infections. Asbestosis, sarcoidosis, and reactions to some drugs also can lead to a pleural effusion.

This chapter includes text excerpted from "Thoracentesis," National Heart, Lung, and Blood Institute (NHLBI), February 24, 2012. Reviewed September 2016.

Diagnosing a Pleural Effusion

Your doctor will diagnose a pleural effusion based on your medical history, a physical exam, and test results.

Medical History

Your doctor will ask about your symptoms, such as trouble breathing, coughing, and hiccups. He or she also may ask whether you've ever:

- had heart disease

- smoked

- traveled to places where you may have been exposed to tuberculosis

- had a job that exposed you to asbestos (a mineral that, in the past, was widely used in many industries)

Physical Exam

Your doctor will listen to your breathing with a stethoscope and tap lightly on your chest. If you have a pleural effusion, your breathing may sound muffled. Your doctor also may hear a dull sound when tapping on your chest.

Diagnostic Tests

You may have one or more of the following tests to diagnose a pleural effusion.

- **Chest X-ray.** This test creates a picture of the structures inside your chest, such as your heart and lungs. A chest X-ray may show air or fluid in the pleural space. The test also may show the cause of the pleural effusion, such as pneumonia or a lung tumor. To get more detailed pictures, the X-ray might be done while you're in various positions.

- **Ultrasound.** This test uses sound waves to create a picture of the structures in your body, such as your lungs. Ultrasound may show the location of fluid in your chest. Sometimes the test is used to find the right place to insert the needle or tube for thoracentesis.

- **Chest computed tomography scan, or chest CT scan.** This test creates a computer-generated picture of the lungs that can show pockets of fluid. A chest CT scan may show fluid even if a chest X-ray doesn't. A CT scan also may show signs of pneumonia or a tumor.

What to Expect before Thoracentesis

Before thoracentesis, your doctor will talk to you about the procedure and how to prepare for it. Tell your doctor:

- whether you're taking any medicines and which ones you're taking
- about any previous bleeding problems you've had
- whether you have allergies to medicines or latex

No special preparations are needed before thoracentesis.

What to Expect during Thoracentesis

Thoracentesis is done at a doctor's office or hospital. The entire procedure (including preparation) usually takes 10–15 minutes, but the needle or tube is in your chest for only a few minutes during that time. If you have a lot of fluid in your pleural space, the procedure may take up to 45 minutes.

You'll sit on the edge of a chair or exam table, lean forward, and rest your arms on a table. You'll be asked to not move, cough, or breathe deeply once the procedure begins.

Your doctor may use ultrasound to find the right place to insert the needle or tube. Ultrasound uses sound waves to create a picture of the structures in your body, such as your lungs.

Your doctor will clean the area on your skin where the needle or tube will be inserted. Then, he or she will inject medicine to numb the area. You may feel some stinging at this time.

Your doctor will insert the needle or tube between your ribs and into the pleural space (the space between the lungs and chest wall). You may feel some discomfort and pressure at this time.

Using the needle or tube, your doctor will draw out the excess fluid around your lungs. You may feel like coughing, and you may feel some chest pain.

Your doctor may take only the amount of fluid needed to find the cause of the pleural effusion. However, if you have a lot of fluid in your pleural space, he or she may take more. This helps the lungs expand and take in more air, which allows you to breathe easier.

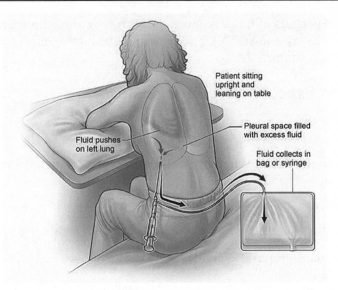

Patient sitting
upright and
leaning on table

Pleural space filled
with excess fluid

Fluid pushes
on left lung

Fluid collects in
bag or syringe

Figure 64.1. *Thoracentesis*

The image shows a person having thoracentesis. The person sits upright and leans on a table. Excess fluid from the pleural space is drained into a bag.

Once the fluid is removed, your doctor will take out the needle or tube. He or she will place a small bandage on the site where the needle or tube was inserted.

What to Expect after Thoracentesis

After thoracentesis, you may have a chest X-ray to check for any lung problems. Your blood pressure and breathing will be checked for up to a few hours after the procedure. This is done to make sure you don't have complications.

Your doctor will let you know when you can return to your normal activities, such as driving, physical activity, and working.

Once at home, call your doctor right away if you have any breathing problems.

What Does Thoracentesis Show?

Your doctor will send the fluid removed during thoracentesis for testing. The fluid will be checked for signs of heart failure, infection, cancer, or other conditions that may cause a pleural effusion (the buildup of fluid between the lungs and chest wall).

Once the cause of the pleural effusion is known, your doctor will talk to you about a treatment plan. For example, if an infection is the cause, you may need antibiotics to fight the infection. If the cause is heart failure, you'll be treated for that condition.

What Are the Risks of Thoracentesis?

The risks of thoracentesis usually are minor. They include:

- **Pneumothorax.** This is a condition in which air collects in the pleural space (the space between the lungs and chest wall). Sometimes air comes in through the needle, or the needle makes a hole in the lung. Usually, a hole will seal itself. If enough air gets into the pleural space, however, the lung can collapse. Your doctor may need to put a tube in your chest to remove the air and let the lung expand again.

- **Pain, bleeding, bruising, or infection where the needle or tube was inserted.** Although rare, bleeding can occur in or around the lungs. Your doctor may need to put a tube in your chest to drain the blood. Sometimes surgery is needed to treat the bleeding.

- **Liver or spleen injuries.** These complications are very rare.

Chapter 65

Lung Transplant

What Is a Lung Transplant?

A lung transplant is surgery to remove a person's diseased lung and replace it with a healthy lung from a deceased donor.

Lung transplants are used for people who are likely to die from lung disease within 1 to 2 years. Their conditions are so severe that other treatments, such as medicines or breathing devices, no longer work.

Other Names for Lung Transplant

- Double-lung transplant
- Living donor lobar lung transplant
- Single-lung transplant

Who Needs a Lung Transplant?

Your doctor may recommend a lung transplant if you have severe lung disease that's getting worse. If your condition is so serious that other treatments don't work, a lung transplant may be the only option.

This chapter includes text excerpted from "Lung Transplant," National Heart, Lung, and Blood Institute (NHLBI), May 1, 2011. Reviewed September 2016.

Lung transplants most often are used to treat people who have severe:

- **COPD (chronic obstructive pulmonary disease).** COPD is the most common reason why adults need lung transplants. COPD is a progressive disease that makes it hard to breathe. "Progressive" means the disease gets worse over time.

- **Idiopathic pulmonary fibrosis (IPF).** IPF is a condition in which tissue deep in your lungs becomes thick and stiff, or scarred, over time.

- **Cystic fibrosis (CF).** CF is the most common reason in children for needing a lung transplant. CF is an inherited disease that causes thick, sticky mucus to build up in the lungs. This leads to repeated, serious lung infections.

- **Alpha-1 antitrypsin deficiency (AAT deficiency).** AAT deficiency is a condition that raises your risk for certain types of lung disease, especially if you smoke.

- **Pulmonary hypertension (PH).** PH is increased pressure in the pulmonary arteries. These arteries carry blood from your heart to your lungs to pick up oxygen.

Applying to a Lung Transplant Program

Lung transplants are done in medical centers (large hospitals) where the staff has a lot of organ transplant experience. If you need a lung transplant, you must apply to a center's transplant program.

Transplant teams at the medical center manage all parts of the center's transplant program. Transplant team members may include a:

- **Thoracic surgeon.** This is a doctor who does lung and chest surgeries.

- **Pulmonologist.** This is a doctor who specializes in lung diseases and conditions.

- **Cardiologist.** This is a doctor who specializes in heart diseases and conditions.

- **Immunologist.** This is a doctor who specializes in immune system disorders.

- **Respiratory technician.** This is a person who cares for people who have breathing and lung problems.

- **Transplant coordinator.** This is a person who arranges the surgery.

Other team members may include a social worker, psychiatrist, financial coordinator, and other specialists and medical personnel, such as a nutritionist and nurses.

The transplant team will need to find out whether you're a candidate for a lung transplant. They will want to make sure you're healthy enough to have the surgery and go through a recovery program.

To do this, they will ask about your medical history. The team will want to know whether you have other serious illnesses or conditions, such as cancer, HIV, or hepatitis. They also will ask whether you've had a major chest surgery. A previous chest surgery may make it hard to do a lung transplant.

The team also will want to know whether you smoke or use alcohol or drugs.

You also will have tests to show whether you're healthy enough for a lung transplant. Tests may include:

- **Lung function tests.** These tests measure how much air you can breathe in and out, how fast you can breathe air out, and how well your lungs deliver oxygen to your blood.

- **Blood tests.** Blood tests help doctors check for certain diseases and conditions. They also help check the function of your organs and show how well treatments are working.

- **Chest CT scan.** This test creates precise pictures of the structures inside your chest, such as your lungs.

- **EKG (electrocardiogram).** This test detects and records the heart's electrical activity.

- **Echocardiography (echo).** Echo uses sound waves to create pictures of your heart.

- **Right cardiac catheterization.** This test measures blood pressure in the right side of your heart. The results give clues about heart valve disease, heart failure, or lung problems.

You'll talk with team members to make sure you're mentally and emotionally willing to accept the risks of the transplant process and later treatment. The team may ask whether you have a good support network of family and friends.

What to Expect before a Lung Transplant

If you get into a medical center's transplant program, you'll be placed on the Organ Procurement and Transplantation Network's

(OPTN's) national waiting list. Your transplant team will work with you to make sure you're ready for the transplant if a donor lung becomes available.

Waiting for a donor lung can be frustrating. However, you can do several things to prepare.

- Go to all of your medical appointments with the transplant team. Take all of your medicines as prescribed.

- Stay as healthy as possible. Don't smoke, and follow your doctor's advice about breathing exercises, physical activity, diet, and drinking alcohol.

- Talk regularly with your transplant team. You and your family should know what to do if a donor lung becomes available. You also should know what to expect before, during, and after the transplant.

- Be ready to go to the transplant center right away if a donor lung becomes available. Make sure the transplant center knows how to reach you at any time, day or night. Your transplant team may give you a pager so they can reach you right away. Make travel and lodging plans in advance. Have a packed suitcase ready to go.

While you wait for a lung, you may feel worried, scared, anxious, or depressed. These feelings are normal in this situation. Talk with your healthcare team about how you feel. They can offer tips for coping with your emotions. Family and friends also can offer support.

When a Donor Lung Becomes Available

OPTN matches donor lungs to recipients based on need. OPTN will consider how severe a person's disease is and how quickly it's worsening. OPTN also will consider whether the transplant will improve the recipient's chances of survival, and by how much.

Organs are matched for blood type and the size of the donor lung and the recipient.

If OPTN and your transplant center think they have a good match for you, the center will ask you to come in as soon as possible.

Once you arrive, your team will do tests to make sure you're healthy enough to have the surgery and that the lung is a good match. If you're healthy enough and the lung is a good match, the team will prepare you for surgery.

What to Expect during a Lung Transplant

Just before lung transplant surgery, you will get general anesthesia. The term "anesthesia" refers to a loss of feeling and awareness. With general anesthesia, you will be asleep during the surgery and not feel any pain.

Once you're asleep, your doctors will make a small incision (cut) in your chest. Next, they will insert a central venous catheter into a vein. This tube allows easy access to your bloodstream. Doctors use it to deliver fluids and medicines to your body.

Your doctors also will insert a tube in your mouth and down your windpipe to help you breathe. They also will insert a tube in your nose and down to your stomach to drain contents from your stomach. A catheter will be used to keep your bladder empty.

The surgeon will make a cut in your chest to open it. He or she will then cut the main airway to your diseased lung and the blood vessels connecting your lung to your heart.

The surgeon will remove your diseased lung and place the donor organ in your chest. Then the surgeon will connect the main airway of the donor lung to your airway and its blood vessels to your heart.

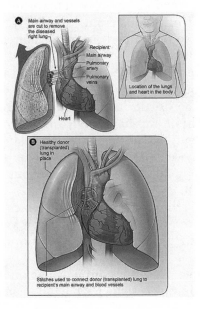

Figure 65.1. *Lung Transplant*

The illustration shows the process of a lung transplant. In figure A, the airway and blood vessels between a recipient's diseased right lung and heart are cut. The inset image shows the location of the lungs and heart in the body. In figure B, a healthy donor lung is stitched to the recipient's blood vessels and airway.

If you're having a double-lung transplant, you may be connected to a heart-lung bypass machine. This machine takes over for your heart and pumps oxygen-rich blood to your body.

During a double-lung transplant, the surgeon will remove your diseased lungs, one at a time, and replace them with the donor lungs.

A single-lung transplant usually takes 4 to 8 hours. A double-lung transplant usually takes 6 to 12 hours.

Some people may need a heart–lung transplant. A heart–lung transplant is surgery in which both the heart and lung(s) are replaced with healthy organs from a deceased donor. For this surgery, you're connected to a heart-lung bypass machine.

What to Expect after a Lung Transplant

Recovery in the Hospital

After lung transplant surgery, you'll go to the hospital's intensive care unit (ICU) for at least several days. The tubes that were inserted before surgery will remain for a few days.

The tube in your windpipe helps you breathe. Other tubes deliver medicines to, and drain fluids from, your body. You also will have sticky patches called electrodes attached to your chest to monitor your heart.

After leaving the ICU, you'll go to a hospital room. The staff will carefully oversee your recovery.

You'll be taught how to do deep breathing exercises with an incentive spirometer. This hand-held device helps you take slow, deep breaths. You also may have lung function tests that use a regular spirometer. This device measures how much air your lungs can hold. It also measures how fast you can blow air out of your lungs after taking a deep breath.

You'll need to cough often. Coughing helps clear fluids from your lungs so they can work well. A nurse will show you how to hold a pillow tightly near your incision site while you cough to help decrease discomfort.

On average, people who have a lung transplant stay in the hospital from 1 to 3 weeks. However, some people have complications and stay much longer.

Recovery after Leaving the Hospital

Before you leave the hospital, your medical team will teach you how to keep track of your overall health. You'll learn how to watch your weight and check your blood pressure, pulse, and temperature. Staff also will show you how to check your lung function.

You'll also learn the signs of the two main complications of lung transplant surgery: rejection and infection.

For the first 3 months after surgery, you'll go to the hospital often for blood tests, chest X-rays, lung function tests, and other tests. After 3 months, if you're doing well, you'll visit less often.

Making healthy lifestyle choices is very important. Not smoking, following a healthy diet, and following your doctor's advice on using alcohol will help you recover and stay as healthy as possible.

A healthy diet includes a variety of fruits, vegetables, and whole grains. It also includes lean meats, poultry, fish, beans, and fat-free or low-fat milk or milk products. A healthy diet is low in saturated fat, *trans* fat, cholesterol, sodium (salt), and added sugar.

Your doctor may recommend pulmonary rehabilitation (PR) after your lung transplant surgery. PR is a broad program that may include exercise training, education, counseling, and more.

Emotional Issues and Support

Having a lung transplant may cause fear, anxiety, and stress. While you're waiting for a lung transplant, you may worry that you won't live long enough to get a new lung. After surgery, you may feel over-whelmed, depressed, or worried about complications.

All of these feelings are normal for someone going through major surgery. Talk about how you feel with your healthcare team. Talking to a professional counselor also can help. If you're very depressed, your doctor may recommend medicines or other treatments that can improve your quality of life.

Support from family and friends also can help relieve stress and anxiety. Let your loved ones know how you feel and what they can do to help you.

What Are the Risks of Lung Transplant?

A lung transplant can improve your quality of life and extend your lifespan. The first year after the transplant is the most critical. This is when the risk of complications is highest.

In recent years, short-term survival after lung transplant has improved. Recent data on single-lung transplants show that:

- About 78 percent of patients survive the first year

- About 63 percent of patients survive 3 years

- About 51 percent of patients survive 5 years

Survival rates for double-lung transplants are slightly better. Recent data show that the median survival for single-lung recipients is 4.6 years. The median survival for double-lung recipients is 6.6 years. Talk with your doctor about what these figures may mean for you.

Complications

The major complications of lung transplant are rejection and infection.

Rejection

Your immune system will regard your new lung as a "foreign object." It will create antibodies (proteins) against the lung. This may cause your body to reject the new organ.

To prevent this, your doctor will prescribe medicines to suppress your immune system. You'll need to take these medicines for the rest of your life.

Rejection is most common in the first 6 months after surgery, but it can happen any time after the transplant. Rejection can happen slowly or suddenly. Your doctor will teach you how to spot possible signs and symptoms of rejection. If you know these signs and symptoms, you can seek treatment right away.

Signs and symptoms of rejection include:

- fever and flu-like symptoms

- chest congestion

- coughing

- shortness of breath

- new pain around the lung

- generally feeling unwell

If you have any of these signs or symptoms, seek medical care. Your doctor may prescribe medicines to treat the rejection and prevent complications.

These medicines may cause side effects, such as headaches, nausea (feeling sick to your stomach), and flu-like symptoms. If you have side effects, tell your doctor. He or she may change your medicines or adjust the doses.

Infection

The medicines you take to prevent the rejection of your new lung may weaken your immune system. As a result, you're more likely to get infections.

While you're in the hospital, staff will take special steps to prevent you from getting infections. After you leave the hospital, you also can take steps to prevent infections:

- Wash your hands often.

- Take care of your teeth and gums.

- Protect your skin from scratches and sores.

- Stay away from crowds and from people who have colds and the flu.

Other Risks

Long-term use of medicines that suppress the immune system can cause diabetes, kidney damage, and osteoporosis (thinning of the bones). These medicines also can increase the risk of cancer. Talk with your doctor about the long-term risks of using these medicines.

Chapter 66

Complementary Health Approaches for Respiratory Disorders

Complementary Health Approaches for Asthma

Most people are able to control their asthma with conventional therapies and by avoiding the substances that can set off asthma attacks. Even so, some people turn to complementary health approaches in their efforts to relieve symptoms. According to the 2002 National Health Interview Survey (NHIS), which included a comprehensive survey on the use of complementary health approaches by Americans, asthma ranked 13th as a condition prompting use of complementary health approaches by adults; 1.1 percent of respondents (an estimated 788,000 adults) said they had used a complementary approach for asthma in the past year. In the 2007 NHIS survey, which included adults and children, asthma ranked eighth among conditions prompting use of

This chapter contains text excerpted from the following sources: Text beginning with the heading "Complementary Health Approaches for Asthma" is excerpted from "Asthma: In Depth," National Center for Complementary and Integrative Health (NCCIH), March 25, 2016; Text under the heading "5 Things to Know about Complementary Health Approaches for Seasonal Allergy Relief" is excerpted from "5 Things to Know about Complementary Health Approaches for Seasonal Allergy Relief," National Center for Complementary and Integrative Health (NCCIH), September 24, 2015.

complementary health approaches by children, but did not appear in a similar ranking for adults.

What the Science Says about Complementary Health Approaches and Asthma

According to reviewers who have assessed the research, there is not enough evidence to support the use of any complementary health approaches for the relief of asthma.

- Several studies have looked at actual or true **acupuncture**—stimulation of specific points on the body with thin metal needles—for asthma. Although a few studies showed some reduction in medication use and improvements in symptoms and quality of life, the majority showed no difference between actual acupuncture and simulated or sham acupuncture on asthma symptoms. At this point, there is little evidence that acupuncture is an effective treatment for asthma.

- There has been renewed patient interest in **breathing exercises** or **retraining** to reduce hyperventilation, regulate breathing, and achieve a better balance of carbon dioxide and oxygen in the blood. A review of seven randomized controlled trials found a trend toward improvement in symptoms with breathing techniques but not enough evidence for firm conclusions.

- A 2011 study examined the placebo response in patients with chronic asthma and found that patients receiving a placebo (placebo inhaler and simulated acupuncture) reported significant improvement in symptoms such as chest tightness and perception of difficulty breathing. However, lung function did not improve in these patients. This is an important distinction because although the patients felt better, their risk for becoming very sick from untreated asthma was not lessened.

NCCIH-Funded Research

NCCIH is currently funding studies to determine whether:

- Mindfulness meditation practices might help manage symptoms or improve quality of life for people with asthma

- Vitamin E might reduce lung inflammation in mice and humans with allergic asthma

- Borage oil or *Ginkgo biloba* might reduce airway inflammation

- Under-the-tongue (sublingual) immunotherapy might build tolerance to substances that trigger allergic asthma.

If You Are Considering Complementary Health Approaches for Asthma

- Conventional medical treatments are very effective for managing asthma symptoms. See your healthcare provider to discuss a comprehensive medical treatment plan for your asthma.

- Do not use any complementary approaches to postpone seeing your healthcare provider about asthma-like symptoms or any health problem.

- Do not replace conventional treatments for asthma with unproven products or practices.

- Keep in mind that dietary supplements can act in the same way as drugs. They can cause health problems if not used correctly or if used in large amounts, and some may interact with medications you take. Your healthcare provider can advise you. If you are pregnant or nursing a child, or if you are considering giving a child a dietary supplement, it is especially important to consult your (or your child's) healthcare provider.

- Tell all your healthcare providers about any complementary health approaches you use. Give them a full picture of what you do to manage your health. This will help ensure coordinated and safe care.

5 Things to Know about Complementary Health Approaches for Seasonal Allergy Relief

Seasonal allergies, also called "hay fever," are triggered each spring, summer, and fall when trees, weeds, and grasses release pollen into the air. When the pollen ends up in your nose and throat, it can bring on sneezing, runny nose, coughing, and itchy eyes and throat. Pollen counts tend to be the highest early in the morning on warm, dry, breezy days and the lowest during chilly, wet periods. People manage seasonal allergies by taking medication, avoiding exposure to the substances that trigger their allergic reactions, or having a series of "allergy shots" (a form of immunotherapy).

People also try various complementary approaches to manage their allergies. According to the 2007 National Health Interview Survey, "respiratory allergy" is among the 15 conditions for which children in the United States most often use complementary approaches. If you are considering any complementary health approach for the relief of seasonal allergy symptoms, here are some things you need to know.

1. **Nasal saline irrigation.** There is reasonably good evidence that saline nasal irrigation (putting salt water into one nostril and draining it out the other) can be useful for modest improvement of allergy symptoms. Nasal irrigation is generally safe; however, neti pots and other rinsing devices must be used and cleaned properly. According to the U.S. Food and Drug Administration (FDA), tap water that is not filtered, treated, or processed in specific ways is not safe for use as a nasal rinse.

2. **Butterbur extract.** There are hints that the herb butterbur may decrease the symptoms associated with nasal allergies. However, there are concerns about its safety.

3. **Honey.** Only a few studies have looked at the effects of honey on seasonal allergy symptoms, and there is no convincing scientific evidence that honey provides symptom relief. Eating honey is generally safe; however, children under 1 year of age should not eat honey. People who are allergic to pollen or bee stings may also be allergic to honey.

4. **Acupuncture.** Only a few small studies have been conducted on acupuncture for relief of seasonal allergy symptoms, and the limited scientific evidence currently available has not shown acupuncture to be beneficial in treating seasonal allergies.

5. **Talk to your healthcare provider.** If you suffer from seasonal allergies and are considering a complementary health approach, talk to your healthcare provider about the best ways to manage your symptoms. You may find that when the pollen count is high, staying indoors, wearing a mask, or rinsing off when you come inside can help.

Chapter 67

Healthcare Professionals Who Treat Respiratory Disorders

Chapter Contents

Section 67.1

Respiratory Therapists: What Do They Do

This section includes text excerpted from "Respiratory
Therapists," Bureau of Labor Statistics (BLS), U.S.
Department of Labor (DOL), December 17, 2015.

Respiratory therapists care for patients who have trouble breathing—for example, from a chronic respiratory disease, such as asthma
or emphysema. Their patients range from premature infants with
undeveloped lungs to elderly patients who have diseased lungs. They
also provide emergency care to patients suffering from heart attacks,
drowning, or shock.

Duties

Respiratory therapists typically do the following:

- interview and examine patients with breathing or cardiopulmonary disorders

- consult with physicians to develop patient treatment plans

- perform diagnostic tests, such as measuring lung capacity

- treat patients by using a variety of methods, including chest
  physiotherapy and aerosol medications

- monitor and record patients progress

- teach patients how to use treatments and equipment, such as
  ventilators

Respiratory therapists use various tests to evaluate patients. For
example, therapists test lung capacity by having patients breathe into
an instrument that measures the volume and flow of oxygen when they
inhale and exhale. Respiratory therapists also may take blood samples
and use a blood gas analyzer to test oxygen and carbon dioxide levels.

Respiratory therapists perform chest physiotherapy on patients
to remove mucus from their lungs and make it easier for them to
breathe. Removing mucus is necessary for patients suffering from lung

diseases, such as cystic fibrosis, and involves the therapist vibrating the patient's rib cage, often by tapping the patient's chest and encouraging him or her to cough.

Respiratory therapists may connect patients who cannot breathe on their own to ventilators that deliver oxygen to the lungs. Therapists insert a tube in the patient's windpipe (trachea) and connect the tube to ventilator equipment. They set up and monitor the equipment to ensure that the patient is receiving the correct amount of oxygen at the correct rate.

Respiratory therapists who work in home care teach patients and their families to use ventilators and other life-support systems in their homes. During these visits, they may inspect and clean equipment, check the home for environmental hazards, and ensure that patients know how to use their medications. Therapists also make emergency home visits when necessary.

In some hospitals, respiratory therapists are involved in related areas, such as diagnosing breathing problems for people with sleep apnea and counseling people on how to stop smoking.

Section 67.2

Working with Your Asthma Doctor

This section includes text excerpted from "So You Have Asthma,"
National Heart, Lung, and Blood Institute (NHLBI), March 2013.

Most people who have asthma experience one or more of the following symptoms: coughing, wheezing, chest tightness, and shortness of breath. The symptoms of asthma are different for different people. And symptoms for one person can change from one time to another. So can the frequency of symptoms.

How often you get symptoms will let you and your doctor know if you need to do more to control your asthma. Call your doctor if—

• You have asthma symptoms more than 2 days a week.

• Your asthma wakes you up 2 or more times a month.

- You are using your quick-relief inhaler more than 2 days a week.

- Your asthma is getting in the way of your usual activities.

These are signs that your asthma is not well controlled and may be getting worse.

With good asthma control, you can:

- Be free from troublesome symptoms day and night:

  - No coughing or wheezing.

  - No difficulty breathing or chest tightness.

  - No nighttime awakening due to asthma.

- Have the best possible lung function.

- Participate fully in any activities of your choice.

- Miss few or no school or work days because of asthma symptoms.

- Have fewer or no urgent care visits or hospital stays for asthma.

- Have few or no side effects from asthma medicines.

Doctors often refer to the list above as the goals of asthma treatment. Most people who have asthma can reach these goals by taking the following four actions:

1. Work closely with your doctor and other healthcare professionals (such as a nurse practitioner, physician assistant, nurse, respiratory therapist or asthma educator) to learn how to manage your asthma and keep it under control. Regular "asthma check-ups" with your doctor will help.

2. Learn which medicines to take, when to take them, and how to use them correctly. For your quick-relief inhaler, ask your doctor if you can add a spacer to make it easier to take the medicine. Then take all of your medicines just as your doctor recommends.

3. Identify the things that bring on your asthma symptoms, also called your asthma triggers. Then avoid them, or at least reduce your contact with them.

4. Watch for changes in your asthma. You need to know when an asthma attack is coming and what to do. If you act quickly and

follow the doctor's instructions, you can help keep your asthma symptoms from getting worse.

Tips for Creating Good, Clear Communication with Your Doctor or Other Healthcare Professional

Speak Up. Tell your doctor or other healthcare professional about what you want to achieve by improving control of your asthma. Ask for his or her help in achieving those treatment goals.

Be Open. When your doctor or other healthcare professional asks you questions, answer as honestly and completely as you can. Briefly describe your symptoms. Include when you started having each symptom, how often you have it, and whether it has been getting worse.

Keep It Simple. If you don't understand something your doctor or other healthcare professional says, ask for a simple explanation. Be especially sure that you understand how to take any medicines you are given. If you are worried about understanding what the doctor or other healthcare professional says, or if you have trouble hearing, bring a friend or relative with you to your appointment. You may want to ask that person to write down instructions for you.

Sample List of Questions To Ask Your Doctor or Other Healthcare Professional

1. Are you sure it's asthma?

2. Do I need other tests to confirm the diagnosis?

3. If I think my medicine isn't working, is it OK to take more right away?

4. What should I do if I miss a dose?

5. Will my medicine cause me any problems, like shakiness, sore throat, or upset stomach?

6. What if I have problems taking my medicines or following my treatment plan?

7. Is this the right way to use my inhaler? How do I use my inhaler with a spacer?

8. Is this the right way to use my peak flow meter?

9. How can I tell if I'm having an asthma attack? What medicines should I take and how much of each should I take? When should I call you? When should I go to the emergency room?

10. Once my asthma is under control, will I be able to reduce the amount of medicine I'm taking?

11. When should I see you again?

Part Seven

Living with Chronic Respiratory Problems

Chapter 68

Living with Asthma

If you have asthma, you'll need long-term care. Successful asthma treatment requires that you take an active role in your care and follow your asthma action plan (AAP).

Learn How to Manage Your Asthma

Partner with your doctor to develop an AAP. This plan will help you know when and how to take your medicines. The plan also will help you identify your asthma triggers and manage your disease if asthma symptoms worsen.

Children aged 10 or older—and younger children who can handle it—should be involved in creating and following their AAPs.

Most people who have asthma can successfully manage their symptoms by following their AAPs and having regular checkups. However, knowing when to seek emergency medical care is important.

Learn how to use your medicines correctly. If you take inhaled medicines, you should practice using your inhaler at your doctor's office. If you take long-term control medicines, take them daily as your doctor prescribes.

Record your asthma symptoms as a way to track how well your asthma is controlled. Also, your doctor may advise you to use a peak flow meter to measure and record how well your lungs are working.

This chapter contains text excerpted from the following sources: Text in this chapter begins with excerpts from "Living with Asthma," National Heart, Lung, and Blood Institute (NHLBI), August 4, 2014; Text under the heading "Your Written Asthma Action Plan" is excerpted from "So You Have Asthma: A Guide for Patients and Their Families," National Heart, Lung, and Blood Institute (NHLBI), March 2013.

Your doctor may ask you to keep records of your symptoms or peak flow results daily for a couple of weeks before an office visit. You'll bring these records with you to the visit.

These steps will help you keep track of how well you're controlling your asthma over time. This will help you spot problems early and prevent or relieve asthma attacks. Recording your symptoms and peak flow results to share with your doctor also will help him or her decide whether to adjust your treatment.

Ongoing Care

Have regular asthma checkups with your doctor so he or she can assess your level of asthma control and adjust your treatment as needed. Remember, the main goal of asthma treatment is to achieve the best control of your asthma using the least amount of medicine. This may require frequent adjustments to your treatments.

If you find it hard to follow your AAP or the plan isn't working well, let your healthcare team know right away. They will work with you to adjust your plan to better suit your needs.

Get treatment for any other conditions that can interfere with your asthma management.

Watch for Signs That Your Asthma Is Getting Worse

Your asthma might be getting worse if:

- Your symptoms start to occur more often, are more severe, or bother you at night and cause you to lose sleep.

- You're limiting your normal activities and missing school or work because of your asthma.

- Your peak flow number is low compared to your personal best or varies a lot from day to day.

- Your asthma medicines don't seem to work well anymore.

- You have to use your quick-relief inhaler more often. If you're using quick-relief medicine more than 2 days a week, your asthma isn't well controlled.

- You have to go to the emergency room or doctor because of an asthma attack.

If you have any of these signs, see your doctor. He or she might need to change your medicines or take other steps to control your asthma.

Partner with your healthcare team and take an active role in your care. This can help you better control your asthma so it doesn't interfere with your activities and disrupt your life.

Your Written Asthma Action Plan

Your AAP should:

- Include the medicines you should take—explaining:
- what they are and what they do
- how much to take
- when to take each of them
- how to take each of them
- what, if any, side effects you should look for
- List your asthma triggers and provide information on ways to avoid or reduce them.
- Show how to monitor your asthma control using symptoms or peak flow readings.
- Show how to recognize and handle worsening asthma:
- what signs to watch for
- how to adjust your medicines in response to these signs
- when to seek emergency care
- what number to call in an emergency

Chapter 69

Using Devices to Treat Asthma

Metered-Dose Inhaler

A metered-dose inhaler is a device that sprays a pre-set amount of medicine through the mouth to the airways. To keep your asthma under control, it is important to take your medicine as prescribed by your doctor or other healthcare professional and to use the proper technique to deliver the medicine to your lungs. If you don't use your inhaler correctly, you won't get the medicine you need.

Here are general steps for how to use and clean a metered-dose inhaler. Be sure to read the instructions that come with *your* inhaler. Ask your doctor, pharmacist, or other healthcare professional (such as nurse practitioner, physician assistant, nurse, respiratory therapist, or asthma educator) to show you how to use your inhaler. Review your technique at each follow-up visit.

1. Take off cap. Shake the inhaler. Prime (spray or pump) the inhaler as needed according to manufacturer's instructions (each brand is different).

2. If you use a spacer or valved holding chamber (VHC), remove the cap and look into the mouthpiece to make sure nothing

This chapter includes text excerpted from "Asthma Tipsheets," National Heart, Lung, and Blood Institute (NHLBI), March 2013.

is in it. Place the inhaler in the rubber ring on the end of the spacer/VHC.

3. Stand up or sit up straight.

4. Take a deep breath in. Tilt head back slightly and blow out completely to empty your lungs.

5. Place the mouthpiece of the inhaler or spacer/VHC in your mouth and close your lips around it to form a tight seal.

6. As you start to breathe in, press down firmly on the top of the medicine canister to release one "puff" of medicine. Breathe in slowly (gently) and as deeply as you can for 3 to 5 seconds.

7. Hold your breath and count to 10.

8. Take the inhaler or spacer/VHC out of your mouth. Breathe out slowly.

9. If you are supposed to take 2 puffs of medicine per dose, wait 1 minute and repeat steps 3 through 8.

10. If using an inhaled corticosteroid, rinse out your mouth with water and spit it out. Rinsing will help to prevent an infection in the mouth.

How to Clean a Metered-Dose Inhaler and Spacer / VHC

Keep your inhaler and spacer/VHC clean so they can work properly. Read the manufacturer's instructions and talk to your doctor, pharmacist, or other healthcare professional about how to clean your inhaler and spacer/VHC (each brand is different). When cleaning your inhaler and spacer/VHC, remember:

• Never put the medicine canister in water.

• Never brush or wipe inside the spacer/VHC.

Dry Powder Inhaler

A dry powder inhaler delivers pre-set doses of medicine in powder form. The medicine gets to your airways when you take a deep, fast breath in from the inhaler. To keep your asthma under control, it is important to take your medicine as prescribed by your doctor or other healthcare professional and to use the proper technique to deliver the medicine to your lungs. If you don't use your inhaler correctly, you won't get the medicine you need.

Here are general steps for how to use and clean a dry powder inhaler. Be sure to read the instructions that come with *your* inhaler. Ask your doctor, pharmacist, or other healthcare professional (such as nurse practitioner, physician assistant, nurse, respiratory therapist, or asthma educator) to show you how to use your inhaler. Review your technique at each follow-up visit.

1. Remove cap and hold inhaler upright (like a rocket). If the inhaler is a Diskus®, hold it flat (like a flying saucer).

2. Load a dose of medicine according to manufacturer's instructions (each brand of inhaler is different; you may have to prime the inhaler the first time you use it). Do not shake the inhaler.

3. Stand up or sit up straight.

4. Take a deep breath in and blow out completely to empty your lungs. Do not blow into the inhaler.

5. Place the mouthpiece of the inhaler in your mouth and close your lips around it to form a tight seal.

6. Take a fast, deep, forceful breath in through your mouth.

7. Hold your breath and count to 10.

8. Take the inhaler out of your mouth. Breathe out slowly, facing away from the inhaler.

9. If you are supposed to take more than 1 inhalation of medicine per dose, wait 1 minute and repeat steps 2 through 8.

10. When you finish, put the cover back on the inhaler or slide the cover closed. Store the inhaler in a cool, dry place (not in the bathroom).

11. If using an inhaled corticosteroid, rinse out your mouth with water and spit it out. Rinsing helps to prevent an infection in the mouth.

How to Clean a Dry Powder Inhaler

- Wipe the mouthpiece at least once a week with a dry cloth.

- Do **not use water** to clean the dry powder inhaler.

Nebulizer

A nebulizer is a machine that delivers medicine in a fine, steady mist. To keep your asthma under control, it is important to take your medicine as prescribed by your doctor or other healthcare professional and to use the proper technique to deliver the medicine to your lungs. If you don't use your nebulizer correctly, you won't get the medicine you need.

Here are general steps for how to use and clean a nebulizer. Be sure to read the instructions that come with your nebulizer. Ask your doctor, pharmacist, or other healthcare professional (such as nurse practitioner, physician assistant, nurse, respiratory therapist, or asthma educator) to show you how to use your nebulizer. Review your technique at each follow-up visit.

1. Wash hands well.

2. Put together the nebulizer machine, tubing, medicine cup, and mouthpiece or mask according to manufacturer's instructions.

3. Put the prescribed amount of medicine into the medicine cup. If your medicine comes in a pre-measured capsule or vial, empty it into the cup.

4. Place the mouthpiece in your mouth and close your lips around it to form a tight seal. If your child uses a mask, make sure it fits snugly over your child's nose and mouth. Never hold the mouthpiece or mask away from the face.

5. Turn on the nebulizer machine. You should see a light mist coming from the back of the tube opposite the mouthpiece or from the mask.

6. Take normal breaths through the mouth while the machine is on. Continue treatment until the medicine cup is empty or the mist stops, about 10 minutes.

7. Take the mouthpiece out of your mouth (or remove mask) and turn off the machine.

8. If using an inhaled corticosteroid, rinse mouth with water and spit it out. If using a mask, also wash the face.

How to Clean and Store a Nebulizer after Each Treatment

- Wash hands well.

- Wash the medicine cup and mouthpiece or mask with warm water and mild soap. Do not wash the tubing.

- Rinse well and shake off excess water. Air dry parts on a paper towel.

Once a Week

Disinfect nebulizer parts to help kill any germs. Follow instructions for each nebulizer part listed in the package insert.

Always remember:

- Do not wash or boil the tubing.
- Air dry parts on a paper towel.

Between Uses

- Store nebulizer parts in a dry, clean plastic storage bag. If the nebulizer is used by more than one person, keep each person's medicine cup, mouthpiece or mask, and tubing in a separate, labeled bag to prevent the spread of germs.
- Wipe surface with a clean, damp cloth as needed. Cover nebulizer machine with a clean, dry cloth and store as manufacturer instructs.
- Replace medicine cup, mouthpiece, mask, tubing, filter, and other parts according to manufacturer's instructions or when they appear.

Peak Flow Meter

Peak flow meters are devices used to measure how well air is moving through your lungs.

Here are some general steps for how to use a peak flow meter. Be sure to read the instructions that come with your peak flow meter. Ask your doctor, pharmacist, or other healthcare professional (such as nurse practitioner, physician assistant, nurse, respiratory therapist, or asthma educator) to show you how to use your peak flow meter. Review your technique at each follow-up visit. This section also tells you what the numbers on the meter mean and how they can help you and your doctor or other healthcare professional keep your asthma under control.

1. Always stand up. Remove any food or gum from your mouth.

2. Make sure the marker on the peak flow meter is at the bottom of the scale.

3. Breathe in slowly and deeply. Hold that breath.

4. Place mouthpiece on your tongue and close lips around it to form a tight seal (do not put tongue in the hole).

5. Blow out as hard and fast as possible.

6. Write down the number next to the marker. (If you cough or make a mistake, do not write down that number. Do it over again.)

7. Repeat steps 3 through 6 two more times.

8. Record the highest of these three numbers in a notebook, calendar, or asthma diary.

Compare the highest number with the peak flow numbers on your written asthma action plan. Check to see which zone the number falls under and follow the plan's instructions for that zone.

GREEN ZONE: 80%–100% of personal best. Take daily long-term control medication, if prescribed.

YELLOW ZONE: 50%–79% of personal best. Add quick-relief medication(s) as directed and continue daily long-term control medication, if prescribed. Continue to monitor.

RED ZONE: Less than 50% of personal best. Add quick-relief medication(s) as directed. Get medical help now.

How to Find Your Personal Best Or Usual Peak Flow

- Follow the steps above to take your peak flow daily for 2 to 3 weeks when your asthma is under good control. Record the highest number each day.

- Take peak flow at the same time every day. Peak flows are lowest in the early morning and highest between noon and 5 p.m. Recording peak flows at the same time daily will give you the most consistent numbers.

- The highest number during this period of time will be your personal best number.

Your doctor or other healthcare professional may also want you to take your peak flow before and after using your quick-relief medicine. Follow his or her instructions.

Find a new personal best with each new peak flow meter (different meters can give different numbers).

Find a new personal best for children every 6 months to allow for growth changes.

Chapter 70

Lifestyle Modifications for Asthma Control

Many people with asthma find that making changes to their lifestyle can help them gain control over their asthma symptoms. Lifestyle modifications range from avoiding allergens and other asthma triggers in the home environment to adjusting nutrition and exercise programs for optimal health. Even minor lifestyle changes can sometimes offer major benefits in reducing the incidence and severity of asthma attacks. Although lifestyle modifications cannot eliminate the need for asthma medications, they can aid in the management of symptoms and thus make treatments work more effectively.

Modifications for a Healthy Environment

Understanding and avoiding asthma triggers in the home environment is a key to controlling symptoms. For half of people with asthma, a common allergen is responsible for triggering most asthma attacks. Although it may be impossible to completely eliminate allergens from the home environment, the following suggestions can help people with asthma limit their exposure to specific allergens:

Pollen and Mold

For people whose asthma is triggered by pollen and outdoor mold, it is important to keep windows closed during peak allergy seasons.

"Lifestyle Modifications for Asthma Control," © 2016 Omnigraphics, Inc. Reviewed September 2016.

Since pollen and mold counts tend to be highest in the morning hours, it is best to remain indoors as much as possible at this time of day. In addition, consider consulting with a doctor to adjust asthma medications during allergy season. To prevent exposure to indoor mold, fix leaky plumbing, attend to poor home drainage issues that could cause flooding, and use a dehumidifier to rid the home of excess moisture. Use a cleanser with bleach to kill mold on hard surfaces.

Dust Mites

Dust mites thrive in carpets, bedding, and upholstery. For people whose asthma is triggered by an allergy to dust mites, it is especially important to avoid prolonged exposure at night. To kill mites in sheets and blankets, the bedding must be washed once a week in water hotter than 130 degrees Fahrenheit. Mattresses and pillows should be encased in dust-proof zippered covers. Stuffed toys should be kept out of the bedroom or washed weekly in hot water. If possible, avoid carpeting and cloth cushions, especially in the bedroom. Finally, use air conditioning or dehumidifiers to keep indoor humidity below 60 percent in order to create inhospitable conditions for dust mites.

Pet Dander

The best way to avoid exposure to pet dander is to keep pets out of the home. If this is not possible, pets should at least be prevented from entering the bedroom or climbing on fabric-covered furniture. Removing carpeting from the home can also help reduce exposure to pet dander.

Pests

Allergies to cockroaches, mice, and other pests can also trigger asthma. To avoid exposure to these pests, put food away promptly in airtight containers and keep garbage receptacles securely closed. Traps, poison baits, or boric acid are good options for pest control, since people with asthma should not inhale pesticide sprays.

Airborne Irritants

Smoke, dust, chemicals, and other forms of indoor air pollution can irritate the airways of people with asthma. It is best to avoid exposure to products with strong smells, such as paints, cleaning solvents, and perfumes, as well as to fumes from wood-burning stoves, fireplaces, or kerosene heaters. People with asthma should also not smoke, permit smoking in their homes or cars, or go places where other people are smoking. Since dust from a vacuum cleaner can be an asthma trigger, it is best to wear a dust mask while vacuuming or have someone else run the vacuum.

Modifications for a Healthy Lifestyle

For people with chronic diseases like asthma, it is especially valuable to maintain overall health through proper nutrition and exercise. Seeing a doctor regularly, following the recommended treatment plan, paying attention to warning signs, and using medication as directed are also important components of controlling asthma through lifestyle choices.

Recognize Asthma Symptoms and Treat Them Promptly

Some of the common warning signs of worsening asthma include increased wheezing, shortness of breath, chest tightness or pain, coughing, difficulty sleeping, and declining expiratory flow measurements. Recognizing these symptoms and beginning treatment immediately can prevent asthma attacks or at least reduce their severity. A number of asthma-management tools are available online—from groups like the American Lung Association and the Asthma and Allergy Foundation of America—to help people track their symptoms and improve their asthma control.

Exercise Safely with Asthma

Regular exercise offers many health benefits, including more efficient heart and lung function, greater muscle strength and endurance, and improvements in mood. Although it can be tricky to avoid asthma triggers outdoors, the benefits of exercise almost always outweigh the risks. In addition, there are many steps people can take to increase their ability to exercise safely with asthma.

The first step in preventing exercise-induced asthma is to ensure that asthma is well managed. Using a reliever medication about fifteen minutes ahead of time and warming up at a low intensity for at least ten minutes before exercising can also help prevent attacks. During exercise, it is important to watch for asthma symptoms, use a reliever medication if they appear, and only return to the activity if the symptoms go away. After completing an exercise session, experts recommend taking time to cool down and remaining alert for asthma symptoms for thirty minutes.

Although asthma should not prevent people from participating in sports, it may be best to avoid exercising outdoors on days when asthma triggers such as air pollution, pollen, high humidity, or cold temperatures are present. If exercise-induced asthma occurs frequently, varying the type, intensity, or duration of activity may be helpful. It is also a good idea to introduce new activities gradually while watching for asthma symptoms.

Follow a Healthy Diet

Although the evidence is unclear about whether eating specific foods can help control asthma, it is well known that good nutrition offers many health benefits. For instance, a healthy, well-balanced diet boosts the immune system, which may enable people with asthma to fight off respiratory viruses and other illnesses that can worsen their symptoms.

Nutritionists generally recommend eating a wide variety of colorful fruits and vegetables, which contain vitamins and antioxidants. Vitamins C, D, and E are especially important in controlling inflammation and supporting immune system function. Experts also suggest consuming foods rich in omega-3 fatty acids—such as salmon, tuna, sardines, and flaxseeds—which help combat inflammation of the airways. Finally, the live bacteria found in yogurt and probiotic supplements have been shown to improve digestion and reduce the likelihood of an inflammatory response in the gut.

Maintain a Healthy Body Weight

Both diet and exercise play a role in maintaining a healthy body weight, which is another important factor in asthma control. Excess weight—especially around the midsection—puts pressure on the lungs and impedes breathing. As a result, studies show that people who are obese have more severe asthma symptoms and need more medication than those who maintain a healthy weight.

Losing weight can also help eliminate gastroesophageal reflux disease (GERD), a condition in which stomach acid flows back into the esophagus, causing an uncomfortable burning sensation in the chest known as heartburn. GERD and asthma are often linked, with an estimated 75 percent of asthma patients also experiencing heartburn symptoms. Eating smaller meals, not eating before bedtime, elevating the head of the bed, and avoiding alcohol, caffeine, chocolate, fatty foods, spicy foods, and acidic foods can help eliminate GERD as well as control related asthma symptoms.

Check for Food Sensitivities

Sensitivities to certain foods can sometimes trigger an inflammatory response in the gut. If the inflammation affects the airways, it can cause an asthma attack. Some of the most common food sensitivities include dairy products, eggs, soy, wheat, shellfish, and sulfites, which are chemicals used as preservatives in wine, condiments, dried fruits, canned vegetables, and other processed foods. If consuming one of these foods seems to be associated with a worsening of asthma symptoms, it may be helpful to eliminate it from the diet for a few weeks to see if symptoms improve.

Take Care of the Airways

People with asthma may also benefit from alternative medical practices intended to clear the sinuses and nasal passages and improve breathing control and lung capacity. Sinus drainage can trigger asthma symptoms, especially at night. To avoid this problem, it may be helpful to use a neti pot or saline spray to clear out congested nasal passages. When the nasal passages are clear, it reduces strain on the airways and eliminates drainage that may trigger asthma attacks.

Practicing steady, rhythmic, deep-breathing techniques has also been found to reduce symptoms of asthma in some studies. Online resources and smartphone apps are available to guide patients through the steps of various techniques, such as the Papworth method, the Buteyeko breathing technique, and pranayama yogic breathing.

References

1. "Asthma and Diet." WebMD Asthma Health Center, 2015.

2. "Asthma and Exercise." Better Health Channel, March 2015.

3. Badash, Michelle. "Lifestyle Changes to Manage Asthma." LifeScript, 2013.

4. Wlody, Ellen. "Lifestyle Changes Can Help Control Asthma." MedShadow Foundation, August 2, 2013.

Chapter 71

Living with Dyspnea

What Is Dyspnea?

Dyspnea is a medical term for difficult or labored breathing. Having dyspnea can be hard to live with. You may get short of breath during daily activities and become anxious when your breathing changes. Medications may help, and, to get the most benefit, you should take them exactly as instructed by your healthcare team.

Experts such as respiratory therapists, physical therapists, respiratory nurses, and pulmonary specialists will work with you to develop ways to help you breathe and manage dyspnea. These methods include pursed-lip breathing, positioning, paced breathing, and desensitization. Pulmonary exercises for dyspnea are specific for each person.

Pursed-Lip Breathing

This method may seem awkward at first, but it eases labored breathing.

- Breathe in through your mouth or nose.

- Purse your lips together (as if you were whistling). Then, breathe out.

- Try to breathe out until all of the air in your lungs is gone. One way to do this is to take twice as long to breathe out as you do

This chapter includes text excerpted from "Living with Dyspnea: How to Breathe More Easily," National Institutes of Health (NIH), May 13, 2015.

to breathe in. For example, count "one...two" as you breathe in. Purse your lips, then count "one...two... three...four" as you breathe out.

Positioning

When your muscles are relaxed, breathing is easier. Positioning helps when you get short of breath while doing activities, such as climbing stairs.

- Rest against the wall and lean forward with your hands on your thighs. This position relaxes your chest and shoulders, freeing them to help you breathe. Use pursed-lip breathing.

- If you can, sit down with your arms resting on your legs. Continue to do pursed-lip breathing.

If you find it hard to relax your muscles, then ask your nurse to show you other ways to do this. Other body positions may also work for you. Try them until you find the best one.

Paced Breathing

Paced breathing prevents or decreases shortness of breath when you walk or lift light objects. When walking, pace yourself, and move slowly.

For walking:

- Stand still, and breathe in.
- Walk a few steps, and breathe out.
- Rest, and begin again.

For lifting:

Before lifting take a deep breath. When carrying something, hold it close to your body while walking and breathing. This saves energy.

Desensitization

Part of living with dyspnea is getting accustomed to it. Desensitization means that you are not so afraid when you are short of breath. These guidelines will help you get "desensitized."

- Do pursed-lip breathing, positioning, and paced breathing. Breathing with these methods will build your confidence. When shortness of breath occurs, you will be able to deal with it.

- Ask friends and family to understand. Let people around you know when you are short of breath. You do not need to feel embarrassed when you cannot join others in some activities. By doing the methods explained here, you will still be able to do what you always did; you may just need to take a little longer or do them differently.

Chapter 72

Caring for a Child with Asthma

Children and Asthma: The Goal Is Control

The news about children and asthma is both good and bad. Better treatments have banished the stereotype of the asthmatic child as frail and inactive, heavily relying on an inhaler to breathe. Children with asthma are now living active, independent lives.

The U.S. Food and Drug Administration (FDA) is working to make sure that the drugs and devices used to treat asthma—a chronic lung disease that inflames and narrows the airways—are safe and effective.

The bad news is that the number of reported cases of asthma in children has been rising. In 2010, there were 7 million children with asthma, 9.4 percent of Americans under 18, according to the Centers for Disease Control and Prevention (CDC), up from 6.5 million, or 8.9 percent, in 2005.

One reason may be that doctors are diagnosing more kids; illnesses once known as bronchitis or a croupy cough are now being

This chapter contains text excerpted from the following sources: Text beginning with the heading "Children and Asthma: The Goal Is Control" is excerpted from "Children and Asthma: The Goal Is Control," U.S. Food and Drug Administration (FDA), June 11, 2012. Reviewed September 2016; Text beginning with the heading "How to Manage Your Child's Indoor Environment?" is excerpted from "If You Have a Child with Asthma, You're Not Alone," U.S. Environmental Protection Agency (EPA), September 1, 2013.

recognized as asthma. Its symptoms may include coughing, wheezing (a whistling sound when you breathe), chest tightness and shortness of breath, according to the National Heart, Lung, and Blood Institute (NHLBI).

Uncontrolled asthma can lead to chronic lung disease and a poor quality of life, and may slow growth. Benjamin Ortiz, M.D., a medical officer in FDA's Office of Pediatric Therapeutics, recommends that parents work with a pediatrician, and an allergist or pulmonologist (lung specialist) if needed, to develop and follow an asthma action plan that details the treatment options when certain symptoms occur.

"Early intervention results in better health into adulthood," he says.

Knowing the Triggers

"We know what makes asthma worse or better, but don't know the primary cause," Ortiz says. The things that make asthma worse are known as "triggers."

They include:

- Season and climate changes

- High levels of air pollutants

- Tobacco smoke

- Mold

- Mites, roaches

- Plant pollen

- Pet dander

- Strong scents, like perfumes

In addition, certain factors may increase a child's risk of developing asthma:

- Family history of asthma

- Multiple episodes of wheezing before age 2

- Living in crowded housing

- A family member who smokes

- Obesity

- Early development of allergies or eczema

Treatment: Not One-Size-Fits-All

What makes asthma better? While asthma is never "cured," a variety of FDA-approved medications can help manage symptoms.

- For quick relief of severe symptoms, doctors will prescribe "rescue" medications, such as albuterol, which open up the bronchial tubes in the lungs. "The goal is not to use it, but have it available—at home, school, camp—just in case," says Anthony Durmowicz, M.D., a medical officer in the FDA's Center for Drug Evaluation and Research.

- To stabilize chronic and persistent symptoms, doctors will prescribe "controller" medications. The most common, safe and effective controller medications are the inhaled corticosteroids (ICS). With regular treatment, they improve lung function and prevent symptoms and flare-ups, reducing the need for rescue medications, according to NHLBI.

- Children whose asthma is triggered by airborne allergens (allergy-causing substances), or who cannot or will not use ICSs, might take a type of drug called a leukotriene modifier. These come in tablet and chewable forms, though for many people they tend to be less effective than ICSs, especially for more severe asthma, Ortiz says.

- For more severe cases that are not controlled with ICSs or leukotriene modifiers alone, adding long-acting beta agonists (LABAs) such as salmeterol or formoterol might be recommended. FDA cautions against using LABAs alone without an ICS, and recommends that if one must be used, it should be for the shortest time possible.

Most asthma medications are inhaled. Babies and toddlers use a nebulizer, a machine that delivers liquid medication as a fine mist through a tube attached to a face mask. Older children can use a metered dose inhaler or dry-powder inhaler.

To ensure that the proper dose of medication gets into a child's lungs, doctors might also prescribe a device called a spacer, or holding chamber which attaches to the inhaler. "There are practical advantages to using (spacers) in younger kids—the timing and coordination needed to use an inhaler is hard for them," Durmowicz says. Once the child can use the inhaler comfortably, it's no longer as critical, he adds. Clinical trials have shown that "the relative dose delivered to the lungs with and without the spacer is the same."

Healthcare providers also might recommend the use of a peak-flow meter to check how well a child's asthma is controlled by treatment over time. Peak flow meters measure the amount of air the child expels from the lungs.

The type and combination of medications and devices a doctor prescribes depends on severity, frequency of symptom flare-ups, the child's age, activity schedule and sometimes cost.

Adolescence Is Challenging

In adolescence, Durmowicz says, childhood symptoms might disappear, but they are likely to return or be different. When they disappear, teens might think they no longer need to pack medicines when they travel, or keep them at school.

Other pitfalls include less parental supervision, and reluctance to be seen by their peers taking medicine. Doctors can help with a medication schedule that allows for privacy. Also, dry powder inhalers may be small enough to tuck in a pocket or purse and use discreetly.

Ortiz says that following prescribed treatment when symptoms are present—at any age—is crucial, telling parents, "Your child will lead a normal life if their asthma is well controlled."

Keys to Preventing Your Child's Attack

- Work with a doctor to develop a written *Asthma Management Plan* that's right for you and your child.

- Learn what triggers your child's asthma and eliminate or reduce your child's exposure to those allergens and irritants.

- Make sure your child takes medications as prescribed and tell your doctor if there are any problems.

- Keep a daily symptom diary and use a peak flowmeter every day to monitor your child's progress.

What Is an Asthma Management Plan?

Written details by your physician should include:

- a list of your child's asthma triggers

- instructions for using asthma medication(s)

- instructions for using a daily symptom diary and peak flow meter
- details about how to stop an asthma attack or episode in progress
- instructions for when to call the doctor

Part Eight

Additional Help and Information

Chapter 73

Glossary of Terms Related to Respiratory Disorders

acute respiratory distress syndrome: A lung condition that leads to low oxygen levels in the blood.

airways: Pipes that carry oxygen-rich air to the lungs. They also carry carbon dioxide, a waste gas, out of the lungs.

allergens: Allergens are a type of asthma trigger, which cause symptoms through an allergic reaction rather than by irritation.

allergy: A type of excessive immune system reaction to a substance in a person's environment. Allergies can be triggered by eating, touching, or breathing in an allergen.

alpha-1 antitrypsin deficiency: A condition that raises the risk for lung disease (especially if you smoke) and other diseases.

alveoli: The millions of tiny compartments within the lungs at the ends of the airways. Alveoli are where gas exchange takes place—that is, where the blood picks up oxygen (from the air a person has breathed in) and releases carbon dioxide (to be breathed out).

anticholinergics: This type of medicine relaxes the muscle bands that tighten around the airways. This action opens the airways, letting more air out of the lungs to improve breathing. Anticholinergics also help clear mucus from the lungs.

This glossary contains terms excerpted from documents produced by several sources deemed reliable.

asbestos: A mineral that, in the past, was widely used in many industries. Asbestos is made up of tiny fibers that can escape into the air. When breathed in, these fibers can stay in your lungs for a long time.

asthma: A chronic disease of the lungs. Symptoms include cough, wheezing, a tight feeling in the chest, and trouble breathing.

breathing pattern: A general term designating the characteristics of the ventilatory activity, e.g., frequency of breathing.

breathing rate: The number of breaths per minute.

bronchi: The airways that lead from the trachea to each lung, and then subdivide into smaller and smaller branches.

bronchiectasis: A condition in which damage to the airways causes them to widen and become flabby and scarred.

bronchitis: Inflammation of the main air passages to your lungs. It causes cough, shortness of breath, and chest tightness.

bronchoalveolar lavage: A clinical technique which removes cell samples from the lower lungs to allow assessment of inflammation and other respiratory conditions.

bronchoconstriction: The reduction in the diameter of the bronchi, usually due to squeezing of the smooth muscle in the walls. This reduces the space for air to go through and can make breathing difficult.

bronchodilator: A medicine that relaxes the smooth muscles of the airways. This allows the airway to open up (to dilate) since the muscles are not squeezing it shut.

bronchopulmonary dysplasia: A serious lung condition that affects infants.

bronchoscopy: A procedure that allows your doctor to look inside your lungs' airways, called the bronchi and bronchioles.

capillaries: Small blood vessels that run through the walls of the air sacs of the lungs.

chronic obstructive pulmonary disease (COPD): It is a progressive disease that makes it hard to breathe. COPD can cause coughing that produces large amounts of mucus, wheezing, shortness of breath, chest tightness, and other symptoms.

cilia: Tiny hairs coated with sticky mucus that trap germs and other foreign particles that enter the airways during breathing.

corticosteroids: A type of medicine used to reduce inflammation. Corticosteroid drugs mimic a substance produced naturally by the body. In asthma, corticosteroids are often taken through an inhaler for long-term control. They may also be taken orally or given intravenously for a short time if asthma symptoms get out of control.

cystic fibrosis: One of the most common serious genetic diseases. Cystic fibrosis (CF) causes the body to make abnormal secretions leading to mucous build-up. CF mucous build-up can impair organs such as the pancreas, the intestine, and the lungs.

deep vein thrombosis: A blood clot that forms in a vein deep in the body.

diaphragm: A dome-shaped muscle located below the lungs. It separates the chest cavity from the abdominal cavity. The diaphragm is the main muscle used for breathing.

dust mites: Very tiny creatures that live in the dust in people's homes. They thrive especially when the air is humid. Many people are allergic to dust mites, and trying to reduce the number of them in the home is part of many asthma control plans.

emphysema: Condition caused by damage to the air sacs in the lungs. This damage keeps the body from getting enough oxygen. Emphysema is usually caused by smoking.

exhalation: The process of breathing out.

expectorant: A drug that stimulates the flow of saliva and promotes coughing to eliminate phlegm from the respiratory tract.

gas exchange: The lungs' intake of oxygen and removal of carbon dioxide.

Haemophilus influenzae **type b:** A bacterial infection that may result in severe respiratory infections, including pneumonia, and other diseases such as meningitis.

inflammation: Used to describe an area on the body that is swollen, red, hot, and in pain.

influenza: It is a respiratory infection caused by multiple viruses. The viruses pass through the air and enter the body through the nose or mouth. The flu can be serious or even deadly for elderly people, newborn babies and people with certain chronic illnesses.

inhalation: The process of breathing in.

inhaled corticosteroid: Anti-inflammatory medicine breathed directly into the lungs. The advantage to this is that the medicine goes directly to where the inflammation is, and has minimal effects on the rest of the body (and therefore fewer side effects than corticosteroids taken orally).

intercostal muscles: Muscles located between the ribs that play a major role in breathing.

irritant: A substance that triggers asthma symptoms by irritating the airway when breathed in. Examples include cigarette smoke, fumes from a harsh cleaning fluid, or strong perfume.

larynx: The voice box.

lung transplant: Surgery to remove a person's diseased lung and replace it with a healthy lung from a deceased donor.

lungs: The organs that lie on either side of the breastbone and fill the inside of the chest cavity. The left lung is slightly smaller than the right lung to allow room for the heart.

mucus: A thick, slippery fluid made by the membranes that line certain organs of the body, including the nose, mouth, and throat.

obesity hypoventilation syndrome: A breathing disorder that affects some obese people.

otitis media: A viral or bacterial infection that leads to inflammation of the middle ear. This condition usually occurs along with an upper respiratory infection. Symptoms include earache, high fever, nausea, vomiting and diarrhea.

pleurisy: A condition in which the pleura is inflamed. The pleura are membranes that consist of two large, thin layers of tissue. One layer wraps around the outside of your lungs. The other layer lines the inside of your chest cavity.

pneumonia: An infection in one or both of the lungs. Many germs— such as bacteria, viruses, and fungi—can cause pneumonia. The infection inflames your lungs' air sacs, which are called alveoli. The air sacs may fill up with fluid or pus, causing symptoms such as a cough with phlegm, fever, chills, and trouble breathing.

pulmonary artery: This artery and its branches deliver blood rich in carbon dioxide (and lacking in oxygen) to the capillaries that surround the air sacs of the lungs.

pulmonary embolism: A sudden blockage in a lung artery. The blockage usually is caused by a blood clot that travels to the lung from a vein in the leg.

pulmonary function tests: A series of tests done to determine whether a person has breathing problems, and precisely what those problems are. These are used to differentiate among different diseases and disorders. It is sometimes hard for a doctor to tell just by a regular exam whether a person has asthma or another condition, and pulmonary function tests can help clarify the diagnosis.

pulmonary hypertension: Increased pressure in the pulmonary arteries.

pulmonary rehabilitation: A broad program that helps improve the well-being of people who have chronic (ongoing) breathing problems.

respiratory failure: A condition in which not enough oxygen passes from the lungs into the blood.

respiratory system: Organs and tissues that help breathing. The main parts of this system are the airways, the lungs and linked blood vessels, and the muscles that enable breathing.

sarcoidosis: An inflammatory disease marked by the formation of granulomas (small nodules of immune cells) in the lungs, lymph nodes, and other organs. Sarcoidosis may be acute and go away by itself, or it may be chronic and progressive.

sputum: Mucus and other matter brought up from the lungs by coughing.

thoracentesis: A procedure to remove excess fluid in the space between the lungs and the chest wall.

trachea: The largest breathing tube in the body, passing from the throat down to the chest (where it connects to the two bronchi leading to the lungs).

tracheostomy: A surgically made hole that goes through the front of your neck and into your trachea. The hole is made to help you breathe.

upper respiratory tract: Area of the body that includes the nasal passages, mouth, and throat.

ventilation: Physiological process by which gas is renewed in the lungs.

ventilator: A machine that supports breathing. These machines mainly are used in hospitals.

wheezing: Breathing with difficulty, with a whistling noise. Wheezing is a symptom of asthma.

Chapter 74

Directory of Organizations That Help People with Respiratory Disorders

Governmental Organizations That Provide Information about Respiratory Disorders

Agency for Healthcare Research and Quality (AHRQ)
5600 Fishers Ln.
7th Fl.
Rockville, MD 20847
Phone: 301-427-1364
Website: www.ahrq.gov

Agency for Toxic Substances and Disease Registry (ATSDR)
4770 Buford Hwy N.E.
Atlanta, GA 30341
Toll-Free: 800-CDC-INFO
(800-232-4636)
TTY: 888-232-6348
Website: www.atsdr.cdc.gov

Centers for Disease Control and Prevention (CDC)
1600 Clifton Rd.
Atlanta, GA 30333
Toll-Free: 800-CDC-INFO
(800-232-4636)
Phone: 404-639-3311
Toll-Free TTY: 888-232-6348
Website: www.cdc.gov
E-mail: cdcinfo@cdc.gov

Resources in this chapter were compiled from several sources deemed reliable; all contact information was verified and updated in September 2016.

Eunice Kennedy Shriver
National Institute of Child Health and Human Development (NICHD)
Information Resource Center (IRC)
P.O. Box 3006
Rockville, MD 20847
Toll-Free: 800-370-2943
Toll-Free TTY: 888-320-6942
Toll-Free Fax: 866-760-5947
Website: www.nichd.nih.gov
E-mail:
NICHDInformationResource
Center@mail.nih.gov

National Cancer Institute (NCI)
NCI Office of Communications and Education (OCE)
Public Inquiries Office (OPI)
Medical Center Dr.
BG 9609 MSC 97609609
Bethesda, MD 20892-9760
Toll-Free: 800-4-CANCER
(800-422-6237)
Toll-Free TTY: 800-332-8615
Website: www.cancer.gov
E-mail: cancergovstaff@mail.nih.gov

National Center for Complementary and Integrative Health (NCCIH)
9000 Rockville Pike
Bethesda, MD 20892
Toll-Free: 888-644-6226
Toll-Free TTY: 866-464-3615
Toll-Free Fax: 866-464-3616
Website: nccih.nih.gov/
E-mail: info@nccih.nih.gov

National Center for Health Statistics (NCHS)
3311 Toledo Rd.
Rm. 5419
Hyattsville, MD 20782
Toll-Free: 800-CDC-INFO
(800-232-4636)
Website: www.cdc.gov/nchs
E-mail: cdcinfo@cdc.gov

National Health Information Center (NHIC)
U.S. Department of Health and Human Services (HHS)
P.O. Box 1133
Washington, DC 20013-1133
Toll-Free: 800-336-4797
Phone: 301-565-4167
Fax: 301-984-4256
Website: www.health.gov/nhic
E-mail: info@nhic.gov

National Heart, Lung, and Blood Institute (NHLBI)
NHLBI Health Information Center
P.O. Box 30105
Bethesda, MD 20824-0105
Phone: 301-592-8573
Fax: 301-592-8563
Website: www.nhlbi.nih.gov
E-mail: nhlbiinfo@nhlbi.nih.gov

National Institute of Allergy and Infectious Diseases (NIAID)
Office of Communications and Government Relations (OCGR)
6610 Rockledge Dr.
MSC 6612
Bethesda, MD 20892-6612
Toll-Free: 866-284-4107
Phone: 301-496-5717
Toll-Free TDD: 800-877-8339
Fax: 301-402-3573
Website: www.niaid.nih.gov
E-mail: ocpostoffice@niaid.nih.gov

National Institute of Environmental Health Sciences (NIEHS)
P.O. Box 12233, MD K3-16
Research Triangle Park, NC 27709-2233
Phone: 919-541-3345
Fax: 301-480-2978
Website: www.niehs.nih.gov

National Institute of Neurological Disorders and Stroke (NINDS)
P.O. Box 5801
Bethesda, MD 20824
Toll-Free: 800-352-9424
Phone: 301-496-5751
TTY: 301-468-5981
Website: www.ninds.nih.gov

National Institute on Aging (NIA)
31 Center Dr., MSC 2292
Bldg. 31, Rm. 5C27
Bethesda, MD 20892
Toll-Free: 800-222-2225
Phone: 301-496-1752
Toll-Free TTY: 800-222-4225
Fax: 301-496-1072
Website: www.nia.nih.gov
E-mail: niaic@nia.nih.gov

National Institutes of Health (NIH)
9000 Rockville Pike
Bethesda, MD 20892
Phone: 301-496-4000
TTY: 301-402-9612
Website: www.nih.gov
E-mail: NIHinfo@od.nih.gov

National Women's Health Information Center
Office on Women's Health (OWH)
200 Independence Ave. S.W.
Rm. 712E
Washington, DC 20201
Toll-Free: 800-994-9662
Toll-Free TDD: 888-220-5446
Fax: 202-205-2631
Website: www.womenshealth.gov

Occupational Safety and Health Administration (OSHA)
U.S. Department of Labor (DOL)
200 Constitution Ave.
Washington, DC 20210
Toll-Free: 800-321-OSHA
(800-321-6742)
Phone: 202-690-7650
Toll-Free TTY: 877-889-5627
Website: www.osha.gov

U.S. Bureau of Labor Statistics (BLS)
2 Massachusetts Ave. N.E.
Postal Square Bldg.
Washington, DC 20212-0001
Phone: 202-691-5200
Toll-Free TDD: 800-877-8339
Website: www.bls.gov/

U.S. Department of Health and Human Services (HHS)
200 Independence Ave. S.W.
Rm. 443 H
Washington, DC 20201
Toll-Free: 877-696-6775
Website: www.hhs.gov

U.S. Environmental Protection Agency (EPA)
1200 Pennsylvania Ave. N.W.
Washington, DC 20004
Phone: 202-272-0167
TTY: 202-272-0165
Website: www.epa.gov

U.S. Food and Drug Administration (FDA)
10903 New Hampshire Ave.
Silver Spring, MD 20993-0002
Toll-Free: 888-INFO-FDA
(888-463-6332)
Website: www.fda.gov

U.S. National Library of Medicine (NLM)
8600 Rockville Pike
Bethesda, MD 20894
Toll-Free: 888-FIND-NLM
(888-346-3656)
Phone: 301-594-5983
Toll-Free TDD: 800-735-2258
Fax: 301-402-1384
Website: www.nlm.nih.gov
E-mail: custserv@nlm.nih.gov

Private Organizations That Provide Information about Respiratory Disorders

Action on Smoking and Health (ASH)
701 4th St. N.W.
Washington, DC 20001
Phone: 202-659-4310
Fax: 202-289-7166
Website: www.ash.org
E-mail: info@ash.org

Allergy and Asthma Network Mothers of Asthmatics (AANMA)
8201 Greensboro Dr., Ste. 300
McLean, VA 22102
Toll-Free: 800-878-4403
Fax: 703-288-5271
Website: www.
allergyasthmanetwork.org

Allergy/Asthma Information Association (AAIA)
17 Four Season Pl.
Ste. 200
Toronto, Ontario M9B 6E6
Canada
Toll-Free: 800-611-7011
Phone: 416-621-4571
Fax: 416-621-5034
Website: www.aaia.ca
E-mail: admin@aaia.ca

American Academy of Allergy, Asthma, and Immunology (AAAAI)
555 E. Wells St.
Ste. 1100
Milwaukee, WI 53202-3823
Phone: 414-272-6071
Website: www.aaaai.org
E-mail: info@aaaai.org

American Academy of Otolaryngology—Head and Neck Surgery (AAO—HNS)
1650 Diagonal Rd.
Alexandria, VA 22314-2857
Phone: 703-836-4444
Website: www.entnet.org

American Association for Respiratory Care (AARC)
9425 N. MacArthur Blvd.
Ste. 100
Irving, TX 75063-4706
Phone: 972-243-2272
Fax: 972-484-2720
Website: www.aarc.org
E-mail: info@aarc.org

American College of Chest Physicians
CHEST Global Headquarters
2595 Patriot Blvd.
Glenview, IL 60026
Toll-Free: 800-343-2227
Phone: 224-521-9800
Fax: 224-521-9801
Website: www.chestnet.org

American College of Physicians (ACP)
190 N. Independence Mall W.
Philadelphia, PA 19106-1572
Toll-Free: 800-523-1546
Phone: 215-351-2400
Website: www.acponline.org

American College of Radiology (ACR)
1891 Preston White Dr.
Reston, VA 20191
Phone: 703-648-8900
Website: www.acr.org
E-mail: info@acr.org

American Lung Association
1301 Pennsylvania Ave. N.W.
Ste. 800
Washington, DC 20004
Toll-Free: 800-LUNG-USA
(800-586-4872)
Phone: 202-785-3355
Fax: 202-452-1805
Website: www.lung.org

American Medical Association (AMA)
515 N. State St.
Chicago, IL 60654
Toll-Free: 800-621-8335
Website: www.ama-assn.org

American Thoracic Society (ATS)
25 Broadway
18th Fl.
New York, NY 10004
Phone: 212-315-8600
Fax: 212-315-6498
Website: www.thoracic.org
E-mail: atsinfo@thoracic.org

Asthma and Allergy Foundation of America (AAFA)
8201 Corporate Dr.
Ste. 1000
Landover, MD 20785
Toll-Free: 800-7-ASTHMA
(800-727-8462)
Website: www.aafa.org
E-mail: info@aafa.org

Cleveland Clinic
9500 Euclid Ave.
Cleveland, OH 44195
Toll-Free: 800-223-2273
Phone: 216-636-5860 (Info Line)
TTY: 216-444-0261
Website: my.clevelandclinic.org

COPD Foundation
20 F St. N.W.
Ste. 200A
Washington, DC 20001
Toll-Free: 866-731-COPD
(866-731-2673)
Website: www.copdfoundation.org
E-mail: info@copdfoundation.org

Cystic Fibrosis Foundation
6931 Arlington Rd.
2nd Fl.
Bethesda, MD 20814
Toll-Free: 800-FIGHT-CF
(800-344-4823)
Phone: 301-951-4422
Fax: 301-951-6378
Website: www.cff.org
E-mail: info@cff.org

March of Dimes
1275 Mamaroneck Ave.
White Plains, NY 10605
Phone: 914-997-4488
Website: www.marchofdimes.com

National Emphysema Foundation (NEF)
128 E. Ave.
Norwalk, CT 06851
Website: www.emphysemafoundation.org

National Environmental Education Foundation (NEEF)
4301 Connecticut Ave. N.W.
Ste. 160
Washington, DC 20008
Phone: 202-833-2933
Website: www.neefusa.org

National Jewish Health
1400 Jackson St.
Denver, CO 80206
Toll-Free: 877-CALL-NJH
(877-225-5654)
Phone: 303-388-4461
Website: www.nationaljewish.org

Nemours Foundation Center for Children's Health Media
1600 Rockland Rd.
Wilmington, DE 19803
Phone: 302-651-4000
Website: www.kidshealth.org
E-mail: info@kidshealth.org

Ontario Lung Association
18 Wynford Dr., Ste. 401
Toronto, Ontario M3C 0K8
Canada
Toll-Free: 888-344-LUNG
(888-344-5864)
Fax: 416-864-9911
Website: www.on.lung.ca
E-mail: info@on.lung.ca

Pulmonary Hypertension Association (PHA)
801 Roeder Rd., Ste. 1000
Silver Spring, MD 20910
Toll-Free: 800-748-7274
Phone: 301-565-3004
Fax: 301-565-3994
Website: www.phassociation.org
E-mail: PHA@PHAssociation.org

Respiratory Health Association (RHA)
1440 W. Washington Blvd.
Chicago, IL 60607
Toll-Free: 888-880-LUNG
(888-880-5864)
Phone: 312-243-2000
Fax: 312-243-3954
Website: www.lungchicago.org
E-mail: info@lungchicago.org

University of Chicago Asthma and COPD Center
5841 S. Maryland Ave.
Chicago, IL 60637
Phone: 773-702-0880
Website: asthma.bsd.uchicago.edu
E-mail: asthma@medicine.bsd.uchicago.edu

Index

Index

674